D1704394

Ocular Bloodflow in Glaucoma

OCULAR BLOOD FLOW IN GLAUCOMA

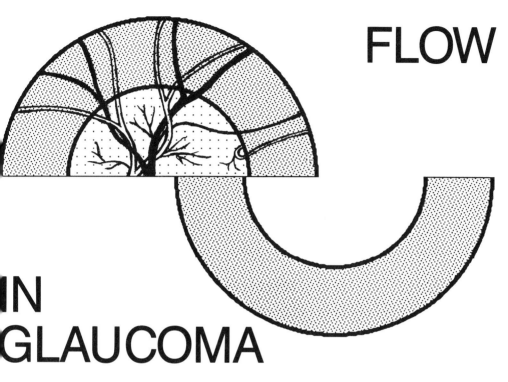

Means, Methods and Measurements

Proceedings of a Meeting held in the Château de Bellinglise near Paris under the auspices of the European Glaucoma Society, September 9–10, 1988

edited by George N. Lambrou and Erik L. Greve

A. Alm	S.S. Hayreh	C.E. Riva
D.R. Anderson	G.N. Lambrou	Y.C.A. Robert
T.J.T.P. van den Berg	M.E. Langham	B. Schwartz
F.C. Delori	L.E. Pillunat	G.L. Spaeth
H.C. Geijssen	C. Prünte	G.O. Sperber
J.E. Grunwald	H.A. Quigley	R. Stodtmeister
H. Hamard	G. Richard	W.-D. Ulrich

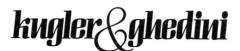

Library of Congress Cataloging-in-Publication Data

Ocular blood flow in glaucoma.

    Includes bibliographical references.
    1. Glaucoma--Congresses. 2. Retina--Blood vessels--
Congresses.   I. Lambrou, George N.   II. Greve, Erik L.
III. Alm, A.   IV. European Glaucoma Society.
RE871.028   1989   617.7'41   89-19833
ISBN 90-6299-053-3

©Copyright 1989 Kugler & Ghedini Publications
All rights reserved. No part of this book may be translated or reproduced in any form by print, photoprint, microfilm, or any other means without the prior written permission of the publisher.

ISBN 90-6299-053-3

Distributors:
For the U.S.A. and Canada:
Kugler Publications
P.O. Box 5794
Berkeley, CA 94705, U.S.A.

For Italy:
Ghedini Editore
Via della Signora, 6
20122 Milano
Telefax (02) 781150

For all other countries:
Kugler Publications bv
P.O. Box 516
1180 AM Amstelveen, The Netherlands
Telefax (+31.20) 380524

The meeting and its publication herein were funded by an educational grant from Chibret International, Ophthalmic Group of Merck, Sharp & Dohme International, Rahway, New Jersey, USA.

This publication reflects the opinion of its authors and not necessarily those of Merck and Co., Inc. or any of its related affiliates and is presented as a service to the medical profession. For detailed prescribing information on any drugs discussed in these proceedings, please consult the Physicians Circular issued by the manufacturer.

FOREWORD

In this book the reader will find the complete proceedings of a meeting of international experts on the subject of ocular blood flow measurements in glaucoma.

Popularized by Bizet's homonymous opera, "l'Arlésienne" is a charming short story by Alphonse Daudet, relating the stir and drama caused in a southern French village by a maiden from Arles, the neighboring town. A rather unusual feature of the plot is that although every character is worried about her influence or speculates about her behavior, the girl herself fails to turn up at any moment in the story.

The disturbances of optic nerve head blood supply have been "l'Arlésienne" of glaucoma research over the past few years. Their involvement - either as a primary or as a secondary phenomenon - has been very much speculated upon, and many attempts have been made to assess them objectively, with methods ranging from the simplest and most elegant to the most elaborate and sophisticated. However, it remains unclear what the clinical significance of many of the reported methods is, and the question remains unanswered: is there a reliable method for measuring ocular blood flow ?

To sum up our present knowledge on the subject, the European Glaucoma Society, in collaboration with Chibret International, instigated a meeting with the purpose of bringing together all the scientists active in basic or clinical research on optic nerve head blood supply, in a setting favorable to extensive discussion and exchange of experience and ideas on future developments in this field.

The meeting was held on September 9th and 10th 1988, in the Château de Bellinglise, near Paris. It was made possible by the stimulating support of Thierry Poirot and Aubrey McWatt of Chibret International, who realized that the problem of optic nerve head blood supply is of major importance for a better understanding of the pathogenesis of glaucoma, and, hopefully, for the management of patients.

From the very beginning, the necessity was stressed to favor the discussions more than the presentations. Rather than giving lectures, the speakers were instructed to discuss their work - including their uncertainties, doubts or lack of understanding - while participants were encouraged not only to ask questions but also to comment freely upon any subject that they considered relevant. As a result, the discussions were very lively and free-flowing, often drifting from specific details to general issues, some of which are of major importance for blood-flow research in glaucoma. Controversies arose of course, and some stern remarks were made at times, but it was generally felt that the success of the meeting was mainly due to what amounted to public debates.

It was considered necessary, therefore, to publish the discussions together with the manuscripts submitted by the authors. They were of course edited to make the debates more concise and coherent, but we have tried to keep as much of their spontaneity and liveliness as possible, reflecting to some extent the atmosphere of the meeting. Even if we have not entirely succeeded in that aspect, we are convinced that the reader will find the debates on the following topics particularly interesting (numbers indicate pages):

- Watershed zones and their possible role in the pathogenesis of glaucoma (49 - 52).
- The importance of frame rate in angiography (49).
- The role of anastomoses in ocular circulation (50 - 52).
- The clinical significance of appearance times in fluorescein angiography (52 - 53 / 275 - 276).
- Receptors on the retinal and optic nerve head vessels (61 - 64).

- Autoregulation of the retinal and optic nerve head vessels (61 - 62 / 151 - 152).
- Does the choroid have autoregulation ? (70).
- Does acute IOP elevation mimick chronic glaucoma ? (85). Can it be dangerous ? (231).
- What is the clinical and histopathological significance of disc pallor ? (86)
- Does redness of the disc really measure the amount of blood present ? (169 - 170)
- What can the role of decreased blood pressure be in glaucoma ? (61 / 88 - 89 / 124)
- Relation between ocular pulses and pathogenesis of glaucoma. (123 - 124)
- How well does blood flow reflect nutritional delivery to the optic nerve head ? (88)
- What exactly does Laser Doppler Velocimetry measure and at what level ? (135 - 136)
- Can the retinal circulation be implicated in the pathogenesis of glaucoma ? (152 - 154)
- Interpretation of the pressure-compliance test and of Electro-Encephalo-Dynamography (191-193 / 221 - 223 / 231 - 233).
- What do fluorescein filling defects really mean ? (88 / 261 - 263)
- Why use video-angiography ? (262 - 263 / 275 - 276)

The editors wish to acknowledge the efforts of Odile-Anne Schumacher of MSD-Chibret France and of Janine Horbacz of Chibret International, who provided efficient and pleasant assistance with every organizational detail.

G.N. Lambrou
E.L. Greve

Amsterdam, May 1989

Table of Contents

Foreword

I. Anatomy, physiology and pathophysiology

Blood supply of the optic nerve head in health and disease *Sohan S. Hayreh*	3
Discussion	49
Anatomy and physiology of ocular blood flow *Douglas R. Anderson*	55
Discussion	61
Microspheres in optic nerve blood flow measurements *Albert Alm*	65
Discussion	69
The 2-deoxyglucose method and ocular blood flow *Göran O. Sperber and Anders Bill*	73
Discussion	81
Histological and clinical features of the optic nerve head in early glaucoma diagnosis *Harry A. Quigley*	83
Discussion	85

II. Ocular pulse measurements

Non-invasive measurement of pulsatile blood flow in the human eye *Maurice E. Langham, Richard A. Farrell, Vivian O'Brien, David M. Silver and Peter Schilder*	93
Ocular perfusion pressure and oculo–oscillo–dynamography *Wulff–D. Ulrich, Christa Ulrich and Gabriele Walther*	101
Ocular pulse measurements in low–tension glaucoma *George N. Lambrou, Peter Sindhunata, Thomas J.T.P. van den Berg, H. Caroline Geijssen, Pietr Vyborny and Erik L. Greve*	115
Discussion	121

III. Laser doppler velocimetry, blue field entoptometry and reflectometry of the optic disc

Noninvasive measurement of the optic nerve head circulation *Charles E. Riva, R.D. Shonat, B.L. Petrig, C.J. Pournaras and G.B. Barnes*	129
Discussion	135
Laser doppler velocimetry and blood rheology; preliminary trials *H. Hamard, A. Parent de Curzon, J. Dufaux and P. Hamard*	137
Discussion	145

Retinal hemodynamics in open-angle glaucoma *Juan E. Grunwald*	147
Discussion	151
Reflectometry measurements of optic disc blood volume *François C. Delori*	155
Discussion	165
Photometry of the optic disc *Yves C. A. Robert and Phillip H. Hendrickson*	167
Discussion	169

IV. Electrodiagnostic tests and ocular blood flow

Pressure tolerance test: I. Clinical technique and specificity *Richard Stodtmeister and Lutz E. Pillunat*	175
Discussion	191
Pressure tolerance test: II. Clinical results and sensitivity *Lutz E. Pillunat and Richard Stodtmeister*	195
Discussion	205
Pattern reversal electro-encephalo-dynamography and pattern reversal electro-retino-dynamography in the assessment of optic nerve head and retinal autoregulation *Wulff-D. Ulrich, Christa Ulrich, Bernd Gerewitz and Helmut Teubel*	207
Discussion	221
Pattern visual evoked potentials under artificial intraocular pressure increase in glaucoma: methodological considerations *Thomas J. T. P. van den Berg, Frans C. C. Riemslag, George N. Lambrou and Hank Spekreijse*	225
Discussion	231

V. Fuorescein angiography

Contributions and limitations of fluorescein angiography in understanding glaucoma; or, "where do we go next?" *George L. Spaeth*	237
Fluorescein angiography: Its contribution to evaluation of the optic disc and the retinal circulation in glaucoma *Bernard Schwartz*	243
Low tension glaucoma ; Correlation between fluorescein angiographic findings and progression *H. Caroline Geijssen and Erik L. Greve*	255
Discussion	261

VI. Video-angiography

Videoangiography: a new technique for the quantification of the retinal circulation   267
Gisbert Richard
Discussion   275

Choroidal angiography   277
Christian Prünte
Discussion   283

Vascular plerometry of the choroid. An approach to the quantification of choroidal blood flow using computer-assisted processing of fluorescein angiograms.   287
George N. Lambrou, Thomas J.T.P. van den Berg and Erik L. Greve
Discussion   295

Index of Authors   297

I. ANATOMY, PHYSIOLOGY AND PATHOPHYSIOLOGY

BLOOD SUPPLY OF THE OPTIC NERVE HEAD IN HEALTH AND DISEASE

Sohan Singh Hayreh

Department of Ophthalmology, University of Iowa, Iowa City, Iowa, USA

The blood supply of the optic nerve head is an important subject because it forms the basis for understanding the pathogenesis of a variety of ischemic disorders of the optic nerve head; these disorders collectively constitute one of the major causes of visual crippling. In view of this, the topic has attracted considerable attention over the past four decades and much conflicting information has been published about it. A critical review of the various studies reveals that, as in other controversial fields of medicine, they have suffered from a variety of problems: most often from incorrect interpretation; some from defective studies using dubious or noncomparable techniques and/or an inadequate sample size; others have been marred by inexperienced investigators (even when one or more of the "authors" of the resultant paper was a person of considerable reputation!); many from application of morphological post-mortem findings to *in vivo* blood flow; still others were marred by the fact that the study was designed (perhaps unintentionally) to prove a dearly cherished notion. Fools have rushed in - in great number - where angels fear to tread. Under these circumstances it is sometimes practically impossible to distinguish fact from fantasy.

I have investigated the blood supply of the optic nerve head in health and disease since 1955, anatomically, physiologically, experimentally and clinically, using a variety of techniques including the following:

1. *Anatomical studies*: These were performed after intra-arterial post-mortem injection of liquid neoprene latex in one hundred human and eight rhesus monkey specimens[1-5].

2. *Histological studies*: These were done after serial sectioning of the anterior part of the normal optic nerve, containing the central retinal vessels (with and without intravascular injection of a dye), in twelve human and eight rhesus monkey specimens[1-6].

3. *Experimental studies*: We investigated the circulation in the optic disc and choroid, using fluorescein fundus angiography, in normal rhesus monkey eyes, and after various types of ocular vascular occlusion (including those of the posterior ciliary arteries (PCAs) and their branches, vortex veins, and central retinal vessels), after raising the intraocular pressure, after experimental malignant arterial hypertension, and after other relevant studies, in over 400 monkey eyes[7-23].

4. *Clinical studies*: We have studied the optic disc and choroidal circulation by fluorescein fundus angiography in about 700 patients with anterior ischemic optic neuropathy[24-28], about 225 patients with glaucoma and allied disorders[7,9,29,30], in a large population of patients with normal optic nerve head and choroidal circulation.

These thirty years of studies have provided a wealth of useful information. Among the most important information revealed, particularly by the *in vivo* studies, is the following:

 a. *Role of posterior ciliary artery circulation*: This is usually the primary source of blood supply to the optic nerve head.

 b. *Disparity between the post-mortem injection and morphological studies and the in vivo studies*: While the post-mortem and morphological studies have been very helpful in some ways, they have provided highly misleading information in others. As regards the actual *in vivo* blood flow and its dynamics in the optic nerve head and the choroid, they have provided little useful information, and some that is downright misleading. The interpretation of *in vivo* ocular circulatory disorders in the light of morphological studies is one of the fundamental reasons for the prevalent conflict on the subject. The pattern of blood supply of the optic nerve head discussed below is based on combined information from all the studies mentioned above, particularly from the *in vivo* fluorescein angiographic studies in normal and diseased states in man and monkeys; our studies have shown that the vascular bed and circulation in man and rhesus monkeys have no recognizable difference.

c. *Marked interindividual variation in the blood supply of the optic nerve head in man*: It has been taken for granted all along that the pattern of blood supply of the optic nerve head in all eyes is identical. On the contrary, our studies have shown clearly that there is a marked interindividual variation in this pattern. These variations are produced by a number of factors, discussed later in this publication.

The following is a brief account of the blood supply of the optic nerve head in health and disease, and the other topics mentioned above.

Blood supply of the optic nerve head:

I have discussed this subject in detail elsewhere[31]. The optic nerve head, for purposes of describing its blood supply, from anterior to posterior perspective, consists of[31]:
i. the surface nerve fiber layer,
ii. the prelaminar region,
iii. the lamina cribrosa region, and
iv. the retrolaminar region.

Figs. 1 and 2 show this division of the optic nerve head diagrammatically, as well as their pattern of blood supply, which is as follows:

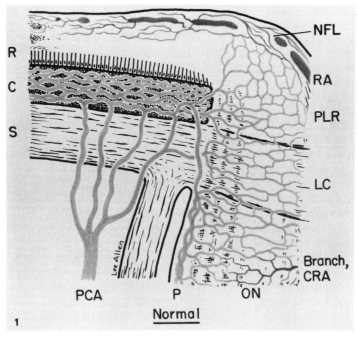

Fig. 1. Schematic representation of blood supply of the optic nerve head and retrolaminar optic nerve. C= choroid, CRA= central retinal artery, LC= lamina cribrosa, NFL= surface nerve fiber layer of the disc, ON= optic nerve, P= pia, PCA= posterior ciliary artery, PLR= prelaminar region, R= retina, RA= retinal arteriole, S= sclera. (Reproduced from Hayreh[31]).

Optic nerve head blood supply in health and disease

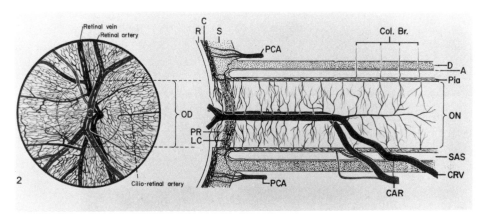

Fig. 2. Diagrammatic representation of blood supply of optic nerve head and intraorbital part of the optic nerve. A = arachnoid, C= choroid, CAR= central retinal artery, CRV= central retinal vein, D= dura, OD= optic disc, ON= optic nerve, PCA= posterior ciliary arteries, R= retina, and S= sclera (Reproduced from Hayreh, SS: Trans Am Acad Ophthalmol Otolaryngol 78:OP240-OP254, 1974)

i. *The surface nerve fiber layer*: This layer is continuous with the adjacent nerve fiber layer of the retina and is mostly supplied by the retinal arterioles (Figs. 3-B, 4). However, in some eyes the temporal part of this layer may instead be supplied by the posterior ciliary circulation from the prelaminar region. When an eye has a cilioretinal artery, the corresponding sector of the surface nerve fiber layer is usually supplied by the posterior ciliary circulation (Fig. 4).

ii. *The prelaminar region*: This part of the optic nerve head lies between the surface nerve fiber layer and the lamina cribrosa. The prelaminar region is supplied by the peripapillary choroid (Figs. 5-9). Centripetal branches arise from the large peripapillary choroidal arteries and supply the adjacent corresponding sector of this region (Fig. 10). Peripapillary choriocapillaris *do not* give any branches to the prelaminar region (Figs. 5-9, 11). The central retinal artery plays no role in its supply. Our fluorescein fundus angiographic studies have revealed a strictly sectoral blood supply.

iii. *The lamina cribrosa region*: This is usually supplied by centripetal branches arising directly from the short PCAs (or from the so-called Circle of Zinn and Haller, when that incomplete circle exists, which is not common), as well as some from the recurrent pial branches from the peripapillary choroid (Figs. 1, 2). The central retinal artery gives no branches here. This is a highly vascular part of the optic nerve head.

iv. *The retrolaminar region*: This part of the optic nerve head lies immediately behind the lamina cribrosa. It is supplied mostly by the recurrent pial branches which arise from the peripapillary choroid and run back on to the pial surface of the retrolaminar region (Figs. 1, 2, 12); these recurrent pial branches give centripetal branches to this part of the optic nerve head. The peripheral pial plexus may also be occasionally supplied to a variable extent by branches from other sources, *e. g.*, central retinal artery and other orbital arteries (Fig. 2). In addition to the peripheral pial centripetal branches, the retrolaminar region may also be supplied in a variable number by axial centrifugal branches from the central retinal artery, when that artery gives out intraneural branches in this region (Figs. 1, 2).

From this account it is evident that the main source of blood supply to the optic nerve head is the PCA circulation, mostly through the peripapillary choroid and to some extent also via the short PCAs.

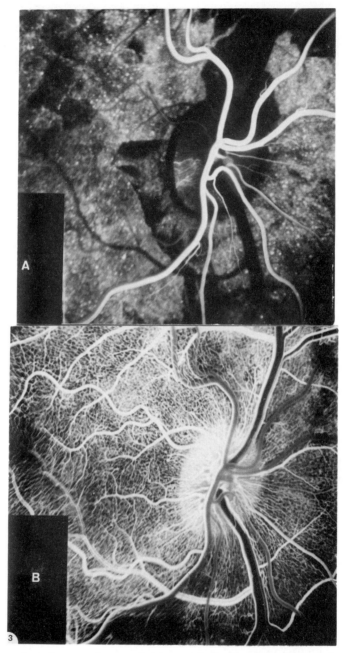

Fig. 3. Fluorescein angiograms of a normal right eye of a healthy Cynomolgus monkey show: (A) . Filling of the choroidal vessels and their distribution to the lower temporal quadrant of the prelaminar region and filling of the retinal arterioles but no filling of the retinal vascular bed. A ring of pigment at the disc margin is masking fluorescence. (B) . During the retinal arteriovenous phase, filling of the capillary bed in the retina as well as the surface layer of the optic disc, resulting in complete masking of the underlying prelaminar vessels. (Reproduced from Hayreh[9])

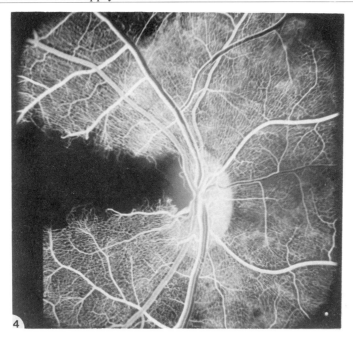

Fig. 4. Fluorescein fundus angiogram of right eye of a normal healthy Rhesus monkey, after experimental occlusion of the lateral PCA. Note the complete absence of filling of the temporal choroid and optic disc and of a sector of the retinal capillary bed supplied by a cilio-retinal artery on the temporal side. (Reproduced from Hayreh[12])

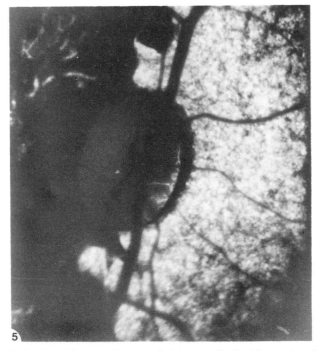

Fig. 5. Fluorescein fundus angiogram of a normal right eye of a healthy monkey during the retinal pre-arterial phase, shows filling of the nasal half of the choroid and early filling of the vessels from the peripapillary choroid in the corresponding prelaminar region. Note filling of the choriocapillaris in the entire nasal half of the choroid without any extension of the filling into the prelaminar region: the choriocapillaris are not continuous with the prelaminar capillaries. Choroidal pigment deposit at disc margin obscures underlying choroidal fluorescence in some places. (Reproduced from Hayreh[9]).

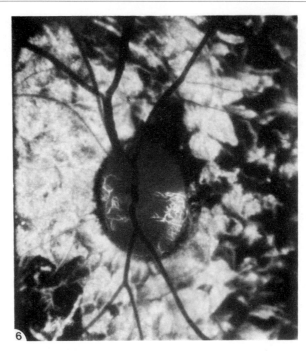

Fig. 6. Fluorescein fundus angiogram of left eye of a normal healthy Cynomolgus monkey (after experimental central retinal artery occlusion to unmask the vessels in the prelaminar region) at normal intraocular pressure shows early filling of the vessels in the prelaminar region from the peripapillary choroid. Choroidal pigment deposit at disc margin obscures underlying choroidal fluorescence in some places. (Reproduced from Hayreh et al. [11])

Angioarchitecture of the optic nerve head: This has been described by a large number of investigators since 1903[6,32-44] on light as well as, more recently, scanning electron microscopy. The vessels in the optic nerve head lie in its septa so that distribution of the septa is really a distribution of the blood vessels. The capillaries form two basic patterns in the retrolaminar part of the optic nerve - longitudinal and transverse (Fig. 13) . The longitudinal capillaries run in between the nerve fiber bundles antero-posteriorly, while the transverse capillaries surround the various nerve bundles at a regular distance and may form a complete or incomplete pentagonal, oval or round network. Collaterals from both the longitudinal and transverse units join to form a complicated capillary plexus. The angioarchitecture in the region of the lamina cribrosa has been described as comprising numerous, small, very close and transversely elongated meshes[34,40], and is very dense[37,38,41]. In my studies I found that in the retrolaminar region the longitudinal and transverse capillaries formed a complicated meshwork, in the lamina cribrosa the capillaries were arranged mostly transversely, like the connective tissue septa there, and in the prelaminar region the arrangement was like that in the retrolaminar region[6]. The peripapillary choriocapillaris *do not* anastomose with the capillary plexus in the prelaminar region (Figs. 5-9, 11) . Like all other investigators in the field, I also found that in the optic nerve head the capillaries form a continuous network throughout its entire length, and are continuous posteriorly with those in the rest of the optic nerve and anteriorly with the adjacent retinal capillaries.

Controversies on the blood supply of the optic nerve head: As pointed out earlier, it is most unfortunate that the subject of the blood supply of the optic nerve head has been plagued for so long by problems and controversies. Interpretation of the findings of any scientific study depends upon one's experience and knowledge of the subject, so that

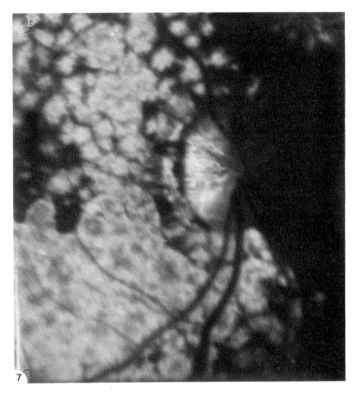

Fig. 7. Fluorescein fundus angiogram of right eye of a normal healthy monkey during the retinal pre-arterial phase, shows early filling of the temporal half of the choroid and of the corresponding prelaminar vessels. Choroidal pigment deposit at disc margin obscures underlying choroidal fluorescence in some places. (Reproduced from Hayreh[10]).

inexperienced investigators with inadequate expertise in the field have inevitably and innocently misinterpreted their findings, resulting in confusion. In the literature, there is overall agreement on the basic pattern of the blood supply described above; however, some papers have described alternative patterns which need to be discussed in order to be placed in their true perspective. These can be divided into the following categories:

a. *The role of peripapillary choroid in blood supply of the optic nerve head*: In the literature, the various post-mortem injection, histological, scanning electron microscopic and fluorescein angiographic studies have overwhelmingly shown that the peripapillary choroid supplies the prelaminar region[31,32,42-59], as I have found in my various studies, and is evident in the various fluorescein fundus angiograms reproduced throughout this paper. However, a few papers, based purely on morphological studies, have claimed that this is not so. I would like to comment on three such papers. Lieberman, Maumenee and Green[33], based on histological study, strongly asserted that the peripapillary choroid has *no* significant role in the blood supply of the optic nerve head. According to these authors, branches from so-called "scleral short posterior ciliary arteries", and not the peripapillary choroidal arteries, supply the prelaminar region, and some of the branches of these arteries formed pial branches to supply the retrolaminar region. At the same time they stated "Insofar as the short posterior ciliary arteries contribute branches to the optic nerve, pial sheath, episclera, and choroid, we henceforth use the term 'scleral short posterior ciliary arteries' instead of Hayreh's 'peripapillary prechoriocapillaris choroidal arteries'". Since they admit that, it is impossible to understand how they can claim that "These branches (of 'scleral short posterior ciliary arteries') usually neither traversed nor originated in the choroid". Later, they claimed to have found, in nearly all specimens, several small

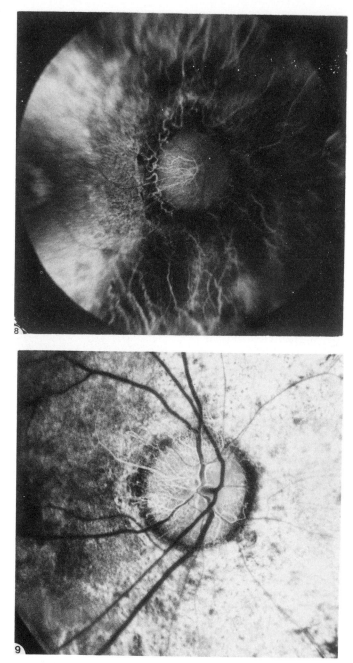

Figs. 8 & 9. Fluorescein fundus angiograms of patients with retinitis pigmentosa during the retinal pre-arterial phase show: (Fig. 8) peripapillary choroidal arterioles and the fine branches arising from them and supplying the temporal part of the prelaminar region (note absence of the choriocapillaris in the peripapillary choroid), and (Fig. 9) prelaminar fine vessels, much more numerous in the temporal part than the nasal part. (Reproduced from Hayreh[9])

capillary vessels arising from the peripapillary choriocapillaris and anastomosing with the vessels of the prelaminar region and surface nerve fiber layer; yet later on in the same paragraph they contradicted themselves, stating "the capillary beds of the optic nerve and

Optic nerve head blood supply in health and disease

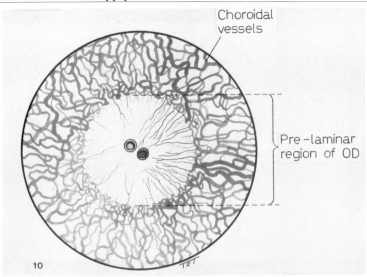

Fig. 10. Schematic representation of the peripapillary choroidal vessels and their centripetal contribution to the prelaminar region of the optic disc, as revealed by fluorescein angiography. The temporal part of the disc has more vessels than the nasal part. (Reproduced from Hayreh[9])

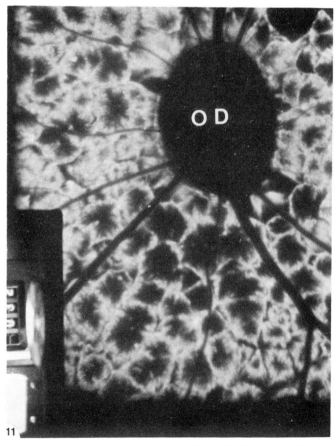

Fig. 11. Fluorescein fundus angiogram of a normal eye of a healthy Rhesus monkey, during the retinal pre-arterial phase showing early filling of the choriocapillaris. Note a sharp inner border of filling of the peripapillary choriocapillaris, which shows no extension into the adjacent prelaminar region of the optic disc (OD).

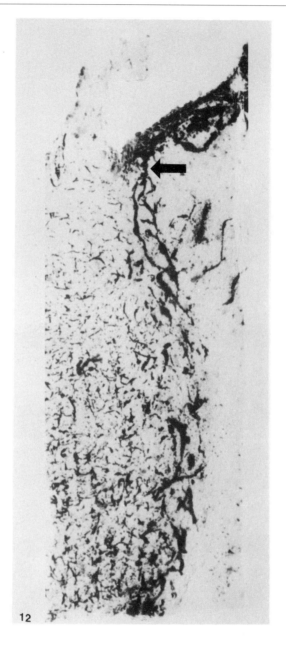

Fig. 12. A longitudinal section of the anterior segment of the intra-orbital part of a human optic nerve and the adjoining part of the eyeball, shows fine angioarchitecture. A recurrent pial branch from the choroidal vessels is seen running backwards in the pia (arrow) . (Reproduced from Hayreh[6])

choriocapillaris were for the most part distinctly separate". All fluorescein angiographic and post-mortem injection cast studies by a large number of authors have clearly demonstrated that choriocapillaris *do not* communicate with the capillaries in the optic nerve head (Fig. 11), thus refuting their earlier statement. If one takes into consideration the difference in semantics between them and the other authors, it seems that they are in fact indirectly stating that the peripapillary choroid does supply the prelaminar region and retrolaminar region of the optic nerve head.

Persons holding the view that the peripapillary choroid does not supply the optic nerve

Optic nerve head blood supply in health and disease

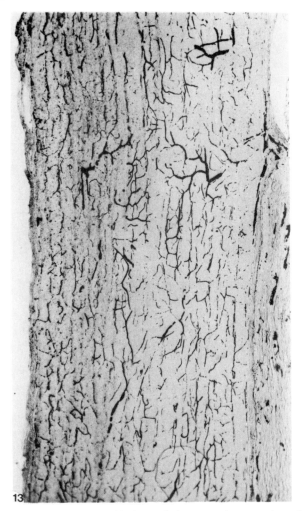

Fig. 13. Longitudinal section of the intra-orbital part of a human optic nerve, shows fine angioarchitecture. (Reproduced from Hayreh[6])

head have argued that if the peripapillary choroid is the main source of blood supply to the optic nerve head, then why, in eyes with ophthalmoscopically seen white peripapillary ring, is there no optic atrophy? It must be pointed out that Bruch's membrane, like many other tissues (e. g., glial tissue, asteroid hyalosis, retinal lipid deposits) is opaque white in appearance to the reflected light of the ophthalmoscope but is transparent to the transmitted light of fluorescein angiography[60]. Thus, the white peripapillary ring seen on ophthalmoscopy is an ophthalmoscopic artifact produced by reflection of incident rays of the ophthalmoscope light from Bruch's membrane (and it does not represent sclera, as has been presumed by many persons) because fluorescein fundus angiography invariably shows the presence of normal large peripapillary choroidal vessels and fine branches arising from them and going to the prelaminar region[9] (Fig. 8) . This phenomenon also explains why redness or pallor of the optic disc on ophthalmoscopy is not a true guide to its vascularity[7,9,60]. Thus lack of awareness of this artifact in the ophthalmoscopic examination is responsible for the erroneous impression mentioned above.

Araki[61], based on his corrosion cast studies, stated that the prelaminar capillaries were not derived from the peripapillary choroid but from branches of the short PCAs. However, study of the two photographs reproduced by the author in support of his conclusion definitely contradicts this. His first picture shows definite branches from the peripapillary choroidal arteries to the prelaminar region and his legend mentions the same in spite of his conclusions to the contrary! His second picture, which he erroneously described as of the prelaminar region, is revealed by a close examination to be an anterior view of the lamina cribrosa, because of its continuity at the margins with the sclera and its morphology; and branches from the short PCAs can be seen piercing the sclera before they ramify in the lamina cribrosa. Thus his contentious conclusions were based on misinterpretation, and on examination of *only one eye*. This is not uncommon in the literature.

A recent paper[62], based on histological, X-ray angiographic and vascular cast scanning electron microscopic studies, made a very dogmatic statement: "The blood supply of the prelaminar layer comes directly from the branches of the short posterior ciliary arteries and Zinn's circle, while the choroidal vessels contribute only a few branches to this area. The above two results are not consistent with Hayreh's idea". A critical review of this paper reveals that this statement is based essentially on wrong interpretation, and the authors have given no details of their scientific data to support their conclusion. My interpretation of the pictures given in support of their findings (invariably the pictures reproduced in any publication represent the best and most representative of that study) would be very different from theirs. For example, what they interpreted as "Circle of Zinn" has been interpreted by me and many others, who have conducted identical studies, as peripapillary choroidal arterial arcade arranged in a circular fashion in the peripapillary region; this peripapillary choroidal arterial arcade is seen clearly in the fluorescein fundus angiogram in Fig. 8 and branches from the arcade to the prelaminar region are also seen in this angiogram. If this arterial arcade were "Circle of Zinn" which lies in the sclera, one would not be able to see it on a fluorescein angiogram. Similarly, the authors stated that "The blood supply to prelaminar region comes from the branches of the short posterior ciliary arteries" but I could not find any illustration in the paper which supports this statement, and there is no data in the paper giving the incidence of branches coming directly from the "short posterior ciliary arteries" and/or from the "Circle of Zinn". The other thing one has to bear in mind is that short PCAs, once they have pierced the sclera, are called the "choroidal arteries" - it seems the authors are calling them "short posterior ciliary arteries" instead of "choroidal arteries"; that is wrong. Thus, I find one of the major causes of the entire confusion in this paper is the definition of the so-called "Circle of Zinn" and of the "short posterior ciliary arteries", and serious problems with the semantics used by the authors. Also in the cast preparation, the authors could not differentiate exactly the prelaminar from the lamina cribrosa region, thereby causing the confusion. Many studies, apart from mine, conducted in man and primates and by highly experienced investigators[42-44,46-50,53], using the same methods as these authors, *i. e.* , post-mortem injection, histological, and scanning electron microscopic techniques, have shown and documented indisputable branches from the peripapillary choroid to the prelaminar region. Also this paper has little scientific validity because it makes generalized statements without giving any specific scientific data about the exact findings and the frequency of distribution of the various patterns. One can find many more problems with this paper to invalidate its conclusions.

Thus a review of these papers demonstrates serious problems with interpretation of their findings rather than with the actual vascular pattern of the optic nerve head.

b. *The nature of the axial vascular system in the optic nerve head*: François and Neetens[37,38,63,64] during the mid-fifties claimed that the "central artery of the optic nerve" formed the axial vascular system, with the central retinal artery playing no role in the blood supply of the optic nerve. They stated that "a central artery of the optic nerve undoubtedly exists"[38] and "the existence of such an artery in the optic nerve is beyond all doubt"[64]; yet neither I[4] nor any other investigator in the field could find any such artery despite careful, detailed studies in much larger samples. It seems that the existence of the central artery of the optic nerve was postulated by François and his colleagues as a prerequisite for explaining the pathogenesis of anterior ischemic optic neuropathy. However, in view of this controversy, in 1977 François reinvestigated the subject with Fryczkowski[65-68], and in their series of 40 optic nerves they *did not* find any central artery of the optic nerve in any specimen, thus confirming findings by me[4] and many others on the subject and finally abolishing the mythical "central artery of the optic nerve" which they had propagated vigorously for almost a quarter of a century. Had I not insisted for almost twenty years that this artery did not exist, we might still be interpreting the ischemic disorders of the optic nerve head and optic nerve as a result of occlusion of the mythical central artery of the optic nerve. In spite of that, Lieberman *et al.*[33] have tried to revive the concept by describing the so-called "central optic nerve artery equivalents" when they stated that "the pial-derived longitudinal arterioles in the retrolaminar nerve qualify as central optic nerve artery equivalents". This statement is totally misleading, because the pial feeders to the optic nerve run in all directions and lie throughout the thickness of the optic nerve in its intraorbital part, without any *in vivo* functional anastomoses; thus these pial-derived vessels in no way deserve the designation of "central optic nerve artery equivalents". Pial branches do not form any worthwhile axial vascular system of the optic nerve which is mostly supplied by the intraneural branches of the central retinal artery (which were presumably seen by Lieberman *et al.*[33] in most of the nerves and misinterpreted). In my studies with liquid neoprene latex,[1,3,4] the central retinal artery gave one to eight prominent branches during its course within the optic nerve in 75% of the specimens (Fig. 2).

c. *Dangers of extrapolating in vivo blood flow pattern in the optic nerve head from morphological studies only*: As discussed above, capillaries in the optic nerve head form a continuous network which is continuous anteriorly with the retinal capillary bed and posteriorly with the adjacent optic nerve. Lieberman *et al.*[33], based on purely histological studies, attached great importance to these capillary anastomoses and stated that because of the free anastomoses in the longitudinal vascular system in the angioarchitecture of the optic nerve, the blood supply to this part of the optic nerve is *not* sectoral, and that the longitudinal system is of great functional importance (indicating thereby that in the event of occlusion of one or more feeders to the system, the blood supply to the involved sector of the optic nerve head can be maintained by these anastomotic capillary channels). This group has argued from purely morphological studies that this freely communicating capillary network (because of presence of the longitudinal vascular system) protects the optic nerve head from developing any ischemia. Unfortunately there is no *in vivo* support at all for this presumption. For example, in the retina, fluorescein angiographic and retinal digest preparations have clearly demonstrated that the retinal capillary network is one freely communicating continuous vascular bed (Figs. 3-B, 4), similar to that in the optic nerve head; in spite of that, occlusion of even a tiny pre-capillary terminal, retinal arteriole always results in the production of a cotton-wool spot and focal non-perfusion of the retinal capillary bed seen on fluorescein fundus angiography and retinal digest studies. Thus, *capillary anastomoses never safeguard the neural tissue in the involved region from ischemic damage, because they are incapable of establishing collateral circulation rapidly enough to protect the neural tissue*. This disparity between the speculation by Lieberman *et al.*[33] (based on morphological studies only) and all *in vivo* studies demonstrates that to extrapolate from morbid anatomical and histological studies to *in vivo* blood flow and circulation is a serious error of judgment. The same criticism holds good where, from morphological studies, the mere presence of capillaries in the optic nerve head[69] or presence of red blood cells in the capillaries[70,71] is interpreted to mean that the circulation is normal - but the simple presence of capillaries or red blood cells in them on histological examination is *no* proof at all that there is normal blood flow in the optic nerve head nor that there is no ischemia. These are a few of the examples where morphological studies are totally misleading about the blood flow in the optic nerve head. Similarly, our experimental occlusion studies on the PCAs and other *in vivo* studies on the choroidal vascular bed[12–18,20] have clearly shown how the various post-mortem injection and morphological studies conducted in the past had misled us into believing that the choroidal vascular bed was one freely communicating system and that it could never develop focal ischemic lesions, when our *in vivo* studies revealed this concept to be totally erroneous and showed that this is a completely end-arterial system (as discussed below). Thus, in conclusion, it is crucial to remember that morbid anatomy and morphology may have no relevance to the physiological *in vivo* blood flow in the eye and optic nerve.

d. *Sectoral distribution of blood supply in the optic nerve head*: In normal eyes, fluorescein fundus angiography reveals a segmental distribution of blood supply in the optic disc. Our studies in about 700 patients with anterior ischemic optic neuropathy have clearly shown a sectoral involvement of the optic nerve head by acute ischemia in all eyes (as shown by the many fluorescein angiograms reproduced below). As discussed above, these findings totally refute the views of Lieberman *et al.*[33] that there is no sectoral distribution of blood supply in the optic nerve head because of the presence of a continuous capillary network.

e. *Watershed areas in the retrolaminar optic nerve*: Rootman and Butler[72] speculated about the presence of a "watershed area" in the retrolaminar optic nerve, without any proof whatsoever. From a knowledge of blood supply of the optic nerve, drawn from more than three decades of studies of the subject in health and disease, I can see no logical reason for the presence of any watershed zone in the retrolaminar region, other than pure armchair philosophy. I would like to stress that the presence of watershed zones between the various PCAs, discussed later on, has nothing to do with what has been speculated by Rootman and Butler[72] and the two should not be confused.

Inter–individual variation in blood supply of the optic nerve head:

Our post-mortem intravascular injection studies as well as *in vivo* studies have shown that there is a marked inter-individual variation in the blood supply of the optic nerve in man. In view of that, the universal impression that all ischemic lesions are explainable on one standard vascular pattern is a fundamental mistake. I have discussed the subject of inter-individual variation in the blood supply of the optic nerve head in detail elsewhere[28]. This variation is produced by the following factors:

I. *Variations in the anatomical pattern of the blood supply of the optic nerve head:*

The pattern described earlier in this paper is very common (Figs. 1, 2). However, there are many variations. For example, the retrolaminar region may be supplied only by the PCA circulation, or, occasionally, the major source of supply to the axial part of the retrolaminar optic nerve may be the central retinal artery; or the two systems may both make contributions, equal or unequal, in different proportions. In still other cases, pial branches from sources other than PCA (*e.g.*, pial branches from the central retinal artery and/or other orbital arteries) may take on a major role. Similarly, the nerve fiber layer, although usually supplied mostly by the retinal arterial circulation, may have a variable contribution from the prelaminar PCA circulation (particularly to the temporal region - Fig. 4).

Thus, the optic nerve head may be supplied to an infinitely variable extent by the PCAs, central retinal artery, and pial branches from sources other than PCA and central retinal artery. Studies based on only a few eyes are likely, therefore, to give skewed information, depending upon what method of investigation was used and what patterns it happened to show in those few specimens - making every investigator believe that the particular pattern he describes is right - which it may well be! This is rather like the old story of the blind

Optic nerve head blood supply in health and disease 17

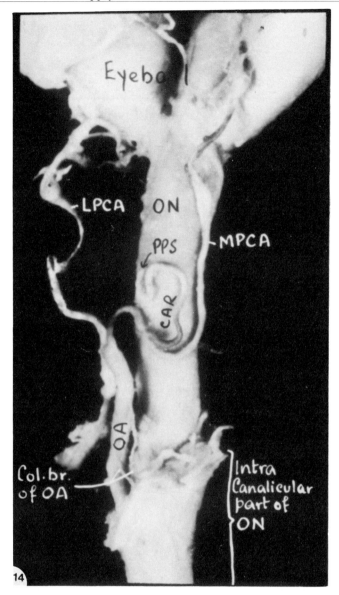

Fig. 14. Photograph of inferior surface of optic nerve (ON) and eyeball, shows ophthalmic artery (OA), central artery of retina (CAR), medial (MPCA) and lateral (LPCA) posterior ciliary arteries filled with Neoprene latex. Also shown are collateral branches (Col. br.) of OA to intracanalicular part of ON. (Reproduced from Singh and Dass[2])

men describing an elephant; each found something different but none could describe the whole. Only a large series such as ours, using a variety of techniques, can give truly accurate information.

II. *Variations in the pattern of posterior ciliary artery circulation*:

As discussed earlier, the PCAs, via the peripapillary choroid or the short PCAs, are the main source of blood supply to the optic nerve head. Therefore, it is natural that variations in the pattern of distribution by the PCAs should influence the pattern of blood supply of the optic nerve head. These variations in the PCAs can be classified into the following categories:

A. *Variations in number of PCAs supplying an eye*: My anatomical studies on the branches of ophthalmic artery in man showed that one to five (one in 3%, two in 48%, three in 39%, four in 8%, five in 2%) PCAs may arise from the ophthalmic artery to supply the eye[73]. I designated the PCAs as "lateral", "medial" and "superior" according to their relation with the optic nerve at their site of entry into the eyeball[73] (Fig. 14) . The lateral PCAs may be none (in 3%) , one (in 75%) , two (in 20%) or three (in 3%) in an eye, with one (in 70%) or two (in 30%) medial PCAs, and an additional one (in 2%) or two (in 7%) superior PCAs.

B. *Variations in the area of the optic nerve head supplied by the various PCAs*: Fluorescein fundus angiography is the only means to obtain definite information about the area supplied by the various PCAs. Our studies have shown that when there are medial and lateral PCAs, there is a marked variation in the area supplied by them (Figs. 15-35) . Our *in vivo* experimental studies after occlusion of the various PCAs [12,13,18,20] and clinical studies in patients with anterior ischemic optic neuropathy have shown that PCAs act as end arteries and the various PCAs neither anastomose with one another nor with the anterior ciliary arteries, so that each PCA has a defined territory of supply in the choroid and the optic nerve head.

1. *When there are only medial and lateral PCAs*: The medial and lateral PCAs supplied the nasal and temporal parts of the choroid respectively (Figs. 15-35) , with the border between the two territories usually vertical, and situated anywhere in the shaded area shown in Fig. 34. In some eyes the border was oriented obliquely.

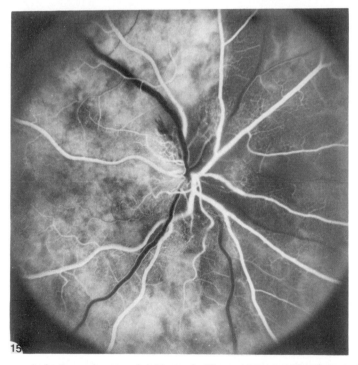

Fig. 15. Fluorescein fundus angiogram, of right eye of a 75-year-old man with anterior ischemic optic neuropathy (negative temporal artery biopsy for giant cell arteritis) , shows normal filling of the area supplied by the lateral PCA (including the temporal half of optic disc) but no filling of the area supplied by the medial PCA (including the nasal half of optic disc) . (Reproduced from Hayreh[28])

Optic nerve head blood supply in health and disease

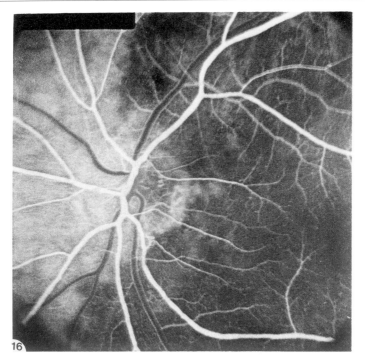

Fig. 16. Fluorescein fundus angiogram, of left eye of a 78-year-old man with anterior ischemic optic neuropathy (negative temporal artery biopsy for giant cell arteritis), shows normal filling of the area supplied by the medial PCA (including the nasal half of disc) but no filling of the area supplied by the lateral PCA (including the temporal half of disc. (Reproduced from Hayreh[28])

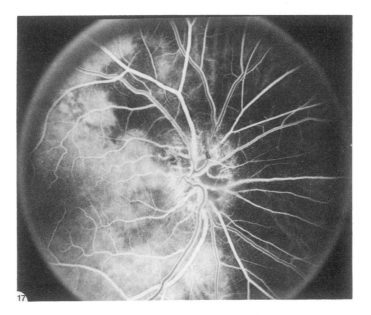

Fig. 17. Fluorescein fundus angiogram, of right eye of an 82-year-old man with arteritic anterior ischemic optic neuropathy, shows normal filling of the area supplied by the lateral PCA (including a small part of the papillomacular bundle in optic disc, with 6/7.5 visual acuity in a tiny island of central vision) but no filling of the area supplied by the medial PCA. (Reproduced from Hayreh, SS: Int Ophthalmol 1:9-18, 1978)

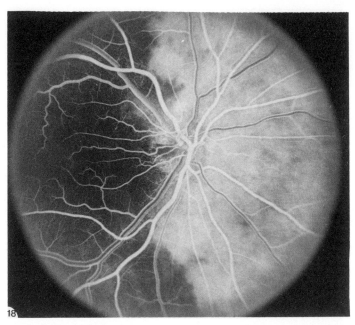

Fig. 18. Fluorescein fundus angiogram, of right eye of a 70-year-old man with anterior ischemic optic neuropathy (negative temporal artery biopsy for giant cell arteritis), shows normal filling of the area supplied by the medial PCA in the choroid and optic disc but no filling of the area supplied by the lateral PCA (including a small sector of the papillomacular bundle in the disc). (Reproduced from Hayreh[28])

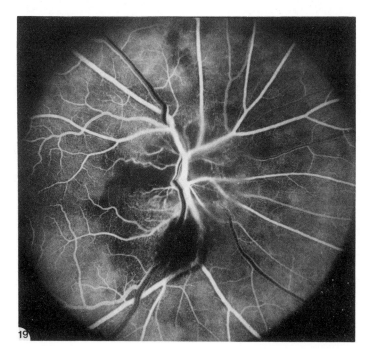

Fig. 19. Fluorescein fundus angiogram, of right eye of a 67-year-old woman with arteritic anterior ischemic optic neuropathy, shows normal filling of the area supplied by the lateral PCA (including a small peripheral part of the superior temporal region of the disc) but no filling of the area supplied by the medial PCA. (Reproduced from Hayreh[28])

Optic nerve head blood supply in health and disease 21

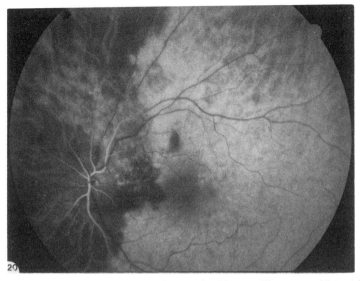

Fig. 20. Fluorescein fundus angiogram, of left eye of a 78-year-old woman with arteritic anterior ischemic optic neuropathy and partial central retinal artery occlusion, shows normal filling of the area supplied by the lateral PCA but much delayed filling of the area supplied by the medial PCA and of the central retinal artery (because of almost complete occlusion of the common trunk of central retinal artery and medial PCA[2,73] at its origin from ophthalmic artery). (Reproduced from Hayreh[28])

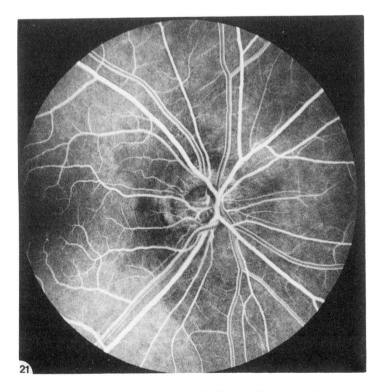

Fig. 21. Fluorescein fundus angiogram, of right eye of a 59-year-old woman with low-tension glaucoma, shows filling of the area supplied by the lateral PCA (temporal to the peripapillary choroid) but no filling as yet of the area supplied by the medial PCA. (Reproduced from Hayreh[80])

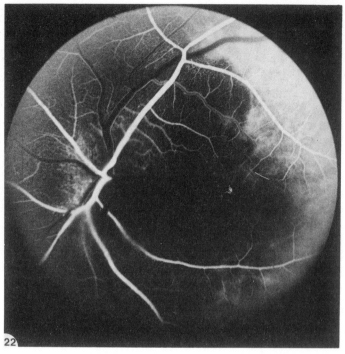

Fig. 22. Fluorescein fundus angiogram, of left eye of a 63-year-old woman with arteritic anterior ischemic optic neuropathy, shows normal filling of the area supplied by the lateral PCA but no filling of the area supplied by the medial PCA (including the entire optic disc, with no perception of light). (Reproduced from Hayreh, SS: Int Ophthalmol 1:9-18, 1978)

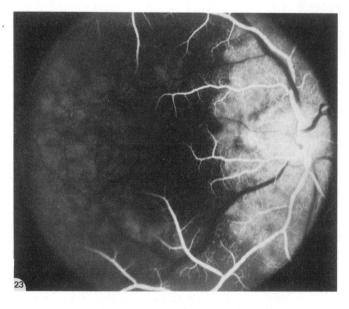

Fig. 23. Fluorescein fundus angiogram, of right eye of a 61-year-old man with internal carotid artery occlusion, shows good filling of the area supplied by the medial PCA (including the entire optic disc) and extremely early patchy filling of the area supplied by the lateral PCA. (Reproduced from Hayreh *et al.* Arch Ophthalmol 100:1585-1596, 1982)

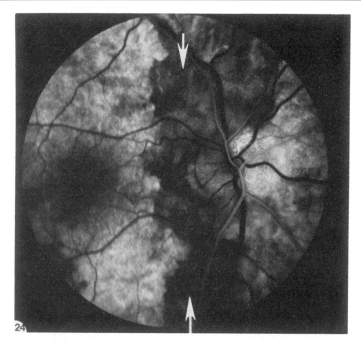

Fig. 24. Fluorescein fundus angiogram, of right eye of a 14-year-old girl with pseudopapilledema, shows the delayed filling of the watershed zone (indicated by arrows) between the lateral and medial PCAs. (Reproduced from Hayreh[28])

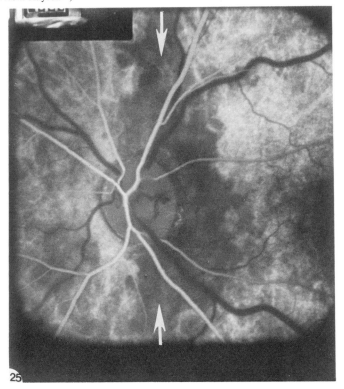

Fig. 25. Fluorescein fundus angiogram of left eye of a 31-year-old woman with resolved non-ischemic central retinal vein occlusion, shows non-filling of the watershed zone (indicated by arrows) between the lateral and medial PCAs. (Reproduced from Hayreh[28])

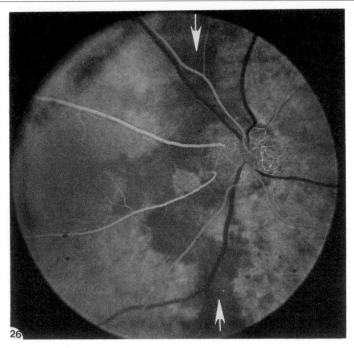

Fig. 26. Fluorescein fundus angiogram, of right eye of a 66-year-old man with old central retinal artery occlusion, shows non-filling of the watershed zone (indicated by arrows) between the lateral and medial PCAs. (Reproduced from Hayreh[18])

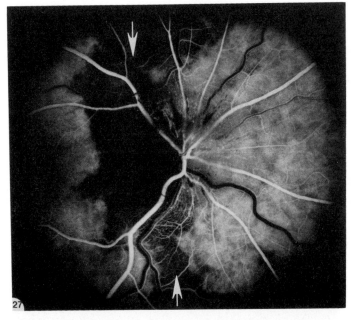

Fig. 27. Fluorescein fundus angiogram, of right eye of a 60-year-old man with non-arteritic anterior ischemic optic neuropathy, shows non-filling of the watershed zone (indicated by arrows) between the lateral and medial PCAs. (Reproduced from Hayreh[28])

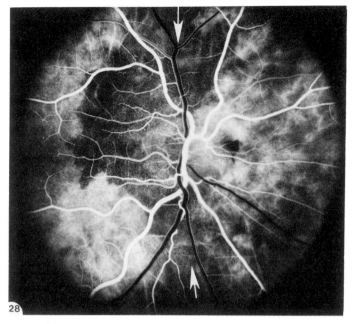

Fig. 28. Fluorescein fundus angiogram, of right eye of a 52-year-old man with non-arteritic anterior ischemic optic neuropathy, shows a non-filling of the watershed zone (indicated by arrows) between the lateral and medial PCAs. (Reproduced from Hayreh[27])

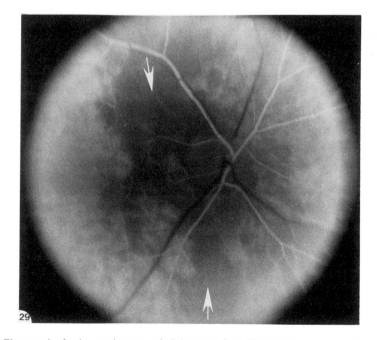

Fig. 29. Fluorescein fundus angiogram, of right eye of an 83-year-old woman with low-tension glaucoma, shows non-filling of the watershed zone (indicated by arrows), and optic disc. (Reproduced from Hayreh[28])

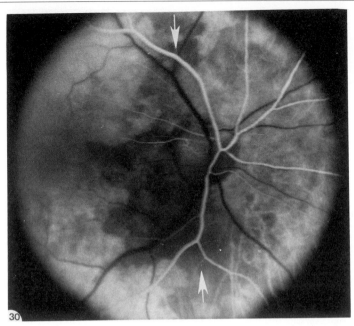

Fig. 30. Fluorescein fundus angiogram, of right eye of a 68-year-old man with low-tension glaucoma, shows poor and patchy filling of the watershed zone (indicated by arrows), optic disc and peripapillary choroid. (Reproduced from Hayreh[28])

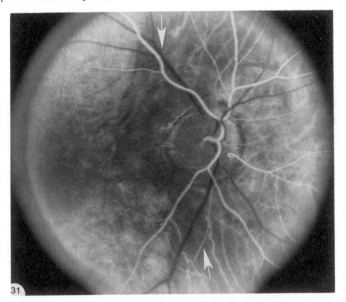

Fig. 31. Fluorescein fundus angiogram, of right eye of a 67-year-old male with low-tension glaucoma, shows filling of the area supplied by the lateral PCA, poor and early filling of the area supplied by the medial PCA and almost no filling of the watershed zone (indicated by the arrows) and the optic disc. (Reproduced from Hayreh[28])

(i) The area supplied by the medial PCA(s) may extend vertically all the way up to almost the nasal border of the fovea (so that the nasal half of the choroid and the entire optic disc is supplied by the medial PCA-system - Figs. 20-23) or the supply may stop short nasal to the nasal peripapillary choroid (so that it may not supply any part of the optic disc - Fig.

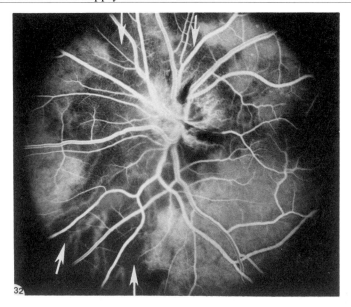

Fig. 32. Fluorescein fundus angiogram, of left eye of a 74-year-old man with arteritic anterior ischemic optic neuropathy, shows non-filling of a watershed zone (indicated by arrows) between the lateral and medial PCAs. (Reproduced from Hayreh[28])

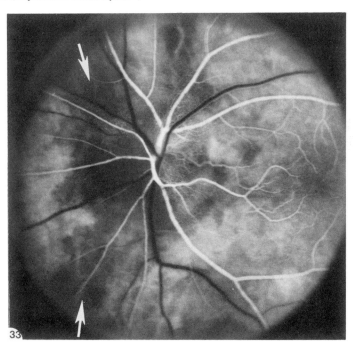

Fig. 33. Fluorescein fundus angiogram, of left eye of a 45-year-old woman with non-arteritic anterior ischemic optic neuropathy, shows non-filling of the watershed zone (indicated by arrow) between the lateral and medial PCAs. (Reproduced from Hayreh[28])

33), or the area of supply may extend anywhere between these two extremes - in that case it may supply variable areas of the optic disc in different eyes (Figs. 15-19) . Because normally the blood flow in the choroidal vascular bed is extremely fast and we cannot routinely take more than one fluorescein fundus angiogram every 0. 5-0. 8 seconds with

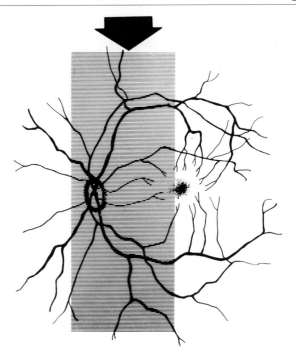

Fig. 34. The shaded area (indicated by arrow) shows the broad area of the choroid between the fovea and nasal peripapillary choroid. The watershed zone between the medial and lateral PCAs may be situated *anywhere* within this area. (Reproduced from Hayreh[28])

the current equipment, it is usually not possible to delineate territorial supply by the various PCAs and their subdivisions; therefore it is not usually feasible to determine whether there are one or more medial PCAs in an eye; the same applies to the lateral PCAs. So it is important to bear this technical limitation of fluorescein angiography in mind when interpreting fluorescein angiograms of the choroid.

(ii) The area supplied by the lateral PCA(s) is reciprocal to that supplied by the medial PCA(s), *i.e.*, if the medial PCA territory extends up to the fovea, then the lateral PCA territory stops short temporal to that so that it takes no part in the blood supply of the optic disc (Figs. 20-33). On the other hand, when the medial PCA territory is nasal to the optic disc (Fig. 33), then the lateral PCA-system supplies the entire optic disc. Thus the medial and lateral PCA-systems share reciprocally the blood supply to the optic disc, with all sorts of combinations.

2. *When there are more than two PCA-systems*: In this case the blood supply to the entire choroid may be like three or more segments of a pie (Figs. 36-39). The area of the optic disc supplied by the various PCAs may vary widely, accordingly.

From this it is evident that the optic disc may be supplied by:
 (i) the medial PCA only,
 (ii) the lateral PCA only,
 (iii) the lateral and medial PCAs in varying proportions, or
 (iv) more than two PCAs in varying extents.

C. *Location of the watershed zone(s) between the various PCAs*: When a tissue is supplied by two or more end-arteries, the border between the territories of distribution of any two end-arteries is called a *"watershed zone"*. The presence of watershed zones

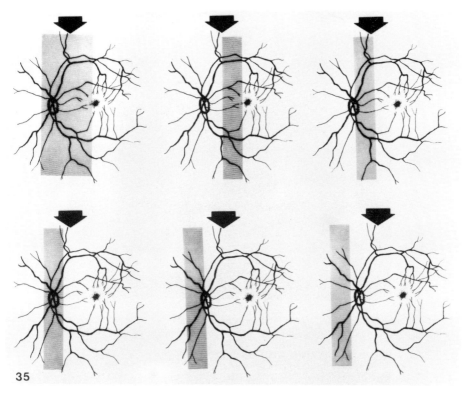

Fig. 35. Diagrammatic representation of some of the locations of the watershed zone (shaded area) between the medial and lateral PCAs in human eyes. In the upper left illustration, the shaded area represents the location where the watershed zone may be situated anywhere within this area (same as Fig. 34). The remaining five illustrations are some examples of the variations in the location. (Reproduced from Hayreh, SS: In: Bernstein EF (ed): Amaurosis Fugax. pp 1–23. New York: Springer-Verlag, 1988)

between the various cerebral arteries is a well-known example. The importance of the watershed zone is that in the event of a fall in perfusion pressure in the vascular bed of one or more end-arteries, the watershed zone, being an area of comparatively poor vascularity, is most vulnerable to ischemia.

Our *in vivo* experimental studies of PCA occlusion[12,13,18,20], as well as clinical studies in anterior ischemic optic neuropathy patients with PCA occlusion or marked stenosis (*e. g.*, in thrombotic occlusion of the PCA seen in patients with giant cell arteritis or in those with embolic occlusion of the PCA - Figs. 15–20, 22)[24–28], we have demonstrated conclusively that the PCAs are end-arteries; this has since been confirmed by other investigators. Our fluorescein angiographic studies have shown the presence of watershed zones between the various PCAs and Figs. 24, 33, 36-39 are some of the examples of the variations seen in its location in different eyes in different conditions. The watershed zone(s) between the various PCAs can only be outlined by a good quality fluorescein fundus angiography but the presently available equipment for angiography has many limitations, as discussed earlier. This is because normally the blood flow in the choroid is so fast that the filling pattern of the areas supplied by the various PCAs and of the watershed zones between them cannot be photographed by the slow speed of angiography equipment available at present; unless, of course, the choroidal circulation is markedly slowed down, as it often is in many eyes with anterior ischemic optic neuropathy, carotid artery insufficiency, and glaucoma and allied disorders. A high resolution videoangiography or cineangiography can provide this information more reliably.

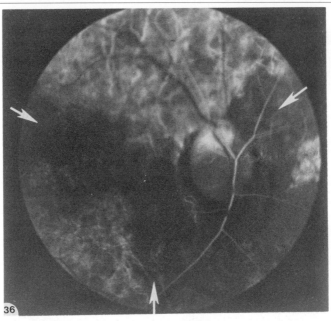

Fig. 36. Fluorescein fundus angiogram, of a normal human right eye, shows a Y-shaped watershed zone (indicated by arrows) between the superior, lateral and medial PCAs. (Reproduced from Hayreh[24])

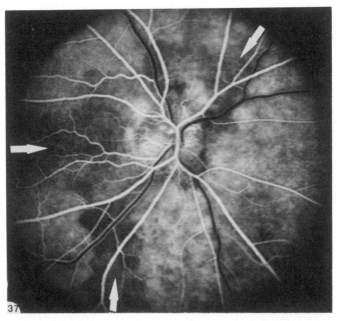

Fig. 37. Fluorescein fundus angiogram, of right eye of a 61-year-old man with non-arteritic anterior ischemic optic neuropathy, shows a markedly delayed filling of a Y-shaped watershed zone (indicated by arrows) between superior, medial and lateral PCAs. (Reproduced from Hayreh[28])

The location of the PCA-watershed zone in relation to the optic disc is an extremely important subject in any discussion of ischemic disorders of the optic nerve head, as revealed by our clinical studies on anterior ischemic optic neuropathy and glaucoma and low-tension glaucoma. This is because our studies indicate that the location of the watershed zone determines the vulnerability of the corresponding part of the optic disc to

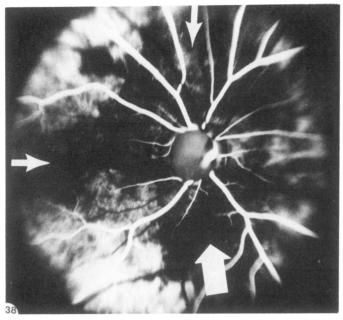

Fig. 38. Fluorescein fundus angiogram of right eye of a 25-year-old woman with primary open-angle glaucoma, total cupping of the optic disc and intraocular pressure of 31 mmHg in the eye, shows non-filling of the watershed zones (indicated by arrows) and peripapillary choroid. (Reproduced from Hayreh[28])

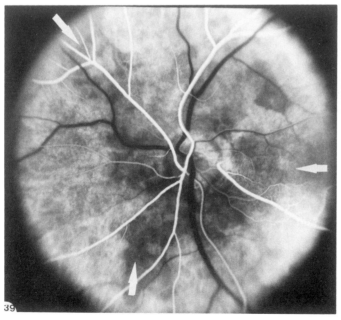

Fig. 39. Fluorescein fundus angiogram, of left eye of a 53-year-old man with ocular hypertension (intraocular pressure 25 mmHg), shows poor and patchy filling of the watershed zone and peripapillary choroid (indicated by arrows). (Reproduced from Hayreh[28])

ischemia. If the watershed zone is located away from the optic disc, the optic nerve head is comparatively less vulnerable to ischemia than if the watershed zone passes through it. The part of the optic disc that lies in the watershed zone is more vulnerable to ischemia than the part that does not. When the entire optic disc lies in the center of a watershed zone,

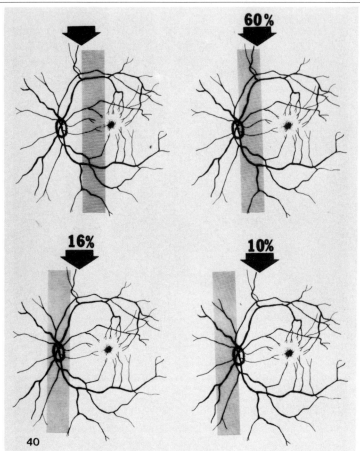

Fig. 40. Diagrammatic representation of some of the locations of the watershed zone (shaded area) between medial and lateral PCAs and their incidence in human eyes with primary open angle glaucoma and low-tension glaucoma.

that disc is most vulnerable to ischemia (Figs. 32, 37, 38) . We have seen this in eyes with anterior ischemic optic neuropathy where the part of the optic disc involved was the part with the watershed zone in it (Figs. 27, 28, 33) . The location of the watershed zone in relation to the optic disc would in turn depend upon the distribution pattern of the various PCAs. I have described above the marked variation in the area supplied by the various PCAs and that, consequently, influences the location of the watershed zone, as is evident from the following:

1. *When there are medial and lateral PCAs*: There is a wide variation in the location of the watershed zone in relation to the optic disc (Figs. 24-35) , so that the watershed zone may be situated:
   (i)   temporal to the peripapillary choroid,
   (ii) pass through the temporal peripapillary choroid,
   (iii) pass through one or the other part of the optic disc,
   (iv) the entire optic disc may lie in the watershed zone,
   (v) pass through the medial peripapillary choroid, or
   (vi) various combinations of the above.

Fig. 35 is a diagrammatic representation of some of the locations of the watershed zone. In our fluorescein angiographic studies in eyes with glaucoma and low-tension glaucoma, where we could outline the watershed zone, we found the incidence of the various

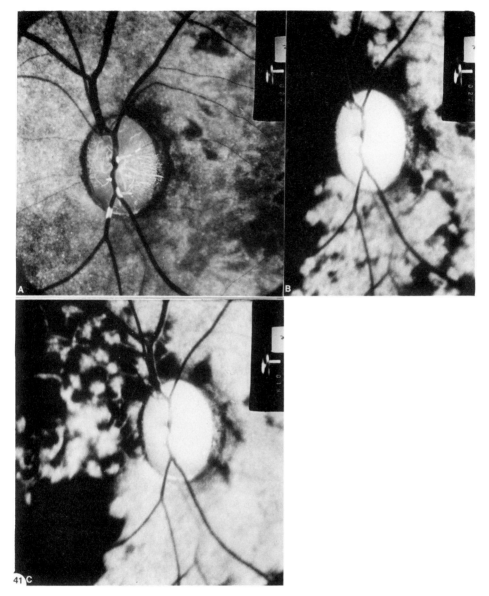

Fig. 41. Fluorescein fundus angiograms, of a normal left eye of a healthy Cynomolgus monkey (after experimental central retinal artery occlusion), at (A) normal, and (B) and (C) 70 mmHg intraocular pressure, show normal choroidal filling in (A), and filling of area supplied only by the lateral PCA in (B) and of additional early filling of area supplied by upper of two medial PCAs a few seconds later in (C). (Reproduced from Hayreh *et al.* [11])

locations of the watershed zone as shown in Fig. 40 - the commonest (60%) site being the temporal part of the optic disc; this may be the reason why nasal step is frequently seen in glaucoma, and why the temporal island of vision is the last to be lost.

2. *When there are three or more PCAs*: The location of the watershed zone varies according to the number of the PCAs and their locations (Figs. 36-39). With three PCAs, usually the watershed zone assumes the shape of the letter "Y", passing through a part of the optic disc (Fig. 36); or the entire optic disc may lie in the watershed zone (Figs. 37-39).

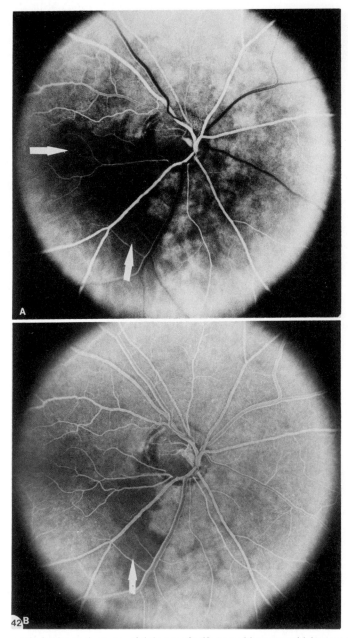

Fig. 42. Fluorescein fundus angiograms, of right eye of a 69-year-old woman with low-tension glaucoma and cupping of the lower half of the optic disc with corresponding visual field defect. A - shows a filling defect (indicated by arrows) in the inferior temporal quadrant of the choroid and lower half of the optic disc. B - (5 seconds after A) shows non-filling of lower half of the watershed zone (indicated by arrow) and the involved lower half of the optic disc. (Reproduced from Hayreh[28])

D. *Difference in blood pressure in various PCAs as well as short PCAs*: Contrary to the generally accepted view, the mean blood pressure in all the major ocular arteries arising from the ophthalmic artery (*e.g.*, central retinal artery and PCAs - Fig. 14) is not always the same, either in health or in disease, as revealed by our experimental and clinical studies (Figs. 41-43). The importance of this is that in the event of a fall of perfusion pressure,

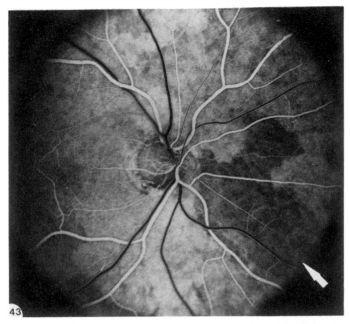

Fig. 43. Fluorescein fundus angiogram, of right eye of a 72-year-old woman with low-tension glaucoma, shows no filling in the distribution of an inferior medial short PCA (indicated by arrow) and involved lower part of the optic disc. (Reproduced from Hayreh[28])

the vascular bed supplied by one artery may be affected earlier and more than others. This is demonstrated by the following examples from our experimental and clinical studies:

In our experimental studies in young, healthy monkeys, with normal eyes, although at normal perfusion pressure the entire choroidal vascular bed filled normally on fluorescein fundus angiography, reduction of perfusion pressure in the PCAs (by experimental elevation of the intraocular pressure) showed much more marked filling defect in the distribution of one PCA than the other. This is demonstrated in Fig. 41 in a case where, at normal intraocular pressure, the entire choroidal vascular bed filled uniformly and simultaneously (Fig. 41A), but on elevation of the intraocular pressure to 70 mm Hg soon after that, angiography showed first filling of the choroid in the territory of the lateral PCA only (Fig. 4lB), with very delayed and slow filling of the medial PCA field later on (Fig. 4lC), indicating that the mean blood pressure in the lateral PCA was higher than in the medial PCA.

In our clinical studies, we have seen many such examples in a variety of conditions. For example, Fig. 23 is an eye with ocular ischemia secondary to complete occlusion of the internal carotid artery. In this eye, fluorescein angiography showed filling of the medial PCA only and even at 43 seconds after injection of the dye there was no filling of the lateral PCA. Similarly, in Fig. 42, an eye with low-tension glaucoma showed a markedly delayed filling of one of the two (inferior) lateral PCAs and the corresponding half of the watershed zone. Fig. 43 is another example of low-tension glaucoma which showed delayed filling of one of the inferior medial short PCAs. This appreciable delayed filling of the choroid in the distribution of one or other PCA or short PCA reflects a lower mean blood pressure in the involved artery as compared to the fellow PCAs in that eye.

E. *Filling defects involving only the upper or lower half of the vertical watershed zone between the PCAs*: I am frequently asked, how can one explain the frequent occurrence of an altitudinal defect in many eyes with anterior ischemic optic neuropathy, when in most of the angiograms shown for the watershed zone, it is usually a complete vertical defect

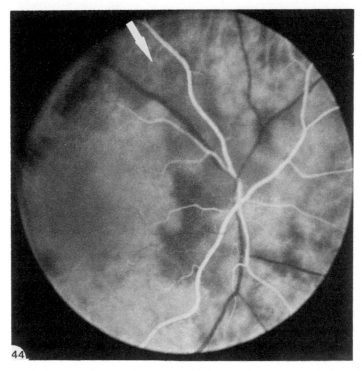

Fig. 44. Fluorescein fundus angiogram, of right eye of a 72-year-old man with arteritic anterior ischemic optic neuropathy, shows a non-filling of the upper half of the watershed zone (indicated by arrows) and involved upper half of the optic disc. (Reproduced from Hayreh[25])

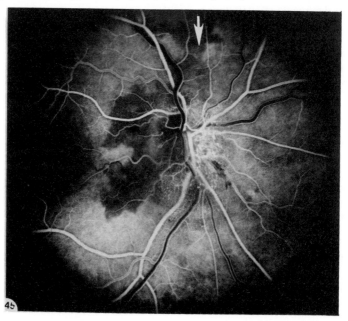

Fig. 45. Fluorescein fundus angiogram, of right eye of a 46-year-old man with non-arteritic anterior ischemic optic neuropathy, shows non-filling of the upper half of the watershed zone (indicated by arrow), superior and temporal peripapillary choroid and the corresponding part of the optic disc. (Reproduced from Hayreh[28])

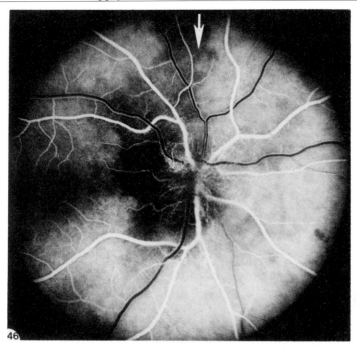

Fig. 46. Fluorescein fundus angiogram, of right eye of a 47-year-old diabetic male with non-arteritic anterior ischemic optic neuropathy, shows non-filling of the upper half of the watershed zone (indicated by arrow), superior and temporal peripapillary choroid and the corresponding part of the disc. (Reproduced from Hayreh[28])

extending all the way from above down? The answer is that watershed zone defects are not always present throughout the vertical length but may be present only in the superior (Figs. 44-46) or inferior (Figs. 42B, 47) half in some eyes.

Naturally the question arises, how can one explain the occurrence of a filling defect involving only one half of the vertical watershed zone? As discussed earlier, an eye can have one or two medial PCAs and up to three lateral PCAs. Let us take the example of an eye which has one medial PCA and two lateral PCAs (superior and inferior), as shown diagrammatically in Fig. 48B; in such an eye, if the inferior lateral PCA has a lower perfusion pressure than the other PCAs, there would be delayed filling of the inferior lateral PCA and a filling defect in the lower half of the watershed zone only - such a situation is shown in Fig. 42 from an eye with low-tension glaucoma. Fig. 49 shows angiograms of a normal monkey eye which had four PCAs - an arrangement similar to that shown diagrammatically in Fig. 48E: Fig. 49B records filling of only the superior medial PCA, and Fig. 49A of both medial and lateral superior PCAs, with the watershed zone located between the two superiorly (indicated by an arrow in Fig. 48B), and no filling of the medial and lateral inferior PCAs. Fig. 48 shows diagrammatically the various combinations which can occur when an eye has more than two PCAs to account for the development of filling defect in only one half of the watershed zone which may be vertically or obliquely oriented. The corresponding part of the optic disc would be involved by ischemia. We have actually seen most of these examples in our clinical studies; the others remain speculative as yet.

III. *Variations in the blood flow in the optic nerve head*:

From the point of view of actual nutrition of the optic nerve head, the essential requirement is the blood flow. As in all the other intraocular vascular beds, the blood flow in the optic nerve head depends upon the following factors:

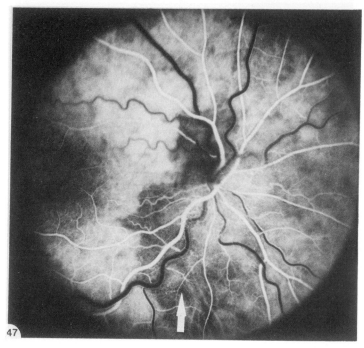

Fig. 47. Fluorescein fundus angiogram, of right eye of a 63-year-old man with internal carotid artery occlusion and non-arteritic anterior ischemic optic neuropathy, shows non-filling of lower half of the watershed zone (indicated by arrow), superior peripapillary choroid and the corresponding parts of the optic disc. (Reproduced from Hayreh[28])

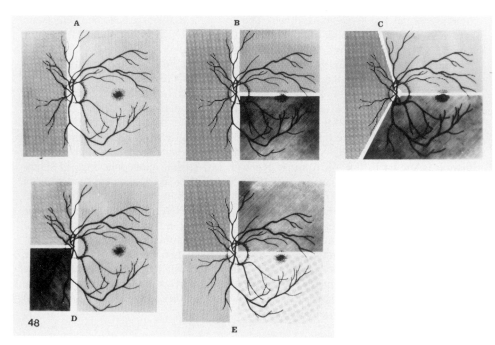

Fig. 48. Diagrammatic representations of some examples of the locations of the borders between the territories of the various PCAs: (A) - with two PCAs: one medial and the other lateral; (B-D) - with three PCAs in different combinations: (B,C) have one medial and two lateral PCAs, and (D) one lateral and two medial; and (E) with four PCAs: two medial and two lateral.

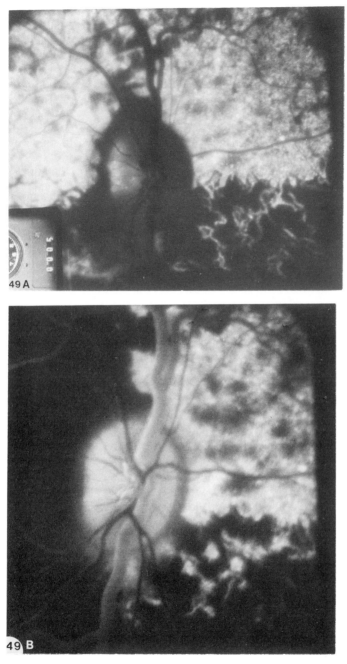

Fig. 49. Fluorescein fundus angiograms of a normal left eye of a healthy Cynomolgus monkey (after experimental occlusion of the central retinal artery to unmask the posterior ciliary vessels in the prelaminar region of the optic disc) with four PCAs (similar to Fig. 48 E) , show: (A) after the first injection of the dye, filling of upper half of the choroid and optic disc with a well-demarcated horizontal border; (B) after the second injection of the dye, filling of superior nasal quadrant before the filling of the superior temporal quadrant of the choroid, indicating that the superior half of the choroid was in fact supplied by two superior PCAs - one medial and the other lateral, and the arrow indicates the watershed zone between the two superior PCAs. The marked fluorescence of the optic disc in (B) was due to the previous injection of fluorescein. (Reproduced from Hayreh[10])

A. *Mean blood pressure*: This is equal to the diastolic blood pressure plus one third of the difference between the systolic and diastolic blood pressures. What matters is the mean blood pressure in the peripapillary choroidal arteries (which are usually the main source of blood supply to the optic nerve head) and the capillaries of the optic nerve head, and not so much the systemic blood pressure measured elsewhere. Indirectly, of course, the mean blood pressure in the optic nerve head depends upon the systemic blood pressure, because that determines to a great extent the blood pressure in the feeding channels of the optic nerve head.

B. *Intraocular pressure*: This plays an important role in determining the perfusion pressure in the intraocular vascular beds, which is calculated by the following formula:

Perfusion pressure = (Mean blood pressure) - (intraocular pressure)

Thus, an increase in intraocular pressure or a fall of mean blood pressure or a combination of the two results in fall of perfusion pressure.

C. *Peripheral vascular resistance*: This also plays an important role in determining the blood flow which can be calculated by the following formula:

$$\frac{\text{Perfusion pressure} \times [(\text{Mean blood pressure}) - (\text{intraocular pressure})]}{\text{Peripheral vascular resistance}}$$

An increase in peripheral vascular resistance must reduce the blood flow, and that can happen in a variety of systemic conditions, including arterial hypertension, arteriosclerosis, and hematologic disorders. Thus, arterial hypertension, although it raises the mean blood pressure, by increasing the peripheral vascular resistance, may ultimately in fact reduce the blood flow in the optic nerve head markedly, as is shown by the development of anterior ischemic optic neuropathy in patients with malignant arterial hypertension[21,22].

D. *Presence or absence of autoregulation*: The object of autoregulation in a tissue is to keep the blood flow relatively constant during changes in its perfusion pressure. Autoregulation is considered a feature of the terminal arterioles although the exact mechanism and site are still not fully understood. With the rise or fall of blood pressure beyond critical levels the arterioles constrict or dilate respectively, to regulate the blood flow. However, autoregulation becomes ineffective when the blood pressure rises or falls beyond certain limits, resulting in *breakthrough of autoregulation*. Thus autoregulation does not protect a tissue all the time but only in a certain range.

It is well-established that the retinal circulation has an efficient autoregulation. Recent studies have shown that optic nerve head vessels also have autoregulation[74-77] although this was denied in earlier studies[78]. The choroid has no autoregulation. If the perfusion pressure rises or falls beyond the critical levels, autoregulation in the optic nerve head fails. For example, the central nervous system has a very efficient autoregulation but still it can develop transient ischemic attacks in the event of a fall of perfusion pressure. Similarly, the optic nerve develops anterior ischemic optic neuropathy because of a transient fall in perfusion pressure during sleep, and these patients classically discover visual loss on waking up in the morning. Thus the mere presence of autoregulation in the optic nerve head does not protect it against ischemic damage. Moreover, it is possible that the autoregulation may not be as efficient in some eyes as others, and with age there may be loss of autoregulation, so that eyes with poor autoregulation may be at much greater risk of developing ischemic damage than those with efficient autoregulation. There are still many unanswered questions on this topic.

Measurement of the blood flow in the optic nerve:

This is evidently the most important parameter we are interested in, for a proper understanding of the pathogenesis of the various ischemic disorders of the optic nerve head. Unfortunately, we have as yet no satisfactory method of measuring the blood flow in the optic nerve head. Of the various factors controlling the blood flow in the optic nerve head, the only parameter we can measure satisfactorily so far is the intraocular pressure. Measurement of systemic blood pressure by the conventional methods may have little relevance to the blood pressure in the optic nerve head capillaries, as discussed above. We have no way of measuring or evaluating the peripheral vascular resistance or the extent of autoregulation in the optic nerve head.

In the literature different methods of obtaining information about the blood flow in the optic nerve head are reported and, very briefly, these include the following:

1. *Morphological studies*: Histological and ultrastructural studies have been employed to learn about the circulation and blood flow in the optic nerve head *in vivo*. The presence of normal capillaries on morphological studies has been interpreted to mean normal circulation in the optic nerve head, but it is well established that this assumption is simply not justified. Morphological studies may actually do more harm than good in this particular context.

2. *Tritiated iodoantipyrine method*: Some authors have used this method to determine the blood flow in the optic nerve head in eyes with raised intraocular pressure[76,79]. The radioactive iodoantipyrine is given intravenously and the amount of its diffusion into the extravascular spaces of the optic nerve head is determined by autoradiography. The validity of the results obtained by this technique in raised intraocular pressure is still doubtful, however, because it gives information on diffusion rather than blood flow in the optic nerve and the two are not necessarily the same thing.

3. *Fluorescein fundus angiography*: This method has been used extensively to determine the blood flow in the optic nerve head. While it has given us a tremendous amount of highly useful information on the subject, its multiple limitations must be kept in mind. I have discussed these in detail elsewhere[30,80]; they include the following:

a. *Unsatisfactory quality of angiograms*: Because of media opacities, inadequate dilatation of the pupil, poor ocular and/or systemic circulation, and poor co-operation, a satisfactory angiogram may not always be obtained.

b. *Limitations of fluorescein angiographic equipment*: As discussed earlier, the current equipment can usually take pictures every 0. 5-0. 8 seconds at its fastest, and that is too slow to catch the various phases in the choroidal filling. Videoangiography with high quality resolution may help to overcome this limitation.

c. *Inadequate resolution of optic disc microvasculature*: Angiography is incapable to resolve microvasculature in the optic disc to demonstrate satisfactorily fine, subtle vascular defects.

d. *Difficulty in outlining the prelaminar disc capillaries*: Once the surface capillaries of retinal origin in the optic disc fill, they completely mask the underlying posterior ciliary circulation in the deeper layers of the disc (Figs. 3, 4).

e. *Optic disc fluorescence on angiography*: We still do not fully understand the origin and importance of disc fluorescence during various phases of the transit of the dye.

f. *Significance of presence or absence of a filling defect on angiography*: There is a good deal of misinformation on this subject among persons who do not have the required expertise in fluorescein angiography of the optic disc, resulting in misinterpretation and wrong conclusions.

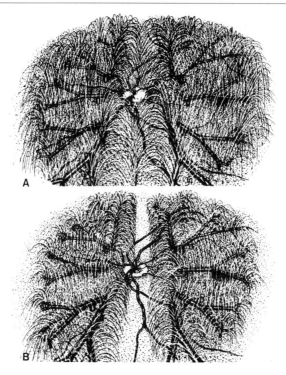

Fig. 50. Two illustrations demonstrating effect of reducing water pressure in garden sprinklers watering a lawn. The sprinklers on two sides of the midline are supplied from two separate sources. (A) Watering with both the sprinklers at normal water pressure. (B) The same area supplied by the sprinklers with reduced water pressure. Note that in the area where water supply by the sprinklers meet in the middle (*watershed zone*), lawn is not being watered now. (Reproduced from Hayreh[80])

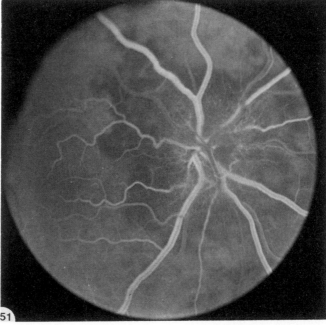

Fig. 51. Right eye of a 72-year-old woman with arteritic anterior ischemic optic neuropathy, and no perception of light. Fluorescein fundus angiogram (three days after the onset of blindness) during the retinal venous phase, shows no filling of the optic disc and peripapillary choroid, with filling of rest of the choroid. (Reproduced from Hayreh[13]).

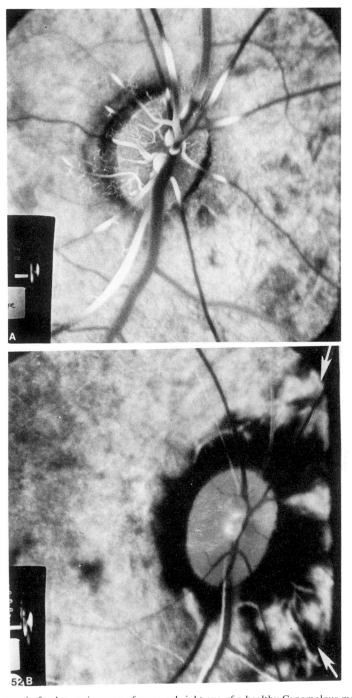

Fig. 52. Fluorescein fundus angiograms of a normal right eye of a healthy Cynomolgus monkey (after experimental central retinal artery occlusion). (A) The entire choroid filled normally at normal intraocular pressure, but, only a few minutes later, (B) at 70 mmHg intraocular pressure, shows no filling of the peripapillary choroid and sparse patchy filling of the watershed zone (indicated by arrows). (Reproduced from Hayreh *et al.*[11])

g. *Reliability of a single angiographic examination*: A single angiographic examination may give quite erroneous and misleading information, because the excitement and worry of visiting the hospital and of angiography, may alter peripheral vascular resistance. Thus, a normal angiogram does not rule out the possibility of circulatory disturbances in the optic disc and/or choroid at other times and *vice versa*.

Therefore, fluorescein angiography has many limitations in providing completely reliable information about the blood flow in the optic nerve head, and one must be fully aware of these when interpreting the results of such a study.

In conclusion: until and unless we have a satisfactory method of measuring the blood flow in the optic nerve head, the current controversies on the various ischemic or presumed ischemic disorders will grind relentlessly on.

Special susceptibility of the choroidal watershed zones and/or peripapillary choroid to non-perfusion or hypo-perfusion in various ischemic disorders:

Our clinical fluorescein angiographic studies in patients with anterior ischemic optic neuropathy (Figs. 27, 28, 32, 33, 37, 44-47, 51), chronic ocular ischemia, primary open angle glaucoma (Fig. 38), ocular hypertension (Fig. 39) and low-tension glaucoma (Figs. 29-31, 42, 43) have commonly demonstrated the special vulnerability of the choroidal watershed zones and/or peripapillary choroid as compared with the rest of the choroidal vascular bed. This was also shown by experimental studies (Fig. 52). The same has been reported in the literature in a large number of clinical and experimental studies on glaucoma[81].

A. *Vulnerability of the choroidal watershed zones to non-perfusion or hypo-perfusion*:

It is well-established that in an end-arterial system, whenever there is a fall in the perfusion pressure, the watershed zone is the most vulnerable to non-perfusion or hypo-perfusion and consequently to ischemia. This has been very well demonstrated in the cerebral circulation, and since the PCA circulation is also an end-arterial system, it has the same basic property. If one were to compare the choroidal vascular bed to a big lawn watered by two sprinklers (lateral and medial PCAs), then the areas watered by the two sprinklers would meet in the middle along a vertical line (the optic disc located on this line in the case of the choroidal vascular bed), as shown in Fig. 50A. When the water pressure in one or both of the sprinklers is reduced, the area watered by the low-pressure sprinkler(s) shrinks away from the midline (Fig. 50B), so that the grass which suffers from lack of water first would be where the areas of the two sprinklers meet (*i.e.* the watershed zone). This is a simplistic explanation of an important phenomenon, of which, unfortunately, most persons in the ophthalmic field are quite unaware. The angiograms in Figs. 24-33, 36-39, 42, 44-47 show the filling defects in the choroidal watershed zones in eyes with anterior ischemic optic neuropathy, low-tension glaucoma, primary open angle glaucoma and ocular hypertension. As discussed above, the location of this watershed zone in relation to the optic disc is an important factor in determining the production and distribution of optic nerve head ischemia.

B. *Special vulnerability of the peripapillary choroid to non-perfusion or hypo-perfusion*:

Since the peripapillary choroid is the main source of blood supply to the optic nerve head (as discussed above), naturally a question arises about the mechanism(s) responsible for this phenomenon. We have as yet no definite explanation for this pattern. One can only speculate. This special vulnerability may be due to a number of factors, including the following:

1. Since the choroidal watershed zone usually passes through the peripapillary choroid, the latter would share the non-perfusion or hypo-perfusion of the watershed zone, as shown in the various angiograms with filling defects of the watershed zone.

2. The following anatomical features of the peripapillary choroid suggest that this part of the choroidal vascular bed is a low-pressure system as compared to the rest of the choroidal circulation[9,80]:

    a. The area of the peripapillary choroid involved lies between the optic disc margin and the sites of entry of the short PCAs into the eyeball. Since the main branches of the short PCAs run forward radially, with the main stream of the blood flow in them directed away from the peripapillary choroid, and the peripapillary choroidal vascular bed itself is presumably formed by small recurrent branches from the main branches, the peripapillary choroid may thus form a backwater and a low-pressure system as compared with the rest of the choroid.

    b. The peripapillary choroid gives out many recurrent pial branches to the retrolaminar optic nerve (Figs. 1, 2, 12) and these branches in their extraocular course are subjected to cerebrospinal fluid pressure in the retrobulbar subarachnoid space around the optic nerve - a pressure much lower than the intraocular pressure. Thus, these recurrent pial branches may act as shunts from the peripapillary choroid which is subjected to the intraocular pressure. This would render the peripapillary choroid a low-pressure system.

These anatomical features of the peripapillary choroidal vessels may render them more prone to non-perfusion or hypo-perfusion in the event of a fall in the perfusion pressure in the choroid than the rest of the choroid, even more than the rest of the watershed zone situated away from the peripapillary choroid.

Clinical applications

From all this discussion, it is clear that the area of the optic nerve head involved by an ischemic disorder would depend upon the following factors:

1. Location of the watershed zone in relation to the optic disc: The part of the optic disc located in the watershed zone is more susceptible to ischemia than the one situated away from it. If the optic disc is situated away from the watershed zone, it would seem to be safe. However, if the optic disc lies in the center of a watershed zone, it is located in the worst possible position and is most vulnerable to ischemia.

2. Distribution of the PCAs in relation to the optic disc and the state of the blood flow in the PCA or the short PCA supplying the optic disc: As discussed earlier, an optic nerve head may be supplied by only one PCA or more than one.

    a. *When the entire disc is supplied by only one PCA* and that PCA has poor blood flow or no blood flow (even if the other PCAs have normal blood flow) , then the optic nerve head is vulnerable to ischemia. On the other hand, if the PCA supplying the disc has good blood flow (even if the other PCAs have poor or no blood flow) the optic nerve head is safe.

    b. *When the optic nerve head is supplied by two or more PCAs*: The area of the optic nerve head supplied by a PCA with poor blood flow is more vulnerable than the rest.

Thus, if the watershed zone is situated away from the optic disc and the PCA supplying the optic disc has a good blood flow, then the disc is safe. The opposite situation makes it highly susceptible to ischemia.

Conclusions

From the above discussion of the various factors which can produce inter-individual variations in the blood supply of the optic nerve head, it is evident that when all the differences are put together, they produce enormous variations. The blood supply pattern of every eye is unique. This makes the subject extremely complex. Many of the current problems in understanding the role of vascular disturbances in ischemic disorders of the optic nerve head are caused by a lack of appreciation of these complexities of its blood supply in health and disease.

Acknowledgments

I am grateful to my wife Shelagh for her help in the preparation of the manuscript, to Mrs. Georgiane Parkes-Perret and Mrs. Ellen Ballas for their secretarial help, and to our photography department for the illustrations. This research was supported by research grants from the National Eye Institute (EY-ll5l, EY-1576, EY-3330) , and in part by unrestricted grants from Research to Prevent Blindness, Inc. and from the Alcon Research Institute.

References

1. Hayreh SS: A study of the central artery of the retina in human beings. Thesis for the Master of Surgery, Panjab University, India, 1958.
2. Singh S, Dass R: The central artery of the retina I. Origin and course. Br J Ophthalmol 44:193-212, 1960
3. Singh S, Dass R: The central artery of the retina II. Distribution and anastomoses. Br J Ophthalmol 44:280-299, 1960
4. Hayreh S: The central artery of the retina - its role in the blood supply of the optic nerve. Br J Ophthalmol 47:651-663, 1963
5. Hayreh SS: The orbital vessels of rhesus monkeys. Exp Eye Res 3:16-30, 1964
6. Hayreh SS: Blood supply and vascular disorders of the optic nerve. Anal Inst Barraquer 4:7-109, 1963
7. Hayreh SS, Perkins ES: Clinical and experimental studies on the circulation at the optic nerve head. Proc Wm MacKenzie Centenary Symposium on the Ocular Circulation in Health and Disease, Glasgow pp 71–86. London: Henry Kimpton 1968
8. Hayreh SS, Perkins ES: The effects of raised intraocular pressure on the blood vessels of the retina and optic disc. Proc Int Symp Fluorescein Angiography, Albi 1969. pp 323–328. Basel: Karger 1971
9. Hayreh SS: Blood supply of the optic nerve head and its role in optic atrophy, glaucoma and oedema of the optic disc. Br J Ophthalmol 53:721-748, 1969
10. Hayreh SS: Pathogenesis of visual field defects - role of the ciliary circulation. Br J Ophthalmol 54:289-311, 1970
11. Hayreh SS, Revie IHS, Edwards J: Vasogenic origin of visual field defects and optic nerve changes in glaucoma. Br J Ophthalmol 54:461-472, 1970
12. Hayreh SS, Baines JAB: Occlusion of the posterior ciliary artery I. Effects on choroidal circulation. Br J Ophthalmol 56:719-735, 1972
13. Hayreh SS, Baines JAB: Occlusion of the posterior ciliary artery III. Effects on the optic nerve head. Br J Ophthalmol 56:754-764, 1972
14. Hayreh SS, Baines JAB: Occlusion of the vortex veins. Br J Ophthalmol 57:217-238, 1973
15. Hayreh SS: The choriocapillaris. Graefes Arch Clin Exp Ophthalmol 192:165-179, 1974
16. Hayreh SS: Submacular choroidal vascular pattern - experimental fluorescein fundus angiographic studies. Graefes Arch Clin Exp Ophthalmol 192:181-196, 1974
17. Hayreh SS: The long posterior ciliary arteries - an experimental study. Graefes Arch Clin Exp Ophthalmol 192:197-213, 1974
18. Hayreh SS: Segmental nature of the choroidal vasculature. Br J Ophthalmol 59:631-648, 1975
19. Hayreh SS, Weingeist TA: Experimental occlusion of the central artery of the retina - I. Ophthalmoscopic and fluorescein fundus angiographic studies. Br J Ophthalmol 64:896-912, 1980
20. Hayreh SS, Chopdar A: Occlusion of the posterior ciliary artery - V. Protective influence of simultaneous vortex vein occlusion. Arch Ophthalmol 100:1481-1491, 1982
21. Kishi S, Tso MOM, Hayreh SS: Fundus lesions in malignant hypertension - II. A pathologic study of experimental hypertensive optic neuropathy. Arch Ophthalmol 103:1198-1206, 1985

22. Hayreh SS, Servais GE, Virdi PS: Fundus lesions in malignant hypertension - V. Hypertensive optic neuropathy. Ophthalmology 93:74-87, 1986
23. Hayreh SS, Servais GE, Virdi PS: Fundus lesions in malignant hypertension - VI. Hypertensive choroidopathy. Ophthalmology 93:1383-1400, 1986
24. Hayreh SS: Anterior ischaemic optic neuropathy - I. Terminology and pathogenesis. Br J Ophthalmol 58:955-963, 1974
25. Hayreh SS: Anterior ischaemic optic neuropathy - II. Fundus on ophthalmoscopy and fluorescein angiography. Br J Ophthalmol 58:964-980, 1974
26. Hayreh SS: Anterior Ischemic Optic Neuropathy. New York: Springer Verlag 1975.
27. Hayreh SS: Anterior ischemic optic neuropathy. Arch Neurol 38:675-678, 1981
28. Hayreh SS: Inter-individual variation in blood supply of the optic nerve head. Its importance in various ischemic disorders of the optic nerve head, and glaucoma, low-tension glaucoma and allied disorders. Docum Ophthalmol 59: 217-246, 1985
29. Hayreh SS, Walker WM: Fluorescent fundus photography in glaucoma. Am J Ophthalmol 63:982-989, 1967
30. Hayreh SS: Factors determining the glaucomatous optic nerve head damage. In: Krieglstein GK (ed) Glaucoma Update-III, pp 40–46. Heidelberg: Springer Verlag 1987
31. Hayreh SS: Structure and blood supply of the optic nerve. In: Heilmann K, Richardson KT (eds) Glaucoma: Conceptions of a Disease. pp 78–96. Stuttgart: Thieme 1978
32. François J, Neetens A: The fine angio-architecture of the anterior optic nerve. In: Cant JS (ed) The Optic Nerve, Proc 2nd Mackenzie Symp, pp 28–39. London: HenryKimpton 1972
33. Lieberman MF, Maumenee AE, Green WR: Histologic studies of the vasculature of the anterior optic nerve. Am J Ophthalmol 82:405-423, 1975
34. Leber T: In :Graefe-Saemisch Handbuch der gesamten Augenheilkunde. 2nd ed vol 2, pt 2. Leipzig: Engelmann 1903.
35. Wolff E: Some aspects of the blood supply of the optic nerve. Trans Ophthalmol Soc UK 59:157-162, 1939
36. Wolff E: The anatomy of the eye and orbit. 3rd edn, pp 265–272. London: Lewis 1948
37. François J, Neetens A, Collette JM: Vascular supply of the optic pathway. II. Further studies by micro-arteriography of the optic nerve. Br J Ophthalmol 39:220-232, 1955
38. François J, Neetens A: Vascularization of the optic pathway. III. Study of intra-orbital and intracranial optic nerve by serial sections. Br J Ophthalmol 40:45-52, 1956
39. Fazio C, Farina P: Sull angioarchitettonica del nervo ottica, del chiasma, della bandelleta. Rev Oto-neuro-oftal 17:38-54, 1940
40. Parsons JH: The Pathology of the Eye, pt 3: pp 949–950. London: Hodder and Stoughton 1906
41. Steele EJ, Blunt MJ: The blood supply of the optic nerve and chiasma in man. J Anat (Lond) 90:486-493, 1956
42. Shimizu K, Ujiie K: Structure of Ocular Vessels, pp 70-79, 108-124, Tokyo: Igaku–Shoin 1978
43. Risco JM, Grimson BS, Johnson PT: Angioarchitecture of the ciliary artery circulation of the posterior pole. Arch Ophthalmol 99:864-868, 1981
44. Fryczkowski AW, Grimson BS, Peiffer RL: Scanning electron microscopy of vascular casts of the human scleral lamina cribrosa. Int Ophthalmol 7:95-100, 1984
45. Anderson DR: Vascular supply to the optic nerve of primates. Am J Ophthalmol 70:341-351, 1970
46. Anderson DR, Braverman S: Re–evaluation of the optic disc vasculature. Am J Ophthalmol 82:165-174, 1976
47. Araki M: Anatomical study of the vascularization of the optic nerve. Nippon Ganka Gakkai Zasshi 79:101-109, 1975
48. Araki M, Honmura S: The collateral communications of the retinal circulation with the choroidal circulation at the optic nerve head. Nippon Ganka Gakkai Zasshi 77:1557-1566, 1973
49. Ernest JT: Pathogenesis of glaucomatous optic nerve disease. Trans Am Ophthalmol Soc 73:366-388, 1975
50. Ernest JT, Potts AM: Pathophysiology of the distal portion of the optic nerve, II. Vascular relationships. Am J Ophthalmol 66:380-387, 1968
51. Evans P, Shimizu K, Limaye S, Deglin E, Wruck J: Fluorescein cineangiography of the optic nerve head. Trans Am Acad Ophthalmol Otolaryngol 77:OP 260-273, 1973
52. François J, Neetens A: Comparative anatomy of the vascular supply of the eye in vertebrates. In: Davson H, Graham P, (eds) The Eye, pt 5, pp 1–70 London: Churchill 1975
53. Henkind P, Levitzky M: Angioarchitecture of the optic nerve - I. The papilla. Am J Ophthalmol 68:979-986, 1969
54. Itoh K: Fluorescein angiographic finding of normal optic disc. Nippon Ganka Gakkai Zasshi 77:1543-1556, 1973
55. Schwartz B, Rieser JC, Fishbein SL: Fluorescein angiographic defects of the optic disc in glaucoma. Arch Ophthalmol 95:1961-1974. , 1977
56. Shimizu K, Yokochi K, Okano T: Fluorescein angiography of the choroid. Jpn J Ophthalmol 18:97-108, 1974
57. Swietliczko I, David NJ: Fluorescein angiography in experimental ocular hypertension. Am J Ophthalmol 70:351-363, 1970

58. Theodossiadis GP: Über die Vaskularisation in der Regio praelaminaris der Papilla optica. Klin Mbl Augenheilkd 158:646-652, 1971
59. Yokochi K, Maruyama H, Sodeno Y: Microcirculation of the disc and peripapillary choroid. Nippon Ganka Gakkai Zasshi 77:1534-1542, 1973
60. Hayreh SS:Colour and fluorescence of the optic disc. Ophthalmologica 165:100-108, 1972
61. Araki M: The role of blood circulation of prelaminar capillaries in producing glaucomatous cupping. Nippon Ganka Gakkai Zasshi 80(4) :201-207, 1976
62. Zhao Y, Li F: Microangioarchitecture of optic papilla. Jpn J Ophthalmol 31:147-159, 1987
63. François J, Neetens A: Vascularization of the optic pathway. I. Lamina cribrosa and optic nerve. Br J Ophthalmol 38:472-488, 1954
64. François J, Neetens A: Central retinal artery and central optic nerve artery. Br J Ophthalmol 47:21-30, 1963
65. François J: Vascularization of the optic nerve. Arch Ophthalmol 95:520, 1977
66. François J, Fryczkowski A: Microcirculation of the anterior part of the optic nerve. Ophthalmologica 175:222-229, 1977
67. François J, Fryczkowski A: The blood supply of the optic nerve. Adv Ophthalmol 36:164-173, 1978
68. François J, Fryczkowski A: A functional importance of central retinal artery anastomoses in the anterior part of the optic nerve. Ophthalmologica 185:15-25, 1982
69. Quigley HA, Addicks EM, Green WR, Maumenee AE: Optic nerve damage in human glaucoma - II. The site of injury and susceptibility to damage. Arch Ophthalmol 99:635-649, 1981
70. Minckler DS, Bunt AH, Johanson GW: Orthograde and retrograde axoplasmic transport during acute ocular hypertension in the monkey. Invest Ophthalmol Vis Sci 16:426-441, 1977
71. Maumenee AE: Causes of optic nerve damage in glaucoma. Ophthalmology 90:741-752, 1983
72. Rootman J, Butler D: Ischaemic optic neuropathy - a combined mechanism. Br J Ophthalmol 64:826-831, 1980
73. Hayreh SS: The ophthalmic artery. III. Branches. Br J Ophthalmol 46:212-247, 1962
74. Ernest JT: Autoregulation of optic-disc oxygen tension. Invest Ophthalmol 13:101-106, 1974
75. Geijer C, Bill A: Effects of raised intraocular pressure on retinal prelaminar, laminar, and retrolaminar optic nerve blood flow in monkeys. Invest Ophthalmol Vis Sci 18:1030-1042, 1979
76. Sossi N, Anderson DR: Effect of elevated intraocular pressure on blood flow; occurrence in cat optic nerve head studied with iodoantipyrine I.-125. Arch Ophthalmol 101:98-101, 1983
77. Weinstein JM, Duckrow RB, Beard D, Brennan RW: Regional optic nerve blood flow and its autoregulation. Invest Ophthalmol Vis Sci 24: 1559-1565, 1983
78. Alm A, Bill A: Ocular and optic nerve blood flow at normal and increased intraocular pressures in monkeys (Macaca irus) : a study with radioactively labelled microspheres including flow determinations in brain and some other tissues. Exp Eye Res 15:15-29, 1973
79. Quigley HA, Hohman RM, Sanchez R, et al: Optic nerve head blood flow in chronic experimental glaucoma. Arch Ophthalmol 103:956-962, 1985
80. Hayreh SS: Pathogenesis of optic nerve damage and visual field defects. In: Heilmann K, Richardson KT (eds) Glaucoma: Conceptions of a disease, pp 104–137. Stuttgart:Thieme 1978

DISCUSSION

Harry A. Quigley : Sohan, you have used angiographic data from anterior ischemic optic neuropathy patients as evidence in favor of a sectorial distribution of blood supply to the optic nerve head. However, from a histopathologic point of view, anterior ischemic optic neuropathy involves all of the disc even though one part of it is usually more affected than the rest: there is loss of nerve fibers, only it is more important in one half than in the other.

Sohan S. Hayreh : I do not dispute that. But from a clinical point of view, as assessed by visual fields, the pattern and amount of loss vary widely. Disc swelling can produce some secondary impairment to the circulation of the initially unaffected part, but the pathogenic mechanism is sectorial.

George L. Spaeth : Is it possible to demonstrate watershed zones in normal eyes?

Sohan S. Hayreh : You realize that the circulation is very fast. If you slow it down in some way then yes, you can demonstrate them. But normal angiograms usually do not pick them out, although very fast angiograms probably would.

Erik L. Greve : Would you expect, then, to demonstrate those watershed zones in normal individuals under acute artificial IOP-elevation with a suction-cup, for instance?

Sohan S. Hayreh : What you would have to do is to slow down the filling of the posterior ciliary arteries, which can probably be achieved by a suction-cup.

Maurice E. Langham : Can the sectorial differences in blood flow be due to variations of vascular resistance?

Sohan S. Hayreh : There may be local variations in vascular resistance but in the cases that I have shown the differences in perfusion are so marked that it is hard to imagine that one part of the choroid will have so much higher vascular resistances than the next.

Erik L. Greve : Sohan, I would like to ask you a more general question: In a clinical setting how do you think that one could best pick up these local variations in blood supply? As you pointed out, standard fluorescein angiography cannot always be relied upon. Do you think that angiograms made in certain particular ways can be of more help, or does the answer not lie in fluorescein angiography at all?

Sohan S. Hayreh : Well, the first thing is that fluorescein angiography must be done very carefully, always by the same person if possible. I have been doing my own angiograms for 25 years to get constant quality material. As far as slowing down the circulation is concerned, I think that there are some important problems. I have tried, with Jean-Jacques DeLaey, artificial acute IOP-elevation, but the quality of the angiograms deteriorates rapidly due to induced astigmatism. This doesn't occur with high-speed or cine-angiography and this is why I am inclined to consider these techniques as more promising for clinical application, and I think that Dr Richard may have something to tell us at this point.

Gisbert Richard : We have examined about 120 healthy human eyes with video-angiography followed by slow-motion analysis of the choroidal filling. Our findings are essentially similar to Dr Hayreh's: First, there can be no more doubts about the fact that choroidal arteries behave as end-arteries. Second, the source of the optic nerve head blood supply can be circular, but this is not very frequent. Finally, in most cases we found watershed zones, usually temporal to the optic nerve head although a number of other patterns do occur: oblique, branching or radiating watershed zones. Sometimes, though, a raster-like filling pattern occurs, which is not consistent with the watershed zone theory. Is it possible that some random parts of a territory supplied by a single artery fill earlier than others?

Sohan S. Hayreh : Such situations do occur in the retinal circulation. Henkind noted radial filling delays in cat eyes, and in my own experiments with monkeys I could see a similar phenomenon, *i.e.* that some parts of the retina fill and empty before others, this filling pattern being the same under acute IOP-elevation. This more-or-less important variation of filling delay might also exist in the choroid.

Harry A. Quigley : Sohan, I have two problems in following your analysis of angiograms from diseased eyes and the way you relate it to physiologic data. The first is that in the majority of cases the watershed zones you describe are vertical, whereas in anterior ischemic optic neuropathy it is usually either the top or the bottom half of the optic nerve head that is involved. The second problem is that the capillaries within the optic nerve head form a continuous plexus, so that in case of reduced flow in the the bottom half of the disc, there's nothing to stop red blood cells in the top part of the optic nerve head from flowing towards the bottom.

Sohan S. Hayreh : I'm glad you have brought this up, Harry, because it gives me the opportunity to stress one thing: Capillaries do not act as arterial branches; the blood supply of the optic nerve head depends directly on the flow in the afferent arteriole. Take the retinal circulation, for instance: a cotton-wool spot is an infarction due to the occlusion of an arteriole. If what you're saying was true, then blood should flow in the infarcted area from the nearby capillaries, since these form a continuous plexus in the retina as well. So cotton-wool spots would never occur, yet they are no uncommon finding.

Erik L. Greve : Harry, you are quoting from histological work, which has provided no evidence for a sectorial blood supply. But don't you think there is evidence from angiograms suggesting that, physiologically at least, the supply is sectorial?

Harry A. Quigley : The only evidence one can collect from a normal angiogram, Erik, is that occasionally fluorescein enters the disc faster from one side than from the other. This simply indicates the flow paths. But we do not know whether the speed with which fluorescein enters the disc has anything to do at all with the true blood flow and with the nutrition of the tissue.

Sohan S. Hayreh : I think it does. When you look at a standard angiogram you can't usually see the pattern of blood supply of the disc because everything fills so fast. But if you had looked at a fast angiogram, you would have seen that each arteriole supplies an individual sector of the disc. And, on the other hand, injury in anterior ischemic optic neuropathy is most of the time segmental.

Discussion

Harry A. Quigley : I agree about the segmental distribution of anterior ischemic optic neuropathy damage, but this isn't necessarily related to the physiologic pattern of blood flow. We don't really know why anterior optic neuropathy is segmental.

Gisbert Richard : With video-angiography, if you have a filling delay in some part of the choroid and you do a very careful slow-motion analysis of the filling pattern of that area, you see that fluorescein comes in from the depth and never from the adjacent areas of the choroid which have filled earlier.

Sohan S. Hayreh : This is indeed the fundamental point that I am trying to make: anastomoses at capillary level serve no useful purpose. They cannot provide a collateral circulation. Tissue perfusion depends only on the terminal arteriole and, again, I think that cotton-wool spots are excellent evidence for this.

Harry A. Quigley : Sohan, if things were as you suggest they are, what would happen if one would isolate a single ciliary artery and inject a dye in it? Would the dye remain in one part of the disc or would it spread throughout its capillary network?

Sohan S. Hayreh : It depends on the situation. In a post-mortem preparation the dye would spread all over the disc, especially if the injection was done with some pressure. Incidentally, this is what happens with choroidal casts, which tend to show that the whole choroid is interconnected, although in the living eye under physiologic conditions there are no anastomoses between the territories of the short posterior ciliary arteries. To come back to your question, if you could manage somehow to inject the dye in a single artery in the living eye, you would see only one sector of the disc become stained. But what you do in an enucleated eye, is push your way through, which gives you erroneous information.

Harry A. Quigley : What you're saying, Sohan, is that in anterior ischemic optic neuropathy for instance, if there is a vertical watershed zone running through the disc, the damage would be limited to either the right or the left disc half. But what usually happens is that it is either the top or the bottom half that is damaged.

Sohan S. Hayreh : There isn't necessarily a contradiction in that. In some angiograms you can see a vertical watershed zone, with its upper part filling earlier than its lower part, or the opposite. Why this happens, I can only speculate: Suppose you have an eye with one medial and two lateral posterior ciliary arteries, one on top of the other, and that the bottom one has a lower pressure; the top part of the watershed zone would fill very fast while the bottom part would fill much slower. At the same time, the tissue perfusion of the lower part of the disc would be more vulnerable. Not all the eyes with highly segmented blood supply get anterior ischemic optic neuropathy, of course. It may well be that they are much more susceptible but we have no evidence on that since we have no way, yet, to determine the blood flow in each of the posterior ciliary arteries.

George L. Spaeth : Scientists tend to abstract, that is to make generalizations out of specific cases. This is of course useful but, if overdone, it may be dangerous too. Maybe we ought to accept that there is a marked interindividual variation and leave things at that, for the time being. I would however like to ask Dr Richard about the percentage of people who show a sectorial distribution of their optic nerve head blood supply in video-angiography. Because if it is just 2%, it might be that these are precisely the eyes at high risk for glaucoma.

Gisbert Richard : No, the percentage is much higher than that: In about 60% of the eyes there is a clear-cut watershed zone. For the rest, such a zone is very hard to demonstrate in about 20% of the eyes. This may mean either that there is no watershed zone or that the arterial territories on either part of it fill at exactly the same rate. In those cases video-angiography can't be of much help.

Douglas R. Anderson : I would first like to make a few comments on what we have just heard: First of all, the appearance time of fluorescein depends not only on the blood pressure in the arterioles but also on the length of the path from the ophthalmic artery to the capillaries. Therefore it does not necessarily reflect the volume flow occurring in a particular vascular bed: The fact that fluorescein arrives later at a given location doesn't necessarily mean that there is a deficient flow; it may mean that the transit path is longer, for instance.

My second comment is on the point raised by Dr Quigley about the anastomotic capillary network and his suggestion that red blood cells should move freely all over it. I think that the diameter of those capillaries is so small that their resistance to flow is very high (even if the overall resistance of the capillary bed is very low, due to the enormous amount of capillaries present). So that if one arteriole is obstructed there may be some extension of the areas supplied by adjacent arterioles, but this is not sufficient to compensate the resulting ischemia and infarction occurs. To all purposes the circulation is of end-artery type, in spite of the capillary anastomoses.

Juan E. Grunwald : Do we have evidence that these anastomoses really exist? It isn't easy to follow capillaries over long distances in serial sections!

Douglas R. Anderson : No, but as Sohan pointed out earlier, if you inject latex under pressure in an enucleated eye the whole capillary network will eventually fill.

Juan E. Grunwald : But the filling may come from the venous side.

Harry A. Quigley : No, there have been casts made from injection in the arteries with the heart cut open so that venous pressure was zero and no reflux was possible showing an interconnected, continuous capillary plexus. The anatomy is clear about that. But I would like to ask you, Dr. Anderson, about the physiological aspect of the circulation: I know that you have done some experiments involving occlusion of the posterior ciliary arteries...

Douglas R. Anderson : Yes, that's right. We did some experiments in which we occluded one or more posterior ciliary arteries. And our results were not the same as Sohan's, which simply means that our experiments weren't identical since we had to occlude a large number of short posterior ciliary arteries to observe some infarction.

Sohan S. Hayreh : I recall your publication*, Doug, from a few years ago. I think that the difference in results comes from a problem that I had also encountered

---

Editors' note : Anderson DR, Davis EB: Retina and optic nerve after posterior ciliary artery occlusion; an experimental study in squirrel monkeys. Arch Ophthalmol 92:422-426, 1974.

in my first studies: The effect of short posterior ciliary artery occlusion is minimized if the vortex veins are obstructed. And when you do a lateral orbitotomy to reach the ciliary arteries, you inadvertently cut the vortex veins unless you are extremely careful not to. This, of course, results in a very increased venous pressure causing a reflux of blood from the venous side into the territories of the occluded arteries, so that ischemia is minimized. But if the vortex veins are left undisturbed, then ischemia is maximal and infarction occurs much easier.

Yves C.A. Robert: There is one more point to consider, I think. If you occlude artificially one of the otherwise healthy ciliary arteries, there is bound to be some collateral supply, at least to a part of that artery's territory. But in the case of a vascular disease, all the arteries are affected, even if some are affected more critically than others. When one of them is occluded in the course of the disease, there will probably be no collateral supply at all because the others have lost their ability to react.

Sohan S. Hayreh : I would like to come back to a point raised by Dr Anderson a few minutes ago. He said that differences in fluorescein appearance time can be due to different flow paths. It is true, of course, that all territories don't fill at the same time. But there are limits to how long these delays can be. In the case of the choroid you can draw the line at two seconds: if you see a delay of one or two seconds, then it can well be a physiologic delay due to a longer flow path. But a delay above two seconds probably reflects lower perfusion.

Harry A. Quigley : Well, there are more things to take into account. Our visualization of the arrival of the fluorescein front is heavily dependent on the form of the front. If there is a lot of turbulence, for instance, the early parts of the front will not be easy to detect. Dr Riva may have something to say about that.

Charles E. Riva : In the early seventies there was a lot of discussion about the respective responsibilities of choroidal and retinal blood flow in glaucoma, based on fluorescein appearance times. And we realized that the relation between the arrival of fluorescein and its first detection depends heavily on pigmentation. So I'm wondering if those watershed zones aren't, to some extent, due to inhomogeneities in pigmentation.

Sohan S. Hayreh : I am fully aware of the work you are referring to; it was done on the rabbit, albino and pigmented. But I don't think that the results were very conclusive. And we have never found any differences in the pigmentation of the eyes with clear-cut watershed zones.

Gisbert Richard : I do not think that either retinal pigment epithelium or choroidal pigmentation make any important difference. Neither does the macular pigment, for that matter, although it is of an entirely different nature. I would like, however, to ask about a peculiar phenomenon, for which I can find no explanation: We have about 1500 angiograms on tape and we have often noticed that if you have an occlusion (or a so-called occlusion) of a retinal arterial branch, then you see a delayed choroidal filling in the same sector. And, conversely, if you have a choroidal so-called occlusion, you often see a delayed retinal filling. Can anyone explain that?

Douglas R. Anderson : With the retinal and choroidal filling defects overlying each other? Well, nothing comes to my mind. Is it only acute or can it also be chronic?

Gisbert Richard : It can be both.

Harry A. Quigley : I guess you have eliminated cases of retinal ischemic edema which could mask the fluorescence coming from the choroid.

Gisbert Richard : Yes, certainly. I can't explain it, except by hypothesizing that there is some connection between the retinal and the choroidal circulations, of which we are unaware yet.

Sohan S. Hayreh : Is it only in one sector, or can it be more diffuse? Because one of the commonest causes of retinal artery occlusion are micro-emboli. And if there is a shower of micro-emboli flowing in, they may obstruct many vascular beds at once.

Erik L. Greve : Yes, this is generally more diffuse than we think.

Douglas R. Anderson : But then the choroidal and retinal territories wouldn't necessarily coincide.

Erik L. Greve : Well, I don't think Dr Richard said they do coincide.

Gisbert Richard : Not necessarily. Take the case of central retinal vein occlusion. We studied the choroidal circulation in about 100 of those patients and we often found a delayed choroidal filling. Besides, this is why they may develop retinal neovascularization. You never get neovascularization after artificial occlusion of the retinal vessels.

Sohan S. Hayreh : This is just an idea, but do you know that about 25 to 30% of all patients with central retinal vein occlusion have either ocular hypertension or glaucoma, which in turn can influence choroidal flow?

Erik L. Greve : I think that we cannot solve this problem now, and that we should move on to the next speaker. It is true that some of the points raised deserve more discussion, but they are bound to come up after the next papers again.

ANATOMY AND PHYSIOLOGY OF OCULAR BLOOD FLOW

Douglas R. Anderson

Bascom Palmer Eye Institute, Miami, Fl 33101, USA

Introduction

There are two reasons for my presentation to be brief. First, the group assembled here is undoubtedly thoroughly acquainted with the standard textbook description of the anatomy and blood flow physiology of the eye (and optic nerve). Secondly, there is little to add to the review publications of Bill and Alm and Bill on this subject[1,2], and my own ideas on optic nerve physiology, including its blood flow, have also recently been reviewed[3]. Therefore I will simply outline and highlight features that may be particularly relevant to the topic of this meeting.

Arterial systems

Among the branches of the ophthalmic artery are the central retinal artery and the ciliary arteries. The central retinal artery penetrates the optic nerve midway in its course through the orbit and travels at the center of the optic nerve forward into the retina. Along the way it provides branches from the core into the substance of the optic nerve as far forward as the lamina cribrosa. It does not provide branches to the optic nerve head, but further in its course again begins to provide branches to the inner layers of the retina and to some extent the superficial-most layers of the optic disc.

There are a variable number of ciliary branches. The short posterior ciliary arteries penetrate the sclera around the optic nerve and break up into choroidal arteries. Other branches of the short posterior ciliary artery and branches of some of the choroidal arteries supply the region of the lamina cribrosa, the optic nerve head, and part of the optic nerve just behind the lamina cribrosa.

In addition to the short posterior ciliary arteries, there are usually two long ciliary arteries that penetrate the sclera posteriorly and traverse forward along the horizontal plane of the globe to the region of the ciliary body. Anterior ciliary arteries travel forward with the extra ocular muscles and penetrate the sclera at the insertion of these muscles. They join with the long posterior ciliary arteries, as well as the choroidal arteries derived from the short posterior ciliary arteries, in an anastomotic system that supplies the ciliary body and iris.

---

*Supported in part by National Glaucoma Research, a program of American Health Assistance Foundation, Rockville, Maryland; in part by U.S. Public Health Service Research Grant RO1-EY-OO031, awarded by the National Institutes of Health, Bethesda, Maryland; and in part by a Senior Scientific Investigators Award to Dr. Anderson by Research to Prevent Blindness, Inc., New York.

Correspondence to: Douglas R. Anderson, M.D., Bascom Palmer Eye Institute, P.O. Box 016880, Miami, FL 33101, USA.

Venous drainage

The central retinal vein drains the area that is supplied by the central retinal artery, except that it also provides the drainage for the optic nerve head. The vortex veins drain the uveal tract, and are an unusual arrangement in vascular systems in that the vein does not travel in close proximity with the corresponding arterial supply. An important feature of the venous drainage is that there is a compression of the veins at the exit from the eye. This results from the fact that the intraocular pressure is higher than the venous pressure in the orbital veins. Because of that, there is a small segment of compression of the vein to produce a resistance that allows the venous pressure inside the eye to be higher than intraocular pressure so that the veins are not completely collapsed, but only partially collapsed locally at the exit from the eye.

Capillary beds

The capillary beds of the retina, optic nerve head, orbital portion of the optic nerve head, and central venous system in general are all very similar. The endothelial cells have tight junctions, and pericytes are embedded within the basement membrane of these vessels. The capillary bed of the retina, optic nerve head, and optic nerve behind the eye are anastomotic at the capillary level, forming one continuous vascular bed. The orientation of the vascular net is in many places dictated by the local architecture, for example forming radial peripapillary capillaries in the nerve fiber layer surrounding the optic disc. They likewise conform to the configuration of the lamina cribrosa and of the longitudinal septa in the orbital portion of the optic nerve.

A separate capillary bed, which is not anastomotic with that of the optic nerve, is the choriocapillaris. This capillary bed differs in its micro-anatomy, having fenestrated vessels aligned in a flat layer against the underside of Bruch's membrane and retinal pigment epithelium, supplied in a lobular fashion by a rather abrupt termination of arterial branches and interspersed venous tributaries.

The capillaries of the ciliary body are fenestrated, leaky capillaries like those of the choroid. Those of the iris have non-fenestrated endothelium with tight junctions between the endothelial cells, though not so firmly sealed as in the retina.

Vascular innervation

Sympathetic innervation accompanies most arteries in the body. However, in the case of the central retinal artery, at least in primates and cats[4,5] the adrenergic innervation continues on the central retinal artery only as far forward as the lamina cribrosa. It does not continue forward into the arterioles of the retina, with rare exceptions (and with the exception of the pre-retinal vessels of the rabbit[6]). Adrenergic innervation does continue intraocularly along the ciliary branches.

Presumably sympathetic branches to control circulation are not required in the retina, where the circulation control occurs primarily by virtue of autoregulation (see below), although in the brain (where autoregulation also exists) adrenergic innervation continues even to vessels of the size of retinal arterioles. It has been hypothesized that in arterial hypertension, sympathetic tone may prevent distension of the arterioles by the high intra-arterial pressure in the brain and choroid, but microaneurysms and other manifestations of hypertensive retinopathy may result from the lack of this innervation in the retina.

Parasympathetic innervation arrives via the third and seventh cranial nerves. The third cranial nerve (oculomotor), through the ciliary ganglion, provides innervation to the uveal blood vessels (and of course to the ciliary muscle and its sphincter). When this nerve is stimulated, acetylcholine release causes vascular constriction as a direct effect on the vascular smooth muscles. The effect is mainly in the anterior uveal tract. (In many arteries, acetylcholine causes constriction if it reaches receptors on the muscle cells, but vasodilation occurs if acetylcholine reaches receptors on the endothelium, which in turn releases a vasodilating substance).

Parasympathetic fibers of cranial nerve seven (facial) through the pterygopalatine ganglion reach the choroid. When this nerve is stimulated, vasodilation occurs, with vasoactive intestinal peptide (VIP) being the apparent mediator.

Sensory nerves (cranial nerve five, trigeminal), when stimulated experimentally, cause vasodilation and other components of an inflammatory response, perhaps in part related to the release of substance P. Prostaglandin release may also be involved in the response. It is not clear how these artificial experimental manipulations of a sensory nerve relate to the normal control mechanisms of blood flow.

Blood ocular barrier

The vessels of the retina and optic nerve all have tight junctions, and there is a barrier to the passage of water-soluble substances from the blood stream into the neural tissue. The retinal pigment epithelial layer and its anterior extension as the epithelial layers on the ciliary body and iris serve to separate the extracellular fluid of the choroid and ciliary body (supplied by leaky blood vessels) from the retina and intraocular fluids (vitreous and aqueous humor). The intraocular fluids are exposed to the extracellular space of the iris through the anterior surface of the iris, but here the blood is separated from the aqueous by the tight junctions of the iris vessels. Leakage of extracellular material anteriorly from the ciliary body into the anterior chamber is prevented by the bulk flow of aqueous humor into the uveal tract (uveoscleral outflow). There remains one place where there is a "defect" in the barrier, namely at the optic nerve head. Here materials can diffuse from the choroid directly into the optic nerve head, as there is no interposing cellular layer with tight junctions.

Autoregulation

Autoregulation is a general phenomenon in which blood flow in the microcirculation is adjusted according to local conditions. Two fundamental mechanisms are thought to be at play. One, the myogenic mechanism, causes an increase in the tone of the smooth muscle whenever there is an increase in transmural pressure. Thus the vessel is protected from stretching whenever the intraluminal pressure becomes high. The second mechanism is metabolic autoregulation, in which the tone of the vessels is adjusted according to local metabolic needs. The chemical messenger to indicate whether or not the local metabolism is adequately supplied may include oxygen tension, carbon dioxide tension, pH, or lactate.

The retina has a reasonably efficient autoregulation, and we see it clinically when the arteries constrict with arterial hypertension or dilate under the influence of carbon dioxide. The choroid does not manifest autoregulation. According to Bill, protection of choroidal vessels from high intra-arterial pressure may occur through a general body-wide increase in sympathetic tone in arterial hypertension instead of through local autoregulation. Metabolic autoregulation may not be called into play in the choroid, because there is a markedly luxuriant flow to the choroid, far in excess of the metabolic needs. Therefore, autoregulation capabilities that might be present would not be manifest until the most severe impairment of choroidal flow had been produced.

The optic nerve head was at one time suspected not to have autoregulation because it shared an arterial supply with the choroid. However efficient autoregulation in the optic nerve head seems to have been shown in several laboratories now. Indeed, even with the severe pressure elevation of acute glaucoma, the optic nerve head damage, if any, is quite minimal, and so clearly the blood flow had been adequately maintained.

The presence of autoregulation has directed attention away from the idea that ischemia participates in the damage to the optic nerve in glaucoma. In our work we have been interested recently in the hypothesis (first mentioned to me informally over coffee by J. Terry Ernest) that perhaps a deficiency in autoregulation of the optic nerve head is a pathologic condition that occurs, for example with age, in certain individuals.[7] Such a pathologic deficiency of autoregulation could account for the minority that suffer damage from intraocular pressure, while the majority of individuals with elevated intraocular pressure do not suffer damage for quite a long time. Right now, this is not much more than a hypothesis, and at this meeting I hope I will learn of methods that might be suitable to study this hypothesis.

Receptors

Recent studies[7-12] show that there are binding sites, presumably receptors, for alpha and beta adrenergic agents, cholinergic agents, and angiotensin in the retinal blood vessels. It seems strange that non-innervated vessels should have receptors for neurotransmitters. Equally strange is that they should have receptors for circulating angiotensin hormone (as well as converting enzyme) when the blood retinal barrier prevents the intraluminal hormone from reaching the reactive muscle coat. We can only presume that perhaps all vessels are endowed during development with receptors for all vasoactive agonists. Then the participation of individual vascular beds in systemic physiologic responses may depend upon (1) the anatomic distribution of adrenergic and cholinergic nervous supply and (2) upon ability of circulating hormones to reach the receptors.

In the present context, a more interesting idea is that circulating vasoconstrictive agonists that normally do not reach CNS vessel walls (because of the endothelial barrier) can reach the vessels of the optic disc through the choroid, from which there is no cellular barrier. In such a case, any vascular tone imparted would translate into an impaired ability to dilate (impaired autoregulation, if you will) leaving the tissue supplied by these vessels vulnerable when blood flow is challenged, for example by arterial hypotension or elevated intraocular pressure. Does this explain how some individuals may have reduced autoregulatory capacity in the optic disc vessels? We have mentioned this theory before[13-16], but accumulation of definitive evidence is slow, and of course the theory may not be true.

References

1. Bill A: Some aspects of the ocular circulation. Invest Ophthalmol Vis Sci 26:410-424, 1985
2. Alm A, Bill A: Ocular circulation. In: Moses RA, Hart WM, (eds): Physiology of the Eye, pp 183–203. St Louis: CV Mosby Company 1987
3. Anderson DR: The optic nerve. In: Moses RA, Hart WM (eds): Physiology of the Eye, pp 491–505. St Louis: CV Mosby Company 1987
4. Laties AM, Jacobowitz D: A comparative study of the autonomic innervation of the eye in monkey, cat, and rabbit. Anat Rec 156:383-396, 1966
5. Laties AM: Central retinal artery innervation. Absence of adrenergic innervation to the intraocular branches. Arch Ophthalmol 77:405-409, 1967
6. Furukawa H: Autonomic innervation of preretinal blood vessels of the rabbit. Invest Ophthalmol Vis Sci 28:1752-1760, 1987
7. Ernest, J.T. Autoregulation of blood flow in the distal segment of the optic nerve. In: Krieglstein GK and Leydhecker W: Glaucoma Update. Berlin: Springer Verlag 1979
8. Rockwood EJ, Fantes F, Davis EB, Anderson DR: The response of retinal vasculature to angiotensin. Invest Ophthalmol Vis Sci 28:676-682, 1987
9. Forster BA, Ferrari-Dileo G, Anderson DR: Adrenergic alpha- and alpha-binding sites are present in bovine retinal blood vessels. Invest Ophthalmol Vis Sci 28:1741-1746, 1987
10. Ferrari-Dileo G, Davis EB, Anderson DR: Angiotensin binding sites in bovine and human retinal blood vessels. Invest Ophthalmol Vis Sci 28-1747-1751, 1987
11. Ferrari-Dileo G, Ryan JW, Rockwood EJ, Davis EB, Anderson DR: Angiotensin-converting enzyme in bovine, feline, and human ocular tissues. Invest Ophthalmol Vis Sci 29:876-881, 1988

12. Ferrari-Dileo G: Beta adrenergic sites in retinal vessels. Invest Ophthalmol Vis Sci 29:695-699, 1988
13. Ferrari-Dileo G, Davis EB, Anderson DR: Biochemical evidence for cholinergic activity in retinal blood vessels. Invest Ophthalmol Vis Sci 30 : 473 - 477, 1989
14. Sossi N, Anderson DR: Blockage of axonal transport in optic nerve induced by elevation of intraocular pressure; effect of arterial hypertension induced by angiotensin I. Arch Ophthalmol 101:94-97, 1983
15. Anderson DR: The posterior segment of glaucomatous eyes. In: Lutjen-Drecol E. (ed): Basic Aspects of Glaucoma Research, pp 167-190. New York: FK Schattauer Verlag 1982
16. Anderson DR: The mechanisms of damage of the optic nerve. In: Krieglstein GK, Leydhecker W (eds): Glaucoma Update II, pp 89-93. New York: Springer-Verlag 1983
17. Anderson DR: Relationship of peripapillary haloes and crescents to glaucomatous cupping. In: Krieglstein GK, (ed): Glaucoma Update III, pp 103–105. Berlin/Heidelberg: Springer-Verlag 1987

DISCUSSION

Peter J. Roylance : What you have just told us about receptors, Dr Anderson, reminds me of some rather surprising and fascinating findings about coronary flow and vasospasm: It was found that in certain conditions vasodilating chemicals have a paradoxical effect on the coronary circulation, causing a vasospasm. It seems that this is due to endothelial damage and that some unexplained deaths of joggers can be explained by that phenomenon.

Douglas R. Anderson : This is very interesting and it fits very well with the idea that there are receptors for acetylcholine both on the pericytes and on the endothelial cells, the first causing vasoconstriction and the second vasodilation, probably through the release of a second messenger. In normal conditions acetylcholine can only reach the receptors on the endothelial cells, and therefore acts as a vasodilator. But if there is endothelial damage or malfunction, then acetylcholine leaks out of the vessels, reaches the pericyte receptors and causes vasospasm. We should investigate for this kind of phenomenon also in the optic nerve head.

Sohan S. Hayreh : Another important factor about autoregulation is that it is efficient only within a small range. Outside that range it has no effect at all, as studies of the circulation of the central nervous system have shown. In pathological conditions this range can be shifted up or down. So that if, in systemic hypertension for instance, this range has been shifted up and you lower the blood pressure by drugs to what is considered as normal level, then you are below the autoregulation range and ischemia is likely to develop. A number of those patients may even go blind.

Douglas R. Anderson : There are two sorts of autoregulation as a matter of fact. The phenomenon that you have just described pertains to the first sort, myogenic autoregulation: this is a response elicited probably by some kind of sensors in the muscle coats of the larger arterioles, which detect when the transmural pressure becomes high and cause a contraction to prevent the vessels from being overstressed and damaged. This is well-documented in the retinal circulation: when the blood pressure is acutely raised in toxemia of pregnancy for instance, the vessels constrict; but if you reverse the hypertension, then the vessels will dilate again. Now if the hypertension is prolonged for years, then the vessels can't dilate any more. They become sclerotic, from a pathologist's point of view, but in terms of physiology you can say that they lose their capacity for autoregulation. When you lower the blood pressure in such patients, the vessels can't dilate to maintain perfusion and, indeed, retinal or optic nerve infarction may occur.

So the first sort of autoregulation, myogenic, is pressure-elicited. The second sort, metabolic, is a response to the local amounts of metabolites: O_2, CO_2, pH or whatever. Maybe someone in this room knows where this autoregulation resides. I do not know, myself, but I wonder if it doesn't reside in the really small vessels. Maybe in the capillaries themselves, which seem to be equipped for such a mechanism, since they have pericytes. So that the myogenic autoregulation would take place in the somewhat larger and the metabolic in the somewhat smaller vessels.

Yves C.A. Robert : Dr Anderson, this last sort of regulation, the only one to deserve the name of autoregulation as I have been told by physiologists, is a slow phenomenon. As I understand it, autoregulation is the ability of an organ to maintain its nutrition constant and, of course, this depends on local metabolite concentrations. But this mechanism is slow: it may take, say, two minutes before it becomes effective. However, there must be some other mechanism involved in the fast reaction of the vessels: if you raise the IOP suddenly, then you can see changes in blood velocities within a few seconds. Maybe the nerves play some role in that, as they do in the heart.

Charles E. Riva : I think we have a problem of terminology to settle before we go on. Guyton, who introduced, I believe, the term "autoregulation" defined it as the maintenance of constant blood flow under varying perfusion pressure. The maintenance of constant metabolite levels, which has nothing to do with constancy of blood flow, he called simply "regulation". Maybe we should stick to those definitions.

Albert Alm : Yes, I think it is very important to use always the terms in the same sense, as Dr Riva has just defined them, for instance. According to those definitions, the choroid doesn't autoregulate. However, this doesn't mean that it is a passive vascular bed. On the contrary, it is very sensitive to nervous influence, as well as to metabolites, and it just seems to lack the myogenic component: it does not react to changes in transmural pressure. To come back to Dr Robert's remark, the myogenic component is probably a fast (though coarse) adjustment to pressure variations, acting before a slower (and finer) metabolic adjustment which becomes effective after one to two minutes. Now if you look at the results of blue field entoptometry, you see that the regulatory changes are complete after about one or one-and-a-half minutes ...

Douglas R. Anderson : ...which is more characteristic of the metabolic response!

Albert Alm : Yes. But as you said, mentioning eclampsia patients, there must also be a response of the retinal vessels to pressure .

Douglas R. Anderson : Not that it couldn't be explained by a metabolic response, too: you can very well imagine that overperfusion will result in high oxygen and low CO_2 levels, which may trigger the reaction.

Albert Alm : But what about the retinal caliber variations in systemic hypertension? This must be a reaction to transmural pressure.

Charles E. Riva : But there has to be some connection between blood flow and metabolites. In our experiments, an increase in IOP results in a decrease in blood flow, but the latter comes up again after about one minute and a half. However, if you breath 100% oxygen you don't have this effect.

Richard Stodtmeister : I do not think there is a contradiction in that: If you increase the IOP, you decrease both the transmural pressure and the perfusion rate. So the two mechanisms may be interconnected.

Bernard Schwartz : I would like to get back to a point you mentioned before, Doug, because I think it is very important. You spoke of receptors in the retinal vessels. What sort of receptors have been demonstrated up to now?

Discussion

Douglas R. Anderson : Well, we have looked for the presence of alpha-1-, alpha-2-, beta-1-, and beta-2-adrenergic receptors, receptors to acetylcholine and to angiotensin in the retinal vessels, even though there is no innervation and therefore no natural source of supply of agonists for those receptors outside the vessels.

Now, I used the term receptors although what we have really found up to now is binding sites, which we have shown to be receptors only in the case of angiotensin. But for angiotensin at least, it is clear: if you apply this substance on the vessels from outside (for instance from the vitreous) rather than from the lumen, they will constrict. And we expect that the other binding sites will prove to be receptors as well. This leads to the idea that most vessels do have receptors as embryological vestiges, even if they have no use for them. In the retina these receptors do not play any significant role under normal circumstances because the vessels aren't innervated, but they might in pathological conditions. Imagine, for instance, a person with systemic hypertension due to excess circulating angiotensin or norepinephrine or whatever. Normally these substances are confined to the vascular lumen, but if there is abnormal leakage, then they can reach the pericytes and cause vasospasm with the ensuing cotton-wool infarction of hypertensive retinopathy.

We haven't yet looked for such receptors in the vessels of the optic nerve head, because those vessels are very small and their study is difficult. But imagine, by analogy, that they have such receptors as well; if that is the case, the blood-brain barrier defect in the optic nerve head becomes very crucial indeed. With ageing, the spectrum of a person's circulating substances may change, and if these substances leak from the choroid into the optic nerve head, they may cause a permanent or occasional tonus in the vessels, so that when a response is required from the latter to compensate for increased metabolic needs, they are unable to respond. Physiologically, this is a loss of autoregulatory capacity. If, through bad luck, the person has forgotten to take his pilocarpine on that day, he may get a micro-infarction with subsequent loss of nerve fibers and visual field. The problem is that it is very difficult to investigate this clinically, because it may happen only occasionally and not on the day that we examine the patient.

Harry A. Quigley : Doug, what you are telling us is extremely interesting. But how can you be so sure that the binding sites you have detected were on the retinal vessels and not in some other of the numerous membranes that tend to get into the preparations?

Douglas R. Anderson : During the preparation the vessels were separated and studied intact, held together by their basal membranes. The rest of the retinal tissue, which came out, was also tested. The binding sites were present in the one and not in the other.

Peter J. Roylance : Was the angiotensin you have been using for testing the receptors angiotensin-1 or angiotensin-2 ?

Douglas R. Anderson : The receptors were tested with an angiotensin-blocker. The physiologic responses occur with both forms of angiotensin. Oddly enough, the converting enzyme seems to be present in massive quantities in the retina and that, too, is a puzzle.

Albert Alm : I think that what Dr Anderson has told us is very important. And he may have a point saying that there may be more receptors than normally needed on cell membranes – after all, even red blood cells do have adrenergic receptors – and that this may be a problem in abnormal situations, such as leakage from the retina or from the choroid.

It also explains why, in the normal person, there is no beta-adrenergic response of the ocular vascular beds: the blood-brain barrier is very effective for catecholamines not only because of the tight junctions but also because of the enzymes that break the catecholamines down. So that beta-blockers wouldn't have any effect on ocular blood flow in a normal person.

Douglas R. Anderson : No, in the normal person any beta-receptors present on a vessel wouldn't be stimulated by beta-agonists, and therefore beta-blockers wouldn't affect that vessel. But we don't know what happens in pathologic conditions.

Charles E. Riva : Has anybody studied vasomotion of the retinal capillaries so far?

Albert Alm : I know that there have been some studies on the subject that failed to demonstrate vasomotion. But the anterior segment had to be removed to observe the retinal vessels and then you can hardly call these conditions physiologic any more.

MICROSPHERES IN OPTIC NERVE BLOOD FLOW MEASUREMENTS

Albert Alm

Department of Ophthalmology, University Hospital, Umeå, Sweden

The question of whether there is autoregulation or not of blood flow through the optic nerve head is obviously important for understanding the relationship between intraocular pressure (IOP) and optic nerve head damage in glaucoma. Since blood flow through the central nervous system, including the retina, is normally autoregulated it is reasonable to expect that this is true for the optic nerve head as well. However, that is not self-evident. The reason is that the vessels to the optic nerve head, with the exception of the surface, are derived from the ciliary circulation, and that they are very small when they enter the optic nerve[9,10]. This means that the main part of the vascular resistance is located in vessels outside the direct influence of the IOP. Autoregulation of blood flow is due to a change in vascular tone in the resistance vessels induced by local events in the tissue, either a reduced transmural pressure (myogenic part) and/or a local accumulation of vasodilatory metabolites (metabolic part). The signal for vasodilation is propagated through the continuous sheet of vascular smooth muscles. Normally the smooth muscle layer becomes discontinuous at the terminal end of the vascular bed. Whether or not the small vessels of the optic nerve head contain a continuous layer of smooth muscles able to communicate with proximal resistance vessels is not clear, and it is quite possible that the vascular anatomy of the optic nerve head could result in a defective autoregulation.

Measuring blood flow in such a small and inaccessible piece of tissue as the optic nerve head raises many problems. Various techniques have been utilized to overcome them, and the use of microspheres as a blood flow indicator is one of them. In this presentation I intend to describe the technique and comment on the results obtained in the few attempts that have been made with this technique to evaluate the effect of increased IOP on optic nerve head blood flow.

The introduction of labelled microspheres provided a break-through for studies on regional ocular blood flow. For the first time it was possible to determine blood flow through the separate tissues of the eye, in fact even to estimate regional differences in blood flow through the retina and the choroid[1]. The technique has since been used in innumerable studies on ocular blood flow in various laboratory animals including monkeys, cats, rabbits and rats. One major advantage of the technique is that no surgical intervention in the eye is necessary before the measurement. The microspheres are injected into the left ventricle of the heart and act as a non-recirculating blood flow indicator. The radioactivity of a tissue sample is proportional to blood flow through the sample. By taking a reference blood sample from one of the major arteries during the first minute after the sphere injection it is possible to calculate tissue blood flow (Fig. 1).

The principle of the method is that the spheres become evenly mixed with blood, follow the blood stream to the various tissues, and become trapped within the capillary beds in proportion to blood flow. Some systematic errors have become evident, to a large extent depending on the size of the spheres. Too large spheres become trapped in vessels proximal to the tissue sample and underestimate blood flow. This has been demonstrated for the brain where 35 µm spheres become trapped in pial vessels and give lower values for regional cerebral blood flow than 15 µm spheres[3]. Too small spheres also underestimate blood flow by passing through the vascular bed. Finally axial streaming, *i.e.* the tendency for the spheres to migrate towards the center of the vessel, may introduce a systematic error. This is caused by a slightly lower sphere concentration in blood entering

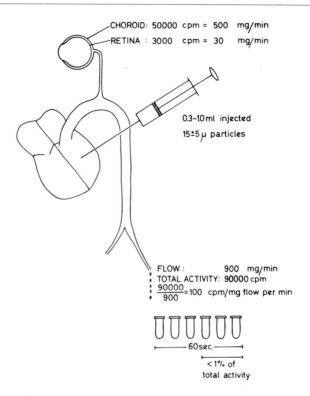

Fig. 1. The general principle of the labelled microsphere method. Spheres are injected into the left ventricle of the heart. Arterial blood is sampled during one minute from a cannulated main artery (as a rule one of the femoral arteries). The reference sample can be divided, *e.g.* in ten second portions, but since more than 99% of the spheres are captured during the first 30 seconds that is not necessary. The radioactivity and weight of the reference blood sample are determined, and the radioactivity/mg is used to calculate blood flow in mg/min to tissues sampled at the end of the experiment.

a small branch compared to blood in the major branch. The tendency to axial streaming depends on sphere size, and is greater with larger spheres. The importance of these systematic errors in determinations of regional ocular blood flow has been estimated in a study on rabbits and monkeys[4]. Since these errors depend on sphere size a mixture of two spheres of different sizes was injected, and blood flow was calulated for each sphere size. In rabbits 9 and 15 μm spheres were used and in monkeys 15 and 35 μm spheres. The findings indicated that 15 μm spheres are the best choice for studies of regional ocular blood flow. 35 μm spheres may underestimate retinal blood flow due to axial streaming in the ophthalmic artery, and 9 μm spheres pass to some extent through the retinal capillary bed and to a larger extent - about 50% - through the vascular beds of the anterior uvea. In the choroid, even 9 μm spheres become trapped, probably due to the fact that the wide choriocapillaries are flat under normal circumstances[6].

Studies with microspheres on blood flow through the optic nerve head pose special problems. The effect of axial streaming is not known but, obviously, too large spheres will not enter the small vessels supplying the prelaminar part of the optic nerve head. Thus a systematic error cannot be excluded, but in a comparison between two eyes in the same animal this would probably be of little consequence. A further problem, due to the small tissue sample, is the limited number of spheres that can be injected. The precision of the measurement depends partly on the number of spheres trapped in the sample[7]. However, this does not prevent measurements in small pieces of tissue. It merely means that more experiments have to be done to achieve the same overall precision. It is the total number of spheres in all experiments rather than the number in the individual experiment that is important[11]. Generally, if a large number of experiments are made, the biological variation in flow is a larger source of error than the error introduced by too few spheres.

The technique described above and in Fig. 1 has been the standard technique for studies on regional ocular blood flow in our laboratory. In one such study on the effect of increased IOP on ocular blood flow in monkeys[2] results were obtained that indicated a lack of autoregulation of optic nerve head blood flow. However, the precision of the measurements was low, suggesting that further studies with microspheres on the optic nerve head would have to be designed specifically for that purpose. The low number of spheres captured in the optic nerve head was one obvious problem but, as mentioned above, one that can be overcome by making more experiments. A larger problem is that the few spheres trapped in the optic nerve head are surrounded by a comparatively dense ring of spheres in the peripapillary choroid which, if inadvertently included in the sample, will have a marked influence on the calculated blood flow. These two problems were overcome by Geijer and Bill[8] who modified the technique for measurements of flow through very small pieces of tissue such as the optic nerve head: they injected a large number of non-labelled 8-10 µm spheres in order to increase the number of spheres trapped in the optic nerve head in each experiment. The actual number of spheres in the optic nerve head was determined by sectioning the frozen eye in 60 µm sections parallell to the long axis of the optic nerve. The sections were dried and the number of spheres within the optic nerve and adjacent retina was counted in each section at a magnificaton of 60x. Thus, not only could the amounts of injected spheres be increased, but the localization of each sphere could also be determined with reasonable precision. The number of spheres in the blood sample was determined by counting in a Bürker chamber.

The difference between the techniques used in the two studies is important, and it is clear that the technique used by Geijer and Bill was a significant improvement on the precision of the technique for studies on the optic nerve head. Their results clearly indicate that blood flow through the optic nerve head is autoregulated. Similar results were obtained by Sperber and Bill[12] in another study on the effect of increased IOP on blood flow and glucose consumption in the eye and brain of monkeys. In this study blood flow was determined with the same technique as in the study of Geijer and Bill[8], and the uptake of 2-deoxy-D-glucose was determined simultaneously. They found no effect of increased IOP on either blood flow or glucose uptake within the autoregulatory range of ocular perfusion pressures, and thus no support for a disturbed circulation or metabolism of the optic nerve head at moderately increased IOP.

In conclusion, it can be stated that blood flow determinations with microspheres have provided valuable information on the effect of changes in ocular perfusion pressure on blood flow through the optic nerve head. In order to provide reliable information it has been necessary to modify the original technique and rely on direct observation and counting of microspheres rather than estimations based on radioactivity. The results obtained with this modified technique strongly support the assumption that blood flow through the optic nerve head is autoregulated to a similar degree as that through the retina. Thus, at least in young healthy eyes, it seems unlikely that reduced blood flow through the optic nerve head is a primary cause of glaucomatous damage at moderately increased IOP.

Acknowledgement

Figure 1 has been reproduced with the permission of the American Physiological Society, Bethesda, MD from Bill, A.: Circulation in the eye. In the Handbook of Physiology. The cardiovascuar system IV, chapter 22, pp. 1001 - 1034. (see ref. 5)

References

1. Alm A, Bill A: The oxygen supply to the retina, II. Effects of high intraocular pressure and of increased arterial carbon dioxide tension on uveal and retinal blood flow in cats. A study with radioactively labelled microspheres including flow determinations in brain and some other tissues. Acta Physiol Scand 84:306-319, 1972
2. Alm A, Bill A: Ocular and optic nerve blood flow at normal and increased intraocular pressures in monkeys (Macaca irus): A study with radioactively labelled microspheres including flow determinations in brain and some other tissues. Exp Eye Res 15:15-29, 1973
3. Alm A: Radioactivelly labelled microspheres in regional cerebral blood flow determinations. A study on monkeys with 15 and 35 µm spheres. Acta Physiol Scand 95:60-65, 1975
4. Alm A, Törnquist P. Stjernschantz J: Radioactively labelled microspheres in regional ocular blood flow determinations. Bibl Anat 16:24-29, 1977
5. Bill A: The circulation in the eye. In: Microcirculation. Part 2. Renkind EM, Michel CC (eds). Handbook of Physiology. Section 2. The American Physiological Society, pp. 1001-1034, 1984
6. Bill A, Sperber G, Ujiie K: Physiology of the choroidal vascular bed. Int Ophthalmol 6:101-107, 1983
7. Buckberg GD, Luck JC, Payne DB, Hoffman JIE, Archie JP, Fixler DE: Some sources of error in measuring regional blood flow with radioactive microspheres. J Appl Physiol 31:598-604, 1971
8. Geijer C, Bill A: Effects of raised intraocular pressure on retinal, prelaminar, laminar, and retrolaminar optic nerve blood flow in monkeys. Invest Ophthalmol Vis Sci 18:1030-1042, 1979
9. Hayreh SS: Blood supply of the optic nerve and its role in optic atrophy, glaucoma, and oedema of the optic disc. Br J Ophthalmol 53:721-748, 1969
10. Henkind P, Levitsky M: Angioarchitecture of the optic nerve. I. The papilla. Am J Ophthalmol 68:979-986, 1969
11. Hillerdal M, Sperber GO, Bill A: The microsphere method for measuring low blood flows: theory and computer simulations applied to findings in the rat cochlea. Acta Physiol Scand 130:229-235, 1987
12. Sperber GO, Bill A: Blood flow and glucose consumption in the optic nerve, retina and brain: Effects of high intraocular pressure. Exp Eye Res 41:639-653, 1985

DISCUSSION

Erik L. Greve: Albert, you mentioned that to be able to communicate with upstream vessels, the vessels of the optic nerve head should have a continuous layer of smooth muscle cells. Can there be no other way of communication?

Albert Alm: There might be, yes, but the question is still open. And we aren't even sure about the smooth muscle cells around the small vessels of the optic nerve head: are they continuous or not? Has anyone looked into that in detail?

Douglas R. Anderson: As far as I know, it is rare to see anything else than capillaries in the optic nerve head, microscopically at least. You almost never see vessels with continuous muscle layers, that you might call arteries. It seems that they break up into capillaries prior to entering the optic nerve head.

Harry A. Quigley: You are absolutely right: in this case 'rare' is as close to 'never' as you can get!

Albert Alm: So in the optic nerve head you only have capillaries with pericytes. But we do not know if the pericytes play any role in regulating vascular resistance.

Douglas R. Anderson: The difference between pericytes and smooth muscle cells is not absolutely clear to me. Pericytes are found around capillaries, are not in contact with one another and are separated with basement membranes; whereas smooth muscle cells are found around arteries and form a continuous sheath without any basal membrane intervening. But apart from that, *i.e.* apart from their location and relationship to neighboring cells, they are identical. In electron microscopy I don't think I can tell the difference between the two without looking at what kind of cells they lie against. So I wonder if they don't have similar roles to play. We know that blood flow through the optic nerve head is somehow autoregulated; this autoregulation could well be the job of the pericytes.

Albert Alm: Yes, that is a possibility.

Charles E. Riva: You mentioned some experiments involving blood flow determination under artificially increased IOP. What was the time-lapse between IOP-elevation and the injection of the microspheres?

Albert Alm: I presume you want to know if there was time enough for the autoregulation to be effective: yes, there was. We didn't control the timing very accurately, since there were a lot of preparations to be done at that moment, but it was about 10 to 20 minutes.

Harry A. Quigley: In our experiments that time-lapse was much longer, around four hours, and the results are essentially the same.

Albert Alm: This time-lapse isn't very critical: the microspheres will spread in the circulation, then get stuck somewhere and stay there. In some experiments, where you inject a second load of microspheres, differently labelled, there might be a 45-minute lapse between the first injection and the sacrificing, but that doesn't alter the results.

Yves C.A. Robert: Some of the studies that you mentioned have provided evidence that the choroid has no autoregulation. Now, why would that be so?

Albert Alm: This is a good question. The answer is that the choroid does have autoregulation, if challenged hard enough. Now as to why this is so hard to demonstrate, my guess is that the myogenic response is either lacking or very short-lasting, so that you can't see it easily. As for the metabolic response, it isn't elicited until there is a very important drop in choroidal perfusion. Take for instance the arteriovenous concentration difference of CO_2 (a potent vasodilator) : it is about 1% – which is very low – because of the overabundance of choroidal blood flow. If that flow is halved, the arteriovenous difference becomes 2%, which is still very low. So the metabolic response will not be triggered until the blood flow is dramatically reduced.

Maurice E. Langham: There is some evidence of choroidal autoregulation in patiets with occlusive disease of the internal carotid. It is common to find perfusion pressures reduced by about two-thirds of the normal value, while the choroidal blood flow has only halved.

Christian Prünte: We have also found signs of autoregulation at choroidal capillary level, even though the arterial supply remained the same. This was done by video-angiography under artificial IOP-elevation in normal eyes.

Charles E. Riva: I have some trouble accepting the explanation you have just given, Dr Alm. There is evidence* that at photoreceptor level, the pO_2 drops almost to zero in the dark; that layer really needs all the oxygen it can get from the choroid. So I wonder what would happen if the choroidal blood flow was indeed reduced by half.

Albert Alm: Well, a few years ago we studied the venous oxygen saturation when the choroidal flow is reduced, and we found that it didn't make any real difference**. The reserve in choroidal blood flow is so huge that it becomes difficult to accept that it is there only for metabolic needs, and I think there is a point in saying that it keeps the temperature of the photoreceptors constant. Moreover, as Dr Langham said, there are patients with greatly reduced choroidal blood flow, sometimes by 50%, and they don't necessarily go blind!

Harry A. Quigley: Dr Riva, you mentioned some experiments showing that in the dark the outer retina needs all the oxygen it can get from the choroid. But were those actual pO_2 measurements or electrophysiological testing?

Editors notes:

* Linsenmeier R.A.: A model of reduced oxygen consumption of the distal retina during systemic hypoxia andelevated intraocular pressure. Suppl Invest Ophthalmol Vis Sci 28(3): 77, 1987 (ARVO abstracts).

** Alm A, Bill A: The oxygen supply to the retina . II. Effects of high intraocular pressure and of increased arterial carbon dioxide tension un uveal and retinal blood flow in cats. A study with radioactively labelled microspheres including flow determinations in brain and some other tissues. Acta Physiol Scand 84: 306-319, 1972

Discussion

Charles E. Riva : pO_2 was actually measured and found to drop to zero when the IOP is raised. But I don't remember if it was also tested electrophysiologically*.

Harry A. Quigley : Because I think it is important to see what the cells will in fact do. If you try to measure $pO2$, you may get an error in your readings. But if there is no oxygen available any more, I would expect - though this is only guesswork - the photoreceptors to drop dead very soon, or at least to stop responding.

Maurice E. Langham : I am not sure that what Charles has reported is in contradiction with Dr Alm's observation about arteriovenous differences in metabolites. It may well be that there is no large surfeit of blood supply to the eye. Because the problem is not getting enough oxygen to the eye; it is delivering it to the tissues. Only a fraction of the oxygen does get delivered: the pO_2 in the anterior chamber is about 40 mmHg whereas it is about 100 mmHg in the arterial blood - and about the same in the vortex veins, for that matter. But if you reduce the choroidal blood flow, then you will get a proportional drop in the amount of oxygen actually delivered. So I think that indeed there is no major excess of O_2 supplied to the eye.

Douglas R. Anderson : One would indeed get a drop in pO_2, I suppose, if the supply was reduced. But we know that even then the eye still sees.

Yves C.A. Robert : But apart from any considerations about autoregulation, it could be that the organ has some tolerance to anoxia.

Sohan S. Hayreh : That could well be; I have seen patients with marked choroidal filling delays, yet with perfectly normal visual function.

---

* *Editors' note*: It was, to some extent. It was found that while the b-wave is only affected by important IOP increases - a fact also known from the literature - the c-wave shows characteristic changes even for mild elevations of the IOP. The authors interpret these changes as signs of hypoxia in the distal retina. See: Yancey S.M. and Linsenmaier R.A. : Differential sensitivity of the components of the cat DC Electroretinagram to moderate increases of intraocular pressure. Suppl Invest Ophthalmol Vis Sci 28 (3) : 407, 1987 (ARVO Abstracts)

THE 2-DEOXYGLUCOSE METHOD AND OCULAR BLOOD FLOW

Göran O. Sperber and Anders Bill

Department of Physiology and Medical Biophysics, University of Uppsala, Sweden

Accurate methods for the determination of blood flow, such as the microsphere method, tend to have a somewhat unsatisfactory spatial resolution. The 2-deoxyglucose method[2,4] has the potential for a much higher spatial resolution. It has been used mainly in the brain, and does not measure blood flow in itself, but glucose consumption. Therefore, the blood flow information obtained from this method is necessarily indirect and must be interpreted with care, especially in pathological situations. However, under normal conditions, there is in the brain a close coupling between blood flow and glucose metabolism[3] and our results so far indicate that this is true for the optic nerve as well[5].

The general principle of this method is that 2-deoxyglucose (2-DG) is injected intravenously, and after a suitable delay (usually 45 min.) the animal is killed and the amount of 2-DG accumulated in tissue is measured. This is usually achieved by using radioactively tagged 2-DG. Alter the animal is killed, the tissues are frozen and sectioned and autoradiograms are made from the sections. The autoradiograms may then be evaluated by densitometry.

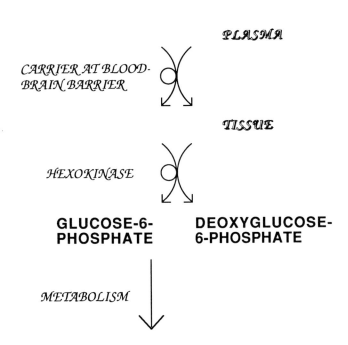

Fig. 1. Schematic representation of the relationships between 2-DG and glucose handling in brain cells.

Correspondence to: Dr Göran Sperber, Department of Physiology and Medical Biophysics, Biomedical Center, Box 572, S–751 23 Uppsala, Sweden

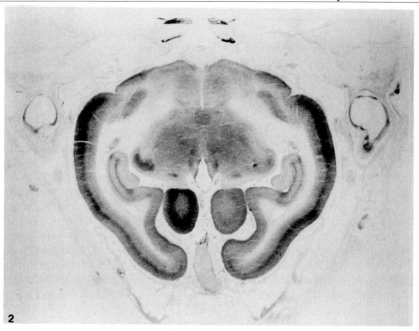

Fig. 2. 2-DG autoradiogram through the brain of a rabbit where one eye was exposed to flashing light while the other eye was kept in darkness.

In the brain, it is well established that 2-DG is transported across the blood-brain barrier by the same mechanism as glucose (Fig. 1), and is metabolized to 2-DG-6-phosphate by the same enzyme as glucose. Therefore, the formation of 2-DG-6-phosphate will be approximately proportional to the rate of glucose consumption. But while glucose-6 phosphate is rapidly metabolized further, 2-DG-6-phosphate is hardly decomposed at all, and may be analyzed at leisure. Since it does not penetrate cell membranes, it tends to remain in place, and the spatial resolution may be limited only by the resolution of the method of analysis, which may be very good if tritium tagging is used.

If quantitative results are needed, glucose and 2-DG concentrations in plasma must be followed, and some tissue constants must be known from previous experiments. These seem to be fairly constant from individual to individual in comparable circumstances, but they may change in abnormal conditions. The most important of these constants is the "lumped constant", the ratio between the steady state fractional extractions of 2-DG and glucose by the tissue.

In the brain, glucose consumption is usually closely coupled to the metabolic rate. Therefore, functional activation of a region results in enhanced 2-DG uptake. Fig. 2 is an autoradiogram from a pigmented rabbit where one eye was exposed to flashing light while the other eye was kept in darkness. In the brain this results in enhanced 2-DG uptake in several regions, most pronounced in the contralateral lateral geniculate body and anterior collicle.

Figs. 3 and 4 show results from two monkeys which were injected with both 2-DG and microspheres. The 2-DG was labeled with C-14 while the spheres were unlabeled and had to be counted by eye in the sections. Fig. 3 shows microsphere distribution along the optic nerve, and Fig. 4 the corresponding distribution of 2-DG. It is seen that both blood flow and 2-DG uptake are much higher in the distal part of the nerve than in its middle part and that both methods indicate higher values in the optic chiasm than in the middle of the nerve. This provides evidence that 2-DG uptake tends to be related to blood flow in the optic nerve as well as the brain. More evidence in this direction has been published[5]. Part of the reason for variations in blood flow and metabolism along the nerve may be that there is also a variation in myelin content (Fig. 5).

Deoxyglucose method 75

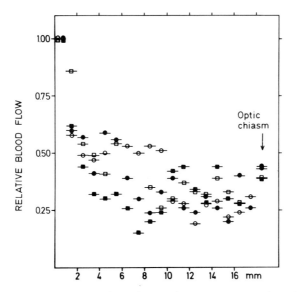

Fig. 3. Distribution of microspheres along the optic nerve in two macaque monkeys. (From Sperber and Bill [5]. © Academic Press Inc. (London) Ltd.)

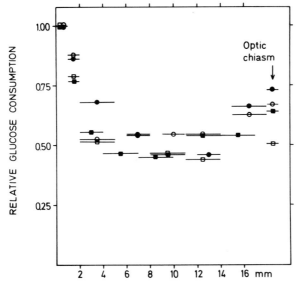

Fig. 4. Distribution of optical density in autoradiograms in the same optic nerves as Fig. 3. (From Sperber and Bill [5]. © Academic Press Inc. (London) Ltd.)

In the ocular tissues, glucose and 2-DG metabolism are not as well charted as in brain, and the use of the method is more risky. In particular, determination of the lumped constant in the eye faces considerable practical problems and has not been carried out so far. It may also be expected to show irregular behavior because of the great differences between the retinal and choroidal circulations. However, semiquantitative results - using the other eye as control - may be quite useful.

We present here some preliminary results using the 2-DG method to study metabolic effects of different lighting conditions on the optic nerve and retina. The experiments are performed with the animals under urethane anesthesia and the 2-DG used is tagged with tritium.

In some experiments, one eye was exposed to constant white light at 200 lux while the other eye was kept in darkness. Autoradiograms of the retina were scanned with a

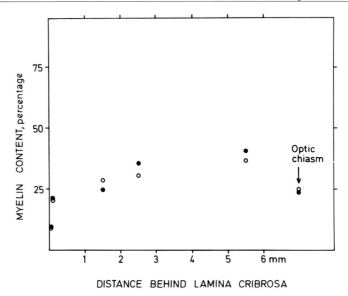

Fig. 5. Distribution of the myelin content along the optic nerves of two monkeys. (From Sperber and Bill [5]. © Academic Press Inc.(London) Ltd)

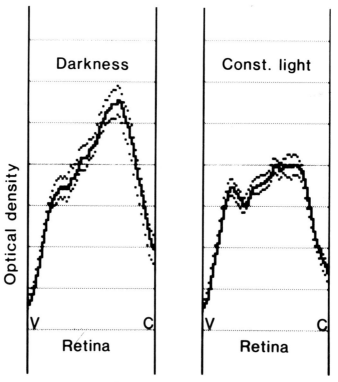

Fig. 6. Optical density profiles through the retina in 2-DG autoradiograms from a monkey with one eye exposed to steady light and one eye in darkness.

Deoxyglucose method

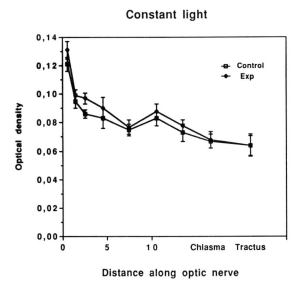

Fig. 7. Distribution of optical density along the optic nerve and tract in the animal shown in Fig. 6 and in another similar experiment.

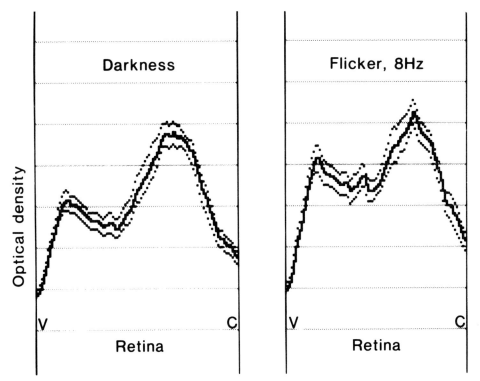

Fig. 8. Profiles analogous to Fig. 6, but with the light flashing at 8 Hz.

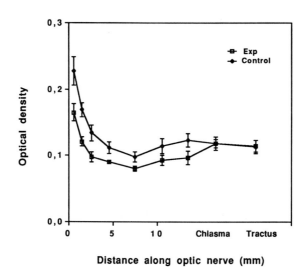

Fig. 9. Distributions analogous to Fig. 7, but with the light flashing at 8 Hz.

microdensitometer from the vitreous side to the choroid and optical density was also determined in large well-defined regions of the optic nerve. In the inner retina, the 2-DG uptake was similar in the two eyes (Fig. 6), indicating that the activity of the ganglion cells was about the same in the light exposed and dark exposed eyes. In the outer parts of the retina corresponding to the photoreceptor layer, the uptake was stimulated in the dark-exposed eye. This suggests that constant light reduces the metabolism of the photoreceptors, most probably as a result of the closure of the sodium channels that is known to take place. With fewer such channels open, one can expect a reduced activity of the sodium pumps in the cell membrane of the inner segments. This raises the possibility that it may be beneficial for patients with marginal perfusion of the retina to remain in moderately lighted surroundings, possibly even during sleep.

The 2-DG uptake in the optic nerve was similar on the two sides as could be expected by a similarity in ganglion cell activity (Fig. 7).

With one eye exposed to light from a stroboscope, flashing at 4-8 Hz, and the other eye kept in the dark, the results were quite different. There was enhanced 2-DG uptake in the inner parts of the retina, indicating that flashing light caused activation of the ganglion cells (Fig. 8). There was enhanced 2-DG uptake in the optic nerve as well (Fig. 9).

This could suggest, for patients with poor ocular perfusion, that lighting conditions should be as steady as possible.

The 2-DG method may also be helpful in finding regions with partial ischemia caused by high intraocular pressure. In a region with partial ischemia, there should be anoxic cells which will switch from aerobic to anaerobic glycolysis. Anaerobic glycolysis requires much more glucose than aerobic (the Pasteur effect), and as a result partial ischemia may cause enhanced 2-DG uptake.

We have tested this idea in monkey eyes which were subjected to such a high intraocular pressure that the perfusion pressure in the eye was reduced to about 20 mm Hg[5]. At such pressures we know from previous experiments[1] with microspheres that the blood flow is reduced by about 50%. There was indeed enhanced 2-DG uptake in the retina as well as in the prelaminar region of the optic nerve (Fig. 10), indicating that the partial ischemia caused the expected metabolic shift.

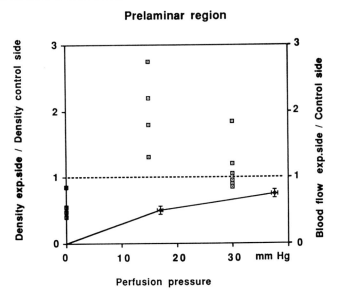

Fig. 10. Blood flow and 2-DG uptake related to ocular perfusion pressure in multiple monkeys.

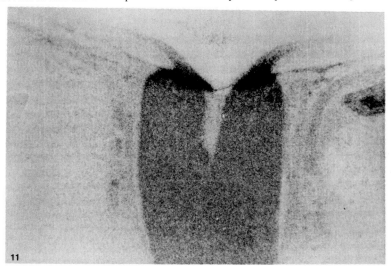

Fig. 11. 2-DG autoradiogram of the papillary region in a monkey eye where intraocular pressure was raised above systemic arterial pressure.

Some experiments were performed with the intraocular pressure adjusted at such a level that the intraocular blood flow was stopped. Somewhat surprisingly, in such experiments 2-DG still accumulated in the prelaminar part of the optic nerve (Fig. 11), most probably by diffusion within the axons from the region of heavy accumulation at the lamina cribrosa. Such diffusion may limit the spatial resolution of the method.

In conclusion, it would seem that the 2-DG method can be used to study, in great spatial detail, the metabolic activity of the optic nerve and retina and alterations in such activity. This also provides information about the circulation and the load on it. The combined use of the microsphere and 2-DG methods permits identification of regions with partial ischemia resulting in anoxia. The results presented may have a bearing on the type of lighting best suited for eyes with poor perfusion.

References

1. Geijer CH, Bill A: Effects of raised intraocular pressure on retinal, prelaminar, laminar and retrolaminar optic nerve blood flow in monkeys. Invest Ophthalmol 18:1030-1042, 1979
2. Sokoloff L, Reivich M, Kennedy C, Des Rosiers MH, Patlak CS, Pettigrew KD, Sakurada O, Shinohara M: The (^{14}C)deoxyglucose method for the measurement of local cerebral glucose utilization: theory, procedure, and normal values in the conscious and anesthetized albino rat. J Neurochem 28:897-916, 1977
3. Sokoloff L: Relationships among local functional activity, energy metabolism, and blood flow in the central nervous system. Fed Proc 40/8:2311-2316, 1981
4. Sokoloff L: Basic principles in imaging of regional cerebral metabolic rates". In: Brain Imaging and Brain Function. Sokoloffl L, (ed). New York: Raven Press 1985
5. Sperber GO, Bill A: Blood flow and glucose consumption in the optic nerve, retina and brain: effects of high intraocular pressure. Exp Eye Res 41:639-653, 1985

DISCUSSION

Harry A. Quigley : First of all one question, Dr Sperber: Have you checked whether the main uptake of deoxyglucose within the optic nerve head is due to the astrocytes or to the axons themselves ?

Göran O. Sperber : No, we haven't.

Harry A. Quigley : Then a remark about your last figure. You suggested that radioactive material is found in the prelaminar portion of the optic nerve, due to diffusion from the lamina cribrosa. But, from the picture, it seems that this diffusion is wholly within the nerve fiber layer and not in the cellular part of the retina. Is it not possible that this is due to retrograde axonal transport?

Göran O. Sperber : It could be possible, yes.

Douglas R. Anderson : But not if the tissue is ischemic; then there would be no axonal transport any more.

Richard Stodtmeister : Except if the axonal transport is not very sensitive to ischemia.

Göran O. Sperber : Or if the energy supply for the axonal transport comes also to some extent from glucose diffusing along the axons. So that at least the first part of the axons still has the capacity for some axonal transport.

Bernard Schwartz : Harry, if you pursue your argument a little further, would you say that metabolism and blood flow are necessary to bring this material across the lamina?

Harry A. Quigley : Well, if there was no metabolism, then you wouldn't see any labelled material. So there must have been some metabolism going on somewhere in the area. And there certainly is in the retrolaminar part, because the experimental data show that blood flow, as well as metabolism, are normal at that level.

Douglas R. Anderson : There is something that is not clear to me about the method: As I understand it, deoxyglucose will enter the cells in parallel with glucose and so reflect glucose delivery. But I don't understand how it can reflect glucose demand.

Göran O. Sperber : Well, there are two steps in the process: first the transportation across the blood-brain barrier and second the phosphorylation of both glucose and deoxyglucose by a single enzyme, hexokinase. It has been shown that hexokinase activity will increase when there is an increased demand for glucose. As for the first step, things aren't so unequivocal, but there is evidence that an increased demand will increase the transportation rate; otherwise the delivery would remain unchanged, whatever the demand. The situation is reasonably clear in the brain. We can't be absolutely certain that it is applicable to ocular tissues, but I see no obvious reason why it shouldn't.

Albert Alm : I am not sure whether the transport capacity across the blood-brain barrier increases, but this is certainly not the rate-limiting step for glucose utilization in the central nervous system. The glucose-extraction rate is very low, so there is a large safety margin.

Douglas R. Anderson : How much would you say the glucose-extraction rate is, Dr Alm ?

Albert Alm : About 10%, I would guess, but I am not sure. It may be higher, but certainly much lower than 100%.

Göran O. Sperber : And the extraction rate for deoxyglucose is approximately half that of glucose.

Douglas R. Anderson : Let's say that the extraction rate for deoxyglucose is 10% in normal conditions. Then let's suppose that by some means you double the volume of flow. Would that reduce the extraction rate to 5%, so that the amount of deoxyglucose present will remain the same – in which case the method does not measure blood flow? Or would the extraction rate remain the same, so that the amount of deoxyglucose present will double – in which case the method reflects blood flow rather than metabolism?

Göran O. Sperber : Well, it's certainly not a direct measure of blood flow. It measures metabolism, rather, though it does reflect blood flow in a way, since the latter is rather well adjusted to the metabolic needs.

Albert Alm : Moreover I think that one shouldn't reason about it in diffusion-related terms. This isn't diffusion, which depends only on partial pressure differences, it is a transport system that carries glucose back and forth across the membrane, and how much is transported back depends on how much is utilized on the cerebral side of the barrier.

HISTOLOGICAL AND CLINICAL FEATURES OF THE OPTIC NERVE HEAD IN EARLY GLAUCOMA DIAGNOSIS

Harry A. Quigley

Johns Hopkins University, School of Medicine, Wilmer Ophthalmological Institute, Glaucoma Service, Maumenee B-ll0, Baltimore, MD 21205, USA

Introduction

I was asked to present in this manuscript material that was discussed at the meeting on Ocular Blood Flow in Glaucoma; but I would like to extend the actual laboratory data with further observations. Specifically, I will point to examples of the importance of understanding histology in order to explain clinical observations. Furthermore, I will comment on the difficulty of separating cause from effect under certain circumstances.

Optic nerve head blood flow in chronic experimental glaucoma

The specific data that I presented at the meeting has already been published[1]. We injected tritiated iodoantipyrine into monkey eyes with unilateral chronic experimental glaucoma to measure blood flow in the optic nerve head with acute and chronic pressure elevation. Elevated pressure and the physical changes induced by glaucoma did not produce any difference between glaucomatous and normal monkey eyes in the amount of blood flow. The method looked at blood flow in the entire optic nerve head, in regional sections, and in small zones (50 µm in diameter). Even within tiny regional areas there was no measurable decrease in flow.

We previously demonstrated that the number of capillary blood vessels in the optic disc in chronic experimental glaucoma eyes per unit volume of the optic nerve head was unchanged from normal fellow eyes. This work indicates that blood vessel structure and blood flow are relatively unaffected by chronically elevated eye pressure in this model.

Clinicopathologic correlation and its usefulness

I study the optic nerve head both as a histologist and a clinician. During the course of the Blood Flow Meeting just concluded, we had the opportunity to hear a number of presentations about clinical findings at the optic disc. Among these were the interesting observations of Drs. Robert[2] and Delori[3] on the measurement of the degree of paleness of the optic disc. In the discussion we heard the proposal by some that pallor of the optic disc, either present spontaneously or induced by pressing on the eye, might be indicative of the amount of blood flow in the eye.

Some years ago, I published a paper describing the histologic basis of optic disc pallor[4]. The optic disc that is spontaneously pale or the normal pale part of the disc that we call the cup are both pale for two major reasons. The normal pinkness of the optic disc comes from light that is conducted to capillaries within the disc rim by normal nerve bundles. Where there is only a thin rim of nerve tissue or a lack of capillaries containing red cells to impart the red color, the disc appears pale. In the optic disc with pallor due to a primary optic atrophy, it is the loss of nerve bundles and the consequent loss of a substantial volume of the nerve rim tissue that leads to pallor. Within such a pale disc rim, there is the normal density of capillaries but the lack of nerve tissue to conduct the light and scatter it amongst these capillaries prevents the generation of a red color. Reflection of incoming light by remaining astrocytes further contributes to a white appearance. In the normal physiologic cup, the height of nerve tissue is so small that light nearly bounces directly off the collagen of the lamina, giving the cup its pallor.

A method of measuring blood flow was presented using the shining of laser light into the nerve rim and measuring the shift of wave length caused by the motion of red blood cells. The authors showed a change in the parameter measured by this laser-Doppler method when optic atrophy is present. However, like pallor of the disc, this may result from a decrease in the total tissue present and hence a decrease in the number of capillaries containing moving red cells, not decrease in blood flow per unit tissue volume. One does not know with this method whether the data are a result of fewer total capillaries being present or from less blood flow per unit volume.

What is cause and what is effect?

In fluorescein angiography of the disc there appears to be an increase in fluorescein visible in the disc's extracellular spaces (so called staining) in glaucoma eyes. In addition, Drs. Schwartz and Spaeth described "filling defects" of the capillary vessels of the disc in glaucoma eyes. Do these two findings represent vascular abnormalities that cause glaucoma optic neuropathy, or are they a result of the loss of tissue and therefore an effect? Certainly, the staining which is observed can be easily understood if one considers the physiology of the extracellular space of the optic nerve head. There is a leak of molecules from the extracellular space of the choroid into the disc rim under normal circumstances. However, because there is normally a thick nerve rim present this fluorescein is minimally visible as one looks at the disc. When, however, glaucoma has caused a substantial loss of nerve rim tissue, fluorescein leaking into the nerve head from the choroid appears more rapidly and is more easily visible to the observer looking at the disc because of the loss of rim tissue. There are no studies that demonstrate that abnormal vascular leakage occurs from optic capillaries in glaucoma.

One explanation for filling defects of the disc is that capillaries that were originally present cease to carry blood, leading to death of nerve tissue. This appears to have been the thesis of Dr. Schwartz and others. On the other hand, it may be that the lack of visible vessels in some areas of the disc results from initial tissue loss rather than causing it. Certainly at an advanced stage of glaucoma damage the total number of capillaries present in the optic disc decreases dramatically, though their density (number per unit area) remains normal.

One way to settle these issues of cause and effect is through prospective study of patients. The initial observation of a possibly useful tool in early glaucoma detection must be tested by following prospectively a large enough group of representative suspect patients in whom a second method of detecting damage is available. This is usually the visual field test. Patients are initially staged as either having or not having a particular finding on the test to be studied (filling defects, induced pallor, etc.) and then this test is repeated to measure its accuracy and reproducibility. The group of patients is followed long enough to determine the rate at which the damage judged by field loss occurs in those with and those without the finding being studied. This develops evidence that the finding is an important indicator of which patient will lose visual function more rapidly.

It may not settle the question of causality, but if the finding to be studied is a good diagnostic indicator it almost does not matter whether it is a cause of glaucoma damage or an effect. In either case, it is clinically useful.

References

1. Quigley HA, Hohman RM, Sanchez R, Addicks EM: Optic nerve head blood flow in chronic experimental glaucoma. Arch Opthalmol 103: 956-962, 1985
2. Robert YCA, Hendrickson PH: Photometry of the optic disc. This volume pp. 167-168
3. Delori FC: Reflectometry measurements of optic disc blood volume. This volume pp.155-164
4. Quigley HA, AndersonDR: Histologic basis of optic disk pallor of optic disc pallor in experimental optic atrophy. Am J Ophthalmol 83: 709-717, 1977

DISCUSSION

Juan E. Grunwald : By what means did you obtain acute IOP elevation in your experiments, Dr Quigley ?

Harry A. Quigley : The short-term IOP elevation in monkey eyes was obtained by placing in the anterior chamber a needle connected to a variable-height reservoir.

Erik L. Greve : The pressure elevations have to be very important, I suppose ?

Harry A. Quigley : Well, this depends on the time you are prepared to wait. For the 4- or 8-hour experiments with monkeys, the IOP was raised to around 65 mmHg. In another study we had one human eye enucleated because of a melanoma which had also caused secondary glaucoma with pressures around 35 or 40 mmHg for the last few days before enucleation.

Douglas R. Anderson : I think that the point raised by Erik is very important. Whether or not, that is, the pathogenic mechanisms involved at pressures, say, above 30 mmHg are the same as those occurring at the low- or mid-20 mmHg range, which is hardly above the normal. It is those last pressures, of course, that are involved in the most common type of POAG. So it is legitimate to ask, do the experiments with an important short-lasting increase really relate to the same disease? We can't take that for granted.

Harry A. Quigley : With all due respect, I would rather disagree. If you do this experiment raising the pressure to 24 or 25 mmHg, you will have to wait a number of years before you see any damage. In our case, when pressures were between 35 and 40 mmHg we had to wait a number of months. It is only a question of timing. You should keep in mind that these were young and healthy animals without the mitigating factors found in the human POAG group: arteriosclerosis, hypertension, medical therapy or whatever and yet the most fascinating thing is that you examine their eyes at the end of the experiment and it looks exactly like what you are seeing every day in your glaucoma patients! I can show you histological preparations of their optic nerve heads and you will see that their nerve fibers die in exactly the same pattern as they do in humans: the same segments of the optic nerve head die first and the same size of fibers. Now whether there is a difference between one group of human glaucoma patients and another in the pattern of optic nerve fiber loss or of visual field loss, it is actually not clear at all. Many studies have been done on that, but it is extraordinarily controversial whether there are differences in the pattern of visual field loss between high-tension and low-tension glaucoma.

Douglas R. Anderson : I happen to think, like you do, that all this is one single mechanism. Yet I have to admit that more and more people, like Stephen Drance or Erik Greve and Caroline Geijssen and before any of them George Spaeth, make a clinical distinction and it seems that there is a difference. There is a hyperbaric type of glaucoma, to use George Spaeth's term, usually secondary, with pressures around 35 or 40 or 45 mmHg, often in younger persons, where you get a generalized enlargement of the cup and a generalized visual field loss that is more prominent than the localized loss although localized loss does occur as well. Incidentally, this seems to be true also in your experimental monkey model. And then there are the low-tension glaucomas or the open-angle glaucomas with pressures in the low- or mid-twenties, usually primary, in older people, with more frequent peripapillary crescents of atrophy or whatever that may be, and with more prominent localized loss. So even if it is a spectrum of conditions due to the same mechanism, it still seems that some distinctions can be made.

Harry A. Quigley : I am not denying that. I simply said that I believe glaucoma to be a disease produced by some mechanism where the IOP is an initiating event. What unifies glaucoma is that there is a physical alteration of the tissues of the disc, and I believe that it is the IOP that induces that alteration, whether it is 22 or 38 mmHg. Of course, there are other mitigating features to the issue, such as blood flow. Why would I be studying blood flow otherwise?

Erik L. Greve : I think, Harry, that for the purpose of this symposium we can distinguish several types of the disease. You spoke about the increased IOP. That can be a mechanism, but there may be more than that. We needn't go deeper in pathogenesis now, this isn't the purpose of the symposium anyway.

Richard Stodtmeister : Dr Quigley, you mentioned that the number of optic disc capillaries per volume of tissue doesn't change in glaucoma. By "tissue", do you mean everything that is in the optic nerve head anterior to the lamina cribrosa, including the glia, or is it just the nerve fibers?

Harry A. Quigley : The only things that we excluded from our measurement were the larger arteries and veins. Therefore, when I spoke of disc tissue volume I meant the total volume of the disc anterior to the myelin lines - with the exception of large vessels - including glial cells, nerve fibers and capillaries with less than two cells in their lining wall. As for the blood vessel area measured, it is only the lumen of the capillaries.

Richard Stodtmeister : But if the number of capillaries per total tissue volume remains the same, how do you explain disc pallor?

Harry A. Quigley : Well, that was the reason why we did the experiment in the first place. If you extrapolate the results, you can conceive that disc pallor is due to two things: First of all when you have optic atrophy, whether from a brain tumor or from glaucoma, there is a tremendous loss of tissue and therefore of capillaries. Which means that there are much fewer capillaries, in absolute number, to intercept white light and reflect back red to give a pink disc rim. The second thing is that when you have lost a substantial number of nerve bundles you have a proportional increase of astrocytes. Nerve bundles do conduct light very well, guiding it deep inside the optic nerve head, but in this case most of them are lost. So the light will hit the astrocytes, arranged perpendicular to your view, and be reflected back to you. In other words, less light will hit the capillaries (a) because there are less of them and (b) because they are surrounded by more astrocytes which will reflect the light before it can reach the capillaries. So if the disc looks pale, it is because there is less tissue there and because the reflecting and scattering characteristics have changed.

Sohan S. Hayreh : Harry, you suggest that capillary dropout is secondary to nerve fiber loss. But this has never been proven: it's a hen-and-egg kind of situation, trying to find which came first. Doing fluorescein angiography in patients with optic atrophy, ascending or descending, I have always found perfectly normal capillaries. Doug Anderson did something similar in experimental optic atrophy and didn't find any reduction in the blood vessels either. So there is no angiographic evidence of your concept that nerve fibers degenerate first and then, since less blood supply is needed, capillaries drop out.

Harry A. Quigley : As you said, Sohan, those studies didn't provide any evidence in favor of that concept, but neither did they against it. They have only shown the weakness of fluorescein angiography, which fails to pick up the loss of as much as 60% of the prelaminar capillary network. It is a nice technique if you wish to visualize the larger vessels on the disc and get a general idea of what is going on there; this is beyond question. But if you compare the angiograms with the histologic preparations, you see that they may not look alike at all. We have done that in monkeys – and though it might be that human eyes are not the same their angiograms aren't that much different – and we found that the number of vessels visible in fluorescein angiography is terribly small compared to the actual number of vessels in the tissue: you can only see the larger vessels on the surface of the disc, which anyway do not atrophy, but not the capillaries which may eventually drop out.

Erik L. Greve : Harry, as I understand it, you found no difference in blood flow between your experimental glaucoma eyes and normal eyes ?

Harry A. Quigley : That's right. Blood flow per volume of tissue is probably the same.

Erik L. Greve : Then you imply that the defects found in fluorescein angiography are simply a reflection of the amount of tissue present ?

Harry A. Quigley : If you take eyes with descending optic atrophy, occurring for instance after optic nerve transection or in a chiasmal tumor, the loss of prelaminar tissue isn't that important: only about 65% of the tissue is lost. So in the angiogram you can see many capillaries because there are enough of them left. But in glaucoma eyes the loss is much more important: practically all the prelaminar tissue is lost. If you do fluorescein angiography in those eyes you see what Drs Schwartz, Spaeth and Hayreh have called a filling defect. But in the scleral lamina of those eyes where I'm proposing you the damage actually happens, there are still many open capillaries providing normal blood flow. The reason you don't see them on the angiograms is that they are surrounded by connective tissue, collagen and astrocytes, while the ones in the prelaminar region were not. The reflectance characteristics of the tissue have changed and the result is that there is less light reaching the fluorescein in the vessels and even less light emitted back for you to detect.

Bernard Schwartz : Looking back, Harry, to some of your results[*] in monkeys with long-term experimental glaucoma, it seems that you have an increase in the area of capillaries per tissue volume, going from the less severe to the more severe cases. In the eyes with mild damage, capillary area per tissue volume expressed as percent of fellow eye, ranges from 91% to 105%. In the severely damaged eyes you have figures from 93% to 120%. The number of cases is

---

[*] *Editors' note*: Quigley HA, Hohman RM, Addicks EM, Green WR: Bloodvessels of the glaucomatous optic disc in experimental primate and human eyes. Invest Ophthalmol Vis Sci 25: 918-931, 1984

probably too small for these differences to be significant, but did you check the regression? And how would you explain such an increase?

Harry A. Quigley : To answer your first question, the regression analysis did not bring out anything significant at all. But even if it had done, it might well be that there is a lag between the loss of nerve tissue and the dropout of capillaries and that I hadn't waited long enough in my experiment. Had I waited one or two more years, the values might have come back to normal. This might be an explanation but I am very hesitant about it all, because the numbers are really much too small to formulate such a suggestion.

Maurice E. Langham : I would like to bring up a technical point, Harry: you can decrease perfusion pressure either by raising IOP or by decreasing blood pressure. But if you are dealing with blood flow in the envelope of the eye as you do in the lamina cribrosa, I think that it is not correct to increase the IOP, since it might induce a bias. Do you have any data on how the results of the two methods compare ?

Harry A. Quigley : I would say they show the same thing.

Maurice E. Langham : This would be rather surprising, from a physiological point of view.

Harry A. Quigley : When I say they show the same thing, I mean that I found a maintenance of blood flow in experimental eyes with increased IOP. And Joël Weinstein, using metaraminol, found that blood flow was maintained despite dramatic lowering or raising of systemic blood pressure. Am I quoting correctly Weinstein's work, Doug ?

Douglas R. Anderson : Yes, Weinstein showed that blood flow was maintained despite a drop in blood pressure, and used this as evidence of autoregulation in the optic nerve head. But I'm not sure I understand why it would matter which way you influence perfusion pressure.

Maurice E. Langham : It does matter, Doug, because if you increase IOP you create a tension in the envelope.

Harry A. Quigley : I agree with Maurice that there might be a difference. But I believe that we should rather think in terms of nutritional delivery to the axons, and not just in terms of blood flow rate.

Charles E. Riva : Still the question of blood flow rate is very important, because the diffusion of metabolites between capillaries and tissue is strongly dependent on it. If you take oxygen diffusion, for instance, it has been shown that slowing down the blood flow increases oxygen delivery because the molecules have more time to diffuse out of the capillaries.

Harry A. Quigley : What Dr Riva is implying is that any of our methods could be flawed because we don't measure the essential phenomenon, nutritional delivery, but other parameters relating more or less to it, such as blood flow. However, when someone uses a microsphere method and a tritiated iodo-antipyrine method and in another laboratory someone uses two differently labelled iodo-antipyrine molecules and in a third laboratory someone else uses deoxyglucose and all these results show the same general picture, then I think we can come to the following conclusion: In the normal eye of a young person, the blood flow in the optic nerve head is held relatively constant against modest variations of blood pressure or IOP. If, therefore, clinically significant changes are induced by increases in IOP, this means that there are other important factors that are overlooked: small, localized changes in blood flow, for instance, or autoregulation abnormalities. But the fact remains that a normal young person with no autoregulation disturbances who develops secondary glaucoma after an injury, shows a very similar picture to the 70-year-old person with multiple vascular problems and with an IOP of 23 mmHg. So the general view is that there may be mitigating features that lead to some differences between the various groups of persons with higher or lower IOP, but the overall mechanism of glaucomatous optic neuropathy is initiated by a change in eye pressure.

II. OCULAR PULSE MEASUREMENTS

NON-INVASIVE MEASUREMENT OF PULSATILE BLOOD FLOW IN THE HUMAN EYE

Maurice E. Langham, Richard A. Farrell[1], Vivian O'Brien[1], David M. Silver[1] and Peter Schilder

The Johns Hopkins University School of Medicine, The Wilmer Eye Institute, 601 North Broadway, Baltimore, MD 21205; [1]The Applied Physics Laboratory, The Johns Hopkins University, Laurel, MD 21207; USA

The flow of blood into the eye is pulsatile and causes a rhythmic fluctuation of the steady-state intraocular pressure (IOP). It is the amplitude and the shape of the IOP pulse that reflects the pulsatile component of the ocular blood flow.

The pulsatile characteristics of the IOP may be measured non-invasively with high fidelity by constant flow pneumatic tonometry. The frequency response of the pneumatic tonometer is dependent on the rate of gas flow, the gas density and on the geometry of the sensor; typically, the frequency response exceeds 100 Hertz, which is well above the fundamental heart rate[28]. Fig. 1 is taken from the paper of these authors and shows the close agreement between recordings of IOP using the Langham pneumatic probe and analog recordings employing a fluid-filled high sensitivity pressure transducer, connected by a cannula to the anterior chamber of an anesthetized rabbit. Note that the pulsatile character of the manometric recording of the IOP is faithfully mirrored by the recording of the non-invasive tonometric system.

In order to quantitate, automate and rapidly analyze the IOP pulsations, the analog signal from the pneumatic probe is digitalized and fed into an IBM PS2/30 system[15]. Using this system representative digital recordings of the IOP in pairs of eyes of a healthy subject are shown in Fig. 2. Each IOP measurement takes 10 microseconds and is repeated at 30 millisecond intervals, giving a total of approximately 30 pressure readings during each

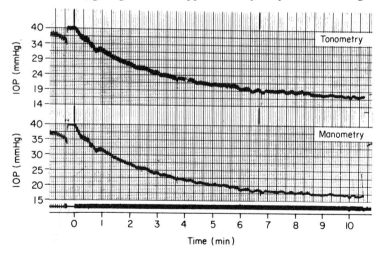

Fig. 1. Comparison of IOP measurements made by the floating tip pneumatic tonometer (top record) and by direct recording from the anterior chamber (lower record) in the anesthetized rabbit. The IOP was increased from its steady state value of 17 mmHg to 40 mmHg by connection of the anterior chamber to a saline reservoir. At T=0 min, the tap to the reservoir was turned off. This figure is taken from Walker, Compton and Langham (1975) with the permission of the publishers.

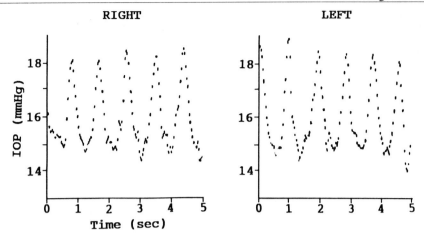

Fig. 2. Representative digital recordings of the IOP's in pairs of eyes of a healthy young adult subject. The diastolic IOP is the mean of the minimal values during the period of diastole; the systolic IOP is the mean of the maximal values during systole. The PA is derived from the minimal and maximal IOP values in each pulse. All values are calculated automatically using the appropriate software.

IOP pulsation. If required, the number of IOP readings may be increased to several thousand per second. The average of all the individual IOP measurements is the steady state IOP (*i.e.* the Goldmann applanation value). The pulsations of the IOP may be observed using both applanation and indentation tonometers; Goldmann[13] recognized the problem of recording a single IOP reading and suggested "prendre la position moyenne!". Thus, the average of the IOP values recorded with the pneumatic tonometer is equivalent to a standardized and correctly executed Goldmann applanation reading[23].

Until the present time the IOP has been defined as the value at which the rates of aqueous humor and outflow are equal (*i.e.* it reflects the steady state aqueous humor dynamics). The ability to define precisely the exact form of the IOP pulsations around the steady state value extends the use of tonometry to the analysis of ocular blood flow. Each contraction of the heart causes a bolus of blood to flow into the ophthalmic artery and to spread rapidly through the retinal and ciliary choroidal vessels. The bolus of blood increases the ocular volume with a proportionate increase of the IOP. Following relaxation of the heart and closure of the aortic valve the IOP decreases to a minimal value. In the cardiovascular system the maximal blood pressure during systole is termed the systolic blood pressure and the minimal pressure occurring during diastole is termed the diastolic blood pressure. In keeping with these definitions, the maximal IOP during systole and the minimal value during diastole are termed the systolic and diastolic IOP's respectively.

Mathematically, the total blood flow into the eye may be considered to be the sum of two different components; namely, the pulsatile (F_P) and the non-pulsatile (F_N). The non-pulsatile component affects the diastolic or minimum IOP, but is otherwise unseen by the pulsatile component. The steady component of blood flow is assumed to be in a steady-state equilibrium with its outflow, so that in the absence of pulsatile flow the IOP and the eye volume would be constant. The pulsatile flow comprises a period of net pulsatile inflow ($0 < t \leq t_{in}$), where the IOP is increasing, and a period of net pulsatile outflow ($t_{in} < t \leq \tau$), where the IOP is decreasing, with τ the complete cycle time. Thus, the duration of the period of net pulsatile inflow is t_{in} and that of net pulsatile outflow is $t_{out} = \tau - t_{in}$. Starting time equal to zero at the time of the minimum IOP, then the total amount of blood that would have flowed into the eye between zero and some subsequent time t is given by

$$V_{in}(t) = \int_0^t dt' [F_p(t') + F_N] \tag{1}$$

At steady state, the continuous (assumed constant) outflow must exceed the non-pulsatile inflow by some amount g, so that the amount of blood that would have flowed out of the eye at time t is simply

$$V_{out}(t) = \int_0^t dt'[F_N + g] \qquad (2)$$

Since the blood and other fluid-filled tissues of the eye are incompressible, the volume of the eye will have increased by an amount

$$\Delta V(t) = V_{in}(t) - V_{out}(t) = \int_0^t dt'[F_p(t') - g] \qquad (3)$$

Because the eye volume does not show significant pulse-to-pulse variations, the total pulsatile flow of blood into the eye during a cardiac pulse is simply

$$\int_0^t dt' F_p(t')$$

which must equal the total pulsatile flow out of the eye, which is $g\tau$. The number of pulses per second (or pulse repetition frequency) is $1/\tau$, so that the rate of pulsatile flow in the eye is $g\tau(1/\tau) = g$. However, the tonometer measures the eye volume changes given by Eq. (3), and not

$$\int_0^t dt' F_p(t')$$

which is the pulsatile component of blood flow. Fortunately, the mathematical analysis described in the paper by Silver et al.,[26] shows that this PBF can be obtained from the characteristics of the eye volume changes measured by the tonometer. In particular, if V_{max}, V_{min} are the eye volumes that correspond to respectively the maximum and minimum IOP, then the PBF rate can be approximated by

$$g = (V_{max} - V_{min})/(\tau - t_{in}) \qquad (4)$$

Thus, the only step that remains is to determine V_{max} and V_{min}, which can be achieved by using the relationship between IOP and eye volume in living human eyes[9,22,30].

An alternate and more exact derivation of the pulsatile blood flow (PBF) is described by Silver et al.[26]. Their approach is illustrated in Fig. 3. The upper curve is the IOP recording in a normal subject, and the middle curve is the volume change of the eye as a function of time. It will be seen that the IOP and volumetric curves are similar in form. The lower curve gives the derivative dV/dt of the volume curve as a function of time. From the assumption of constant outflow and the condition that the eye volume does not vary significantly from pulse–to–pulse, one can determine the average PBF rate from the latter curve. In this subject the flow rate exceeded by about 10% that derived by the alternate procedure described above.

The pressure gradient maintaining the ocular blood flow is the ophthalmic arterial pressure (OAP) less the IOP, *i.e.* the ocular perfusion pressure (OPP). Retinal ophthalmodynametric measurements of the OAP's are difficult to make and the published results have shown wide disparities[8]. The most detailed studies are those of Weigelin and Lobstein[29] who reported the mean OAP to be 75 mmHg in normal subjects (brachial blood pressure 120/80 mmHg). An objective and more simple measurement has been developed based on the relation between the amplitude of the IOP pulse and IOP[18]. Controlled increments of the IOP are induced using a scleral cup connected to a vacuum system, and simultaneous recordings taken of the IOP and PA. The PA values change in a non-linear manner with increased IOP, and the PA is extinguished at an IOP equal to the ophthalmic

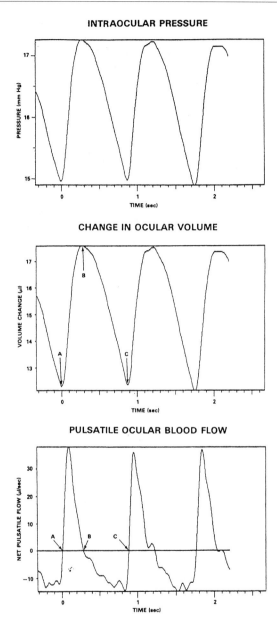

Fig. 3. The net pulsatile ocular blood flow in a normal healthy subject. The top figure shows instantaneous IOP measurements taken at 10 millisecond intervals. The middle figure gives the change in ocular volume relative to a reference ocular volume at 10 mmHg. The data corresponds to the IOP measurements of the upper figure. The region from A to B represents expansion of the eye; the region from B to C represents contraction of the eye. The lower figure gives the net pulsatile ocular blood flow corresponding to the above figures. The region from A to B represents net inflow of blood; the region from B to C represents net outflow; the points A, B and C are synchronous respectively with points A, B and C.

arterial systolic pressure[18]. At this IOP blood flow into the eye ceases and vision fades rapidly, inwards from the periphery. In young subjects the PA/IOP relation is frequently sigmoid in form, whereas in older subjects the relation is more often parabolic in form[14,17–19].

The measurements of the OAP by traditional ophthalmo-dynamometry and by the ocular pulse procedure differ fundamentally from the procedures of Gee et al.,[12] and that described by Ulrich in this symposium[27]. In traditional ophthalmodynamometry the IOP that induces pulsations of the retinal artery is the diastolic pressure and the IOP that extinguishes the pulse is the systolic pressure in the ophthalmic artery. In the procedure of Langham and To'mey[18] the ophthalmic arterial systolic pressure is derived from the IOP/PA relation (i.e., is based on the decrease of the PA with increased IOP). In the Gee procedure the initial step is to increase the IOP to a level that eliminates ocular pulsations, and then to slowly decrease the IOP until the pulse reappears (Gee et al.,[12] Ulrich and Ulrich[27]). Thus, this technique examines the IOP required to allow the blood vessels to reopen. The interesting observation of Ulrich (this symposium) that there is an abnormally large pressure differential between the opening pressures of the retinal and ciliary choroidal arteries in patients with low tension glaucoma means that the vascular resistance of the ciliary vessels was abnormally high. The observations of Ulrich appear analogous to those of Langham and Maumenee[16] that the intrascleral vessels failed to reopen at a normal rate in glaucomatous eyes after the aqueous drainage vessels had been occluded by application of suction to a perilimbal suction cup. The possibility that the ciliary choroidal system has an abnormally low ocular perfusion pressure in glaucomatous eyes, including low tension cases, is not supported by the findings of Langham[14].

The hemodynamics of eyes of a small group of healthy adult subjects (mean age 65 ± 3 yrs) evaluated from IOP measurements is summarized in Table 1. The average PBF of 724 $\mu l \, min^{-1}$ greatly exceeds the total retinal blood flow of 50 $\mu l \, min^{-1}$ [24,25]. This means that the major proportion of the PBF is ciliary choroidal. The negligible contribution of retinal blood flow to the IOP pulse is seen clinically in the constancy of the pulse following occlusion of the central retinal artery (Dobbie[7]; author's unpublished observations) and in the complete loss of the pulse in patients with severe choroidal ischemia (Dobbie, personal communications).

The proportion of the total ocular blood flow that is pulsatile remains unresolved, but comparison of pulsatile and total ocular blood flow measurements indicate it to be substantial. For example, an approximate measure of the total ocular blood flow may be derived from a knowledge of the ocular blood flow when the IOP is raised to the diastolic ophthalmic arterial pressure. At this IOP the non-pulsatile blood flow is zero and consequently the residual pulsatile component is the total blood flow. The mean blood flow at the diastolic pressure is 200 $\mu l \, min^{-1}$ and the corresponding ocular perfusion pressure 15 mmHg based on the data published by Langham and To'mey[18]. Using these values and the assumption that the ciliary choroidal vascular resistance remains constant with change of IOP, the total ocular blood flow in the undisturbed eye would be 900 $\mu l \, min^{-1}$ compared to the observed mean PBF of 724 $\mu l \, min^{-1}$ (Table 1). The assumption of a constant vascular resistance is in agreement with experimental evidence that the uveal blood flow is directly proportional to the OPP over a wide range of values[1,2,4,11,20,31]

Table 1. Ocular hemodynamics in healthy eyes of adult subjects (mean age – 65 yr)

Parameter	Right eye	Left eye	Difference	
Pulsatile blood flow $\mu l \, min^{-1}$	724 ± 42(8)	718 ± 37(8)	6.6	± 6.5(8)
Diastolic IOP mmHg	15.5 ± 1.0(8)	15.6 ± 0.8(8)	0.43	± 0.2(8)
Systolic IOP mmHg	17.9 ± 1.0(8)	18.1 ± 0.9(8)	0.45	± 0.2(8)
Ophthalmic arterial pressure mmHg*	87 ± 2.3(8)	–	0	
Anticipated OAP	87	–	–	
Diastolic brachial arterial pressure mmHg	73 ± 4(8)	–	–	
Systolic brachial arterial pressure mmHg	130 ± 3.3(8)	–	–	

* The ophthalmic arterial pressures were evaluated from the relation between IOP and PA (Langham and To'mey[18]).

The probability that a major proportion of the total ocular blood flow is pulsatile in the undisturbed eye gains further support from transcranial Doppler studies in man and from ocular blood flow studies in animals. Aslid[3] used a high resolution 8 MHz ultrasound Doppler probe to measure the blood velocity in the ophthalmic artery. The results on 24 healthy subjects revealed a peak velocity of 45 ± 8 cm sec^{-1} during systole, which fell to nearly zero in diastole. A zero velocity means that the blood flow was completely pulsatile. The total blood flow in eyes of rabbits has been measured directly from sectioned vortex veins and by tracer procedures. Fisher (1936) reported an ocular blood flow of ca 1000 µl min^{-1} in anesthetized rabbits based on vortex vein measurements; subsequently, in similar studies on anesthetized rabbits values as high as 1800 µl min^{-1} [20] and 2000 µl min^{-1} [5] were reported. Radio active labelled microsphere entrapment procedures on anesthetized rabbits gave an average total ocular blood flow of 1300 µl min^{-1} [21]. A similar value was found in conscious rabbits by Bill[6]. In order to undertake microsphere studies on the conscious rabbit Bill occluded one common carotid artery to allow placement of a catheter prior to the measurement of the blood flow. Because carotid ligation increases the systemic blood pressure and blood flow to the contralateral carotid artery, the value of 1300 µl min^{-1} is probably high by 10-20%. By comparison, analysis of the IOP pulse in the eyes of conscious rabbits gave a PBF of 950 ± 22 µl min^{-1} (author's unpublished observations).

In conclusion, a system has been developed for recording with high fidelity the IOP pulse. A mathematical theory is described for evaluating the pulsatile component of the ocular blood flow. The application of this technology to the healthy eyes of human subjects indicates a ciliary choroidal pulsatile blood flow of 700 to 800 µl min^{-1}. This blood flow represents the major proportion of the total ocular blood flow, but the exact relation between the pulsatile and non-pulsatile components in healthy and diseased eyes remains to be clarified.

References

1. Alm A, Bill A: Blood flow and oxygen extraction in the cat uvea at normal and high intraocular pressures. Acta Physiol Scand 80:19-28, 1970
2. Alm A, Bill A: Ocular and optic nerve blood flow at normal and increased intraocular pressure in monkeys (Macaca iris): A study with radioactive labelled microspheres including flow determinations in brain and some other tissues. Exp Eye Res 15:15-29, 1973
3. Aslid E: Transcranial Doppler Sonography. Astid (ed) Springer-Verlag 1986
4. Bill A: Intraocular pressure and blood flow through the uvea. Arch Ophthalmol 67:90-102, 1962a
5. Bill A: Quantitative determinations of uveal blood flow in rabbits. Acta Physiol Scand 55:l0l-ll0, 1962b
6. Bill A: Effects of acetazolamide and carotid occlusion on the ocular blood flow in unanesthetized rabbits. Invest Ophthalmol 13:954-958, 1974
7. Dobbie JG: Circulatory changes in the eye associated with retinal detachment and its repair. Trans Am Ophthal Soc LXXCVIII: 503-566, 1980
8. Duke-Elder S: The physiology of the eye and vision. System of Ophthalmology. Vol IV, pp 19-23. St. Louis: CV Mosby 1968
9. Eisenlohr J, Langham ME, Maumenee AE: Manometric studies of the pressure/volume relations in living and enucleated eyes of individual subjects. Br J Ophthalmol 46:536-548, 1962
10. Fischer FP: Ein Versuch, den Energiewechsel des Auges zu bestimmen. Ber Dtsch Ophthalmol Ges 48:95-99, 1936
11. Friedman E: Choroidal blood flow. Arch Ophthalmol 83:95-99, 1970
12. Gee W, Smith CA, Hinsen CE, Wylie EJ: Ocular plethysmography in carotid artery disease. Med Instruments 8:244-248, 1974
13. Goldmann H: Un nouveau tonomètre à aplanation. Bull Soc Fr Ophtalmol 67:474-478, 1954
14. Langham ME: Visual sensitivity to intraocular pressure. In: Glaucoma Update II, p 161-167. Krieglstein GK, Leydhecker W. (eds). Berlin/Heidelberg: Springer-Verlag 1983
15. Langham ME: Ocular blood flow and visual loss in glaucomatous eyes. Glaucoma Update III. GK Krieglstein, Berlin/Heidelberg: Springer–Verlag 1987
16. Langham ME, Maumenee AE: The diagnosis and treatment of glaucoma based on a new procedure for the measurement of intraocular dynamics. Trans Am Acad Ophthalmol Otolaryngol 68:277-300, 1964

17. Langham ME, Preziosi TJ: Non-invasive diagnosis of mild to severe stenosis of the internal carotid artery. Stroke 15/4:614-620, 1984
18. Langham ME, To'mey KF: A clinical procedure for the measurement of ocular pulse-pressure relationship and the ophthalmic arterial pressure. Exp Eye Res 27:17-25, 1978
19. Langham ME, To'mey KF, Preziosi T: Carotid occlusive disease: The effect of complete occlusion of the internal carotid artery on the intraocular pulse/pressure relation and on the ophthalmic arterial pressure. Stroke 12:759-765, 1981
20. Nakamura Y, Goulstine D. The effect of intraocular pressure on the vortex vein blood flow. Exp Eye Res 15:461-466, 1973
21. O'Day DM, Fish MB, Aronson SB, Pollycove M and Coon A: Ocular blood flow measurement by nuclide labelled microspheres. Arch Ophthalmol 86:205-209, 1971
22. Prijot E: Contribution à l'étude de la tonométrie et de la tonographie en ophtalmologie. Docum Ophthalmol 15:1-226, 1966
23. Quigley HA, Langham ME: Comparative intraocular pressure measurements with the pneumatonograph and Goldmann tonometer. Am J Ophthalmol 80:266-273, 1975
24. Riva CE, Feke GT: Laser Doppler velocity in the measurement of retinal bloodflow. In: Goldmann L (ed): The Biomedical Laser: Technology and Clinical Applications, pp 135–161. New York: Springer-Verlag, 1981
25. Riva CE, Grunwald JE, Sinclair SH, Petrig BL: Blood velocity and volumetric flow rate in human retinal vessels. Invest Ophthalmol Vis Sci 26:1124-1132, 1985
26. Silver D, Farrell R, Langham, ME, O'Brien V, Schilder, P: Ocular pulsatile blood flow. Acta Ophthalmol Scand (Suppl) 1988, in press
27. Ulrich WD, Ulrich CH: Oculo-oscillo-dynamography: A diagnostic procedure for recording ocular pulses and measuring retinal and ciliary arterial blood pressures. Ophthalmic Res 17:308-317, 1985
28. Walker RE, Compton GA, Langham ME: Pneumatic applanation tonometer studies. IV: Analysis of pulsatile response. Exp Eye Res 20:245-253, 1975
29. Weigelin E, Lobstein A: In Opthalmodynomometry (Transl Daily RK, Daily, L). New York: Hafner Co Inc 1963
30. Ytteborg J: The rate of intraocular blood volume in rigidity measurements on human eyes. Acta Ophthalmol (Kbh) 38:410-436, 1960
31. Yu DY, Alder VA, Cringle SJ, Brown MJ: Choroidal blood flow measured in the dog eye in-vivo and in-vitro by local hydrogen clearance polarography: Validation of a technique and response to raised intraocular pressure. Exp Eye Res 46:289-303, 1988

This paper is discussed together with the other papers on ocular pulse measurements, on page 121 ff.

OCULAR PERFUSION PRESSURE AND OCULO–OSCILLO–DYNAMOGRAPHY

Wulff–D. Ulrich, Christa Ulrich and Gabriele Walther

Department of Experimental Ophthalmology, Eye Clinic of the Karl–Marx–University, Leipzig, GDR

Abstract

Oculo-Oscillo-dynamography (OODG) is a method to determine noninvasively ocular perfusion pressures (retinal and ciliary), ocular pulse blood volumes, pulse parameters (inclination time, pulse peak delay time, pulse ascending time, pulse descending time, anacrotic angle, catacrotic angle), and pulse propagation times (relative to the ECG or other pulses). The OODG principle is described and negative pressures to IOP conversion curves are given. The OODG curve is interpreted by comparison with findings in occlusion of the central retinal artery, and by perfusion pressure video angiography (PVA). OODG measuring points are discussed and an attempt to summarize the theory of the OODG method is made. Examples of OODG applications in the diagnosis, therapy control and management of stenosis and occlusion of extracranial cerebral arteries and ocular arterial vessels, of temporal arteritis (Morbus Horton) and of primary open angle and low tension glaucoma are given.

It is pointed out that ocular perfusion pressures are basic parameters in the assessment of ocular circulation and its regulation.

1. Introduction

The last two decades have considerably widened our knowledge of the anatomy and physiology of ocular circulation[1-4]. Physiological results were obtained almost exclusively from experimental studies on animals since invasive techniques had to be used. It was only by fluorescence angiography that progress was made in the study of ocular circulation in humans, which, however, was mainly restricted to the retinal and iris vessels.

What was needed to obtain further insights into the ocular circulation in healthy persons and in patients was the use of noninvasive methods that would be easy to perform and well tolerated by the subject.

In recent years, therefore, we endeavored to develop methods for blood pressure measurement and pulse recording as well as procedures for the assessment of the regulatory behavior (autoregulation) of ocular and optic nerve head circulation.

In the following the oculo-oscillo-dynamographic method (OODG) will be described, which permits measurements of:
- ocular perfusion pressures (retinal systolic, pp$_{sret}$, ciliary systolic, pp$_{scil}$, ocular diastolic, pp$_{doc}$),
- ocular pulse blood volume,
- pulse parameters (inclination time, pulse peak delay time, pulse ascending time, pulse descending time, anacrotic angle, catacrotic angle),
- pulse propagation times (relative to the ECG or other pulses, *e.g.* the carotic pulses).

2. Principle of the OODG method

OODG combines a method of producing defined increases in IOP (*i.e.*, the suction cup method) with a procedure for ocular pulse recording.

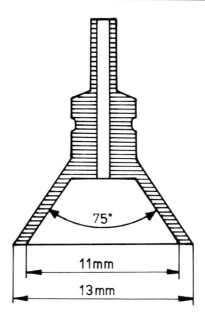

Fig. 1. Cross section and dimensions of an 11 mm suction cup according to Ulrich and Ulrich.

2.1. Suction cup method

The suction cup method according to Ulrich & Ulrich[5-8] uses plastic suction cups of very low weight (about 0.2 to 0.3 g) that easily adhere to the eye even at low negative pressures and need not be held in place manually. Suction cups are available in three sizes, the diameter of the aperture being 11, 12 and 13 mm, respectively. As the device can generate negative pressures of up to 600 mm Hg, ocular arterial pressures up to approx. 160 mm Hg can be determined using a suction cup of 13 mm diameter. The other dimensions of the cups are shown in Fig. 1.

2.2. Conversion of negative pressure to IOP values

2.2.1. Conversion curves: The relation between the negative pressure applied and the resulting IOP is of paramount importance in the OODG method. Though conversion curves were available[9-11] we made studies of our own to determine conversion curves for 11, 12 and 13 mm diameter suction cups (Fig. 2). The curves were established[12] for healthy volunteers of normal ocular refraction allowing deviations within + 2.0 and – 2.0 diopters. The standard deviations of the IOPs are not low and rise with rising pressures. Some typical values are (11 mm suction cup) 0.86, 1.35, 1.77, 2.98 at negative pressures of 25, 50, 100, 300 mm Hg, respectively. For ocular refractions exceeding ± 2 diopters, corrections of the conversion curves have to be made in accordance with Table 1.

2.2.2. Individual conversion: Though the accuracy of the conversion curves is fully satisfactory for measurements in biological and medical practice, IOP can be determined individually, if desired, at any time simultaneous with OODG by using applanation tonometry since the cornea remains free during the OODG procedure. Further details of suction cup methods are described elsewhere[5-8,13,14].

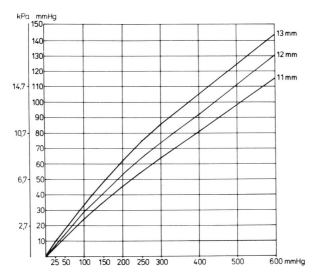

Fig. 2. Negative pressure to IOP conversion curves for 11, 12 and 13 mm diameter suction cups.

Table 1. Correction values for refraction errors. The corresponding correction value is to be added to the measured value.

Refraction error (dioptry)	Negative pressure (mm Hg)					
	50–100	100–200	200–300	300–400	400–500	500–600
−2.5 to −5.0	−0.5	−1.0	−1.0	−1.5	−2.0	−2.0
−5.5 to −8.0	−1.0	−2.0	−2.0	−3.0	−4.0	−4.0
+2.5 to +5.0	+0.5	+1.5	+2.5	+3.5	+4.5	+5.5
+5.0 to +8.0	+1.0	+2.0	+3.5	+5.0	+6.5	+8.5

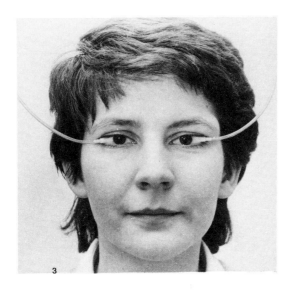

Fig. 3. The suction cups are placed temporally 0.5 -1 mm paralimbally on the eye and fixed by suction.

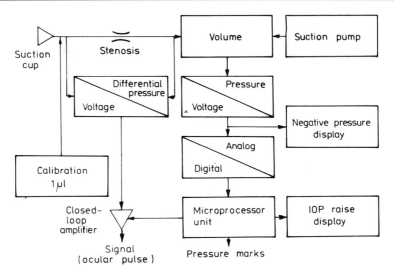

Fig. 4. Block diagram of the OODG device.

2.3. Pulse curve recording:

After drop anesthesia of both eyes the two suction cups are placed temporally on the globes (Fig. 3) and are made to adhere by applying a slight negative pressure to the cups. The suction cups are connected through a plastic hose to a suction pump, and two modified highly sensitive infrasound transducers and a volume calibrating system. The pulse blood volume variations of both eyes are transferred to the elastically deformable capacitive infrasound transducers, amplified and recorded. In this way an ocular pulse oscillogram (oculo-oscillogram - OOG) can be obtained for any artificially elevated IOP (static mode).

If the ocular pulse is recorded at falling IOP, starting from suprasystolic values, an oculo-oscillo-dynamogram (OODG) is obtained (dynamic mode). The main functions of the OODG device are represented in a simplified block diagram (Fig. 4).

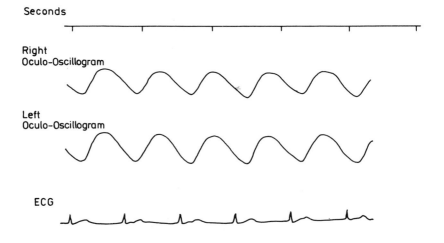

Fig. 5. Oculo-oscillogram (OOG) of both eyes taken at an IOP of 30 mm Hg and ECG.

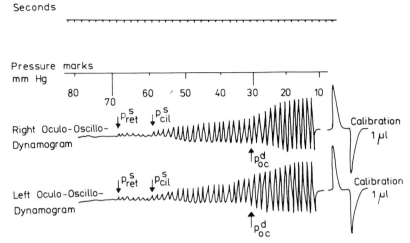

Fig. 6. Oculo–oscillo–dynamogram (OODG) of both eyes. p_{sret} systolic retinal perfusion pressure, p_{scil} systolic ciliary perfusion pressure, p_{doc} diastolic ocular perfusion pressure.

2.3.1. Static mode – OOG: Fig. 5 shows an oculo-oscillogram taken at an IOP of 30 mm Hg simultaneously with the ECG. Oculo-oscillograms can be analyzed with respect to both time and amplitude. Amplitude measurements are facilitated by the 1 µl volume calibration provided in the OODG device. It is thus possible to compare the ocular pulse blood volumes intraindividually and interindividually. Analysis of other pulse parameters and determination of pulse wave propagation times can be performed as described elsewhere[5–7].

The ocular pulse is an integral pulse curve of the uveal and retinal circulatory systems. As the retina takes up only 4 to 5% of the total circulation of the eye, the ocular pulse is predominantly of uveal origin.

2.3.2. Dynamic mode – OODG: Fig. 6 shows an oculo-oscillo-dynamogram (OODG) of both eyes from a healthy person. The pressure marks denote the respective ocular perfusion pressures. The first pulse variation to be seen corresponds to the systolic retinal perfusion pressure (pp_{sret}), and, on allowing the pressure to fall further, the first distinctly higher pulsation which clearly surpasses the retinal oscillations, represent the systolic ciliary perfusion pressure (pp_{scil}). In the range of ocular diastolic pressures it is not possible to separate retinal from ciliary diastolic perfusion pressure. Ocular diastolic perfusion pressure (pp_{doc}) can be detected: (1) from the change of pulse form (the first pulse with a peaked footpoint occurring at falling pressure) and (2) from the postdiastolic rise of pulse amplitude.

To obtain the ocular arterial pressures (such as the retinal arterial pressure, the ciliary arterial pressure), the initial IOP P_0 has to be added to the respective perfusion pressures determined by the OODG method.

3. Interpretation of the OODG curve

At first we had considerable difficulties interpreting the OODG curves. However, clinical findings and video angiography helped us on.

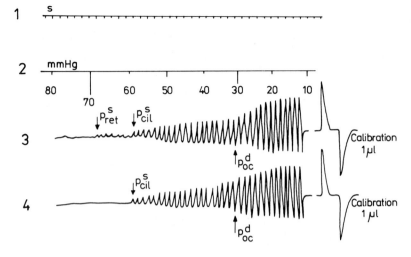

Fig. 7. OODG of a patient with occlusion of the left central retinal artery. Abbreviations as in Fig. 6.

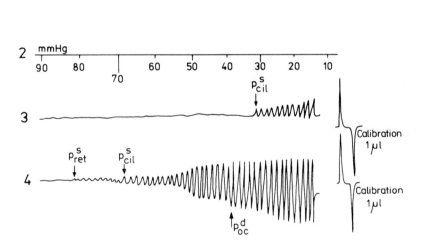

Fig. 8. OODG of a patient with occlusion of the right central retinal artery and, additionally, the right internal carotid artery. Abbreviations as in Fig. 6.

3.1. Oculo-oscillo-dynamogram in central retinal artery occlusion

OODGs taken from patients with occlusion of the central retinal artery are characterized by the complete lack of the very low amplitude oscillations at the onset of the dynamic mode curve[15]. An example is shown in Fig. 7. In cases of isolated central retinal artery occlusion the systolic ciliary perfusion pressure is not changed, *i.e.*, it is on the same level as that obtained from the other eye where there is no occlusion process. In cases of additional proximal stenosis or occlusion (*e.g.*, of the ophthalmic artery or the internal carotid artery) the ciliary perfusion pressure and pulse blood volume are reduced, again with lacking retinal oscillations (Fig. 8). Evidently the first small oscillations to be observed under OODG conditions are of retinal origin.

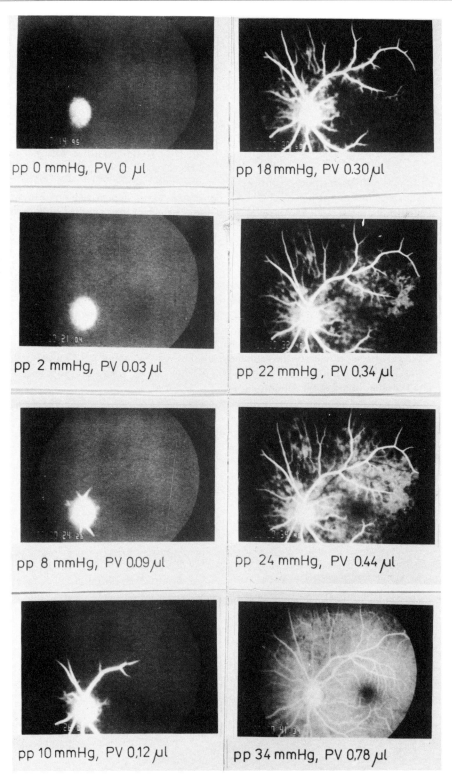

Fig. 9. Perfusion pressure video angiograms of a 20-year old female volunteer. The respective perfusion pressures (pp) and ocular pulse blood volumes (PV) are stated.

3.2. Combined OODG and video angiography – perfusion pressure video angiography (PVA)

Perfusion pressure video angiography (PVA), a method combining OODG and video angiography[16], associates video recordings (50 frames per second) of retinal and choroidal filling with the respective ocular perfusion pressures and the corresponding ocular pulse blood volume. PVA records the gradual filling not only of the retinal but also of the choroidal vascular beds that are thus made visible in great detail.

Fig. 9 shows a few filling situations in the PVA of a 20-year old female volunteer at different perfusion pressures starting from 0 mm Hg. At suprasystolic IOP, *i.e.*, zero perfusion pressure, neither retinal nor ciliary vessels are seen to be filled; however, there is a distinctly translucent fluorescence on the papilla nervi optici. The retinal and ciliary vessels located in front of it are not filled. The retinal vessels appear as a quasi negative print against the fluorescent background. This fluorescence of the papilla at suprasystolic IOP is due to the filling of the retrolaminar vessels that are not directly influenced by high IOP. At a perfusion pressure of 2 mm Hg the retinal vessels on the papilla are filled with fluorescein and at a perfusion pressure of 8 mm Hg, this filling exceeds the border of the papilla. In addition, branches from the ciliary system begin to spread out around the optic nerve head. With further rises in perfusion pressure the other choroidal regions are also filled and displayed.

In the 120 PVA recordings that have been made so far the same filling pattern has been observed in healthy subjects. Under the conditions of OODG, with rising perfusion pressure the retinal system is the first that starts filling. The choroidal system starts filling when the perfusion pressure of the retinal system has reached about 8–12 mm Hg. Up to this point only retinal pulses are seen in the PVA which are in close correspondence with the small oscillations at the beginning of the OODG curve.

4. Measuring points of the OODG method

According to classical circulatory physiological theory, sphygmomanometric and sphygmographic methods measure the blood pressure above the congested or obstructed vascular region where the blood is free to flow off. Table 2 gives a survey of various

Table 2. Noninvasive measuring of the blood pressure gradient across the eye.

Method	Measuring point
Brachial blood pressure measurement (p_{br})	Subclavian artery at its origin from the aorta
Orbital dynamography (p_{orb})	Internal carotid artery at the origin of the ophthalmic artery
Impression dynamometry (p_{oph})	Ophthalmic artery anywhere between its origin from the internal carotid artery and the origin of the central retinal artery
Oculo-oscillo-dynamography (OODG), (p_{ret}, p_{cil})	Central retinal artery close to its origin from the ophthalmic artery, and ciliary arteries
Entopto-capillaro-dynamometry (EDM)	Paramacular retinal capillaries, minute retinal arterioles
Applanation tonometry	Intraocular veins
Episcleral venous pressure measurement	Episcleral veins

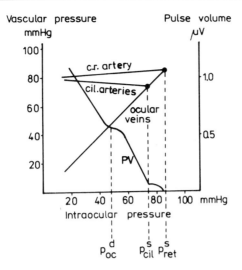

Fig. 10. Retinal arterial, ciliary arterial, ocular venous pressures and pulse blood volume versus IOP, schematic diagram PV pulse (blood) volume, p_{sret} systolic retinal arterial pressure, p_{scil} systolic ciliary arterial pressure, p_{doc} diastolic ocular arterial pressure. The difference between retinal arterial and ocular venous pressures gives the retinal perfusion pressure depending on IOP, that between ciliary arterial and ocular venous pressure the ciliary perfusion pressure, which will be more strongly reduced with rising IOP than the retinal perfusion pressure.

noninvasive methods of measuring the blood pressure with their respective points of measurement including those used in OODG. But here the question arises: how can one explain why the pressures measured in the ciliary system are lower than those measured in the central retinal artery considering that both the central retinal artery and the main ciliary vessels originate from the same ophthalmic artery? And here we are reduced to speculation: It can be assumed that the OODG curve reflects the vascularization pattern. The pressure difference may be due to the special vascular structure of the uveal arterial system. There are numerous branches of the ciliary arteries outside the eye while there are few and only minute branches of the central retinal artery along its way to the eyes as Hayreh already showed in 1962[1]. The more ciliary branches there are outside the eye and the greater the possibility of shunts, the greater will be the pressure difference between the retinal and the ciliary circulatory systems, because the tissue pressure of the eye is higher than that outside, with a corresponding difference in vascular resistance. Thus the blood will be shunted into the ciliary vessels outside the eye. As the pressure difference between central retinal artery and ciliary arteries will become wider with rising IOP the ciliary system will tend to become a low pressure system relative to the retinal system as Hayreh suggested from his anatomical and angiographic studies[17].

OODG permits to detect the functional results of such anatomic variations. An attempt to summarize the theory of the OODG method is made in Fig. 10.

With rising IOP the ocular venous pressure rises accordingly. Central retinal arterial pressure remains uninfluenced or rises slightly. Ciliary arterial pressure decreases with rising IOP. The perfusion pressure of the retinal system (difference between central retinal arterial and ocular venous pressure) is higher than that of the ciliary system. With rising IOP the ciliary perfusion pressure (difference between ciliary arterial and ocular venous pressure) decreases more strongly relative to the perfusion pressure of the central retinal artery. The retinal–ciliary perfusion pressure difference increases with increasing IOP and the pulse blood volume (PV) decreases with rising IOP in a characteristic manner. It can be inferred from the diagram that rising IOP will first affect the ciliary circulatory system.

5. Clinical application of OODG

OODG can make major contributions to the assessment of ocular circulatory disturbance. Only a few brief remarks on practical applications can be made here.

5.1. OODG in stenoses and occlusion of extracranial cerebral arteries

Stenoses or occlusion of the internal carotid artery proximal to the origin of the ophthalmic artery, stenoses or occlusion of the common carotid artery, and stenosis or occlusion of the brachial cephalic trunk, if hemodynamically effective, will also alter ocular circulation[18,19]. In such cases the OODG is characterized by a reduced ocular pulse blood volume and a decrease mainly of the systolic retinal and ciliary perfusion pressures, with the difference between these pressures remaining unchanged. In comparison with other methods that have been used successfully in the diagnosis of occlusion processes of the internal carotid artery[18–20], OODG has distinct advantages:

- systolic ocular pressures (retinal and ciliary), which are the first to be altered significantly in occlusion processes of the carotid artery, can be measured easily;
- along with the perfusion pressures ocular pulse parameters are recorded. In occlusion processes of the carotid artery the OODG shows reduced ocular pulse blood volumes and further characteristic changes such as pulse peak delay time prolongation, lessening of the anacrotic angle α, increase of pulse ascending time. Simultaneous recording of the ECG permits measuring the pulse wave propagation time, which is prolonged;
- simultaneous examination of both eyes saves much time and facilitates assessment and comparison.

By combining OODG with other methods (battery of tests) such as Doppler sonography, orbital dynamography, temporal dynamography, one obtains a high specificity (100%, no false positive data), a high sensitivity (96%) and an overall accuracy of 96%.

5.2. OODG in occlusion of ocular arterial vessels

OODG permits to assess and differentiate occlusions of the central retinal artery, the ophthalmic artery and ciliary arteries. In occlusion of the central retinal artery the low amplitude retinal oscillations disappear as described above (chapter 3.1). In occlusion of ciliary circulatory regions the retinal pulse oscillations are not changed, while the ciliary oscillations, depending on the kind and extent of the occlusion processes involved, will be more or less reduced or disappear completely. In occlusion of the ophthalmic artery both circulatory regions (retinal and ciliary) are involved. Retinal and ciliary pulse blood volumes as well as retinal and ciliary perfusion pressures are reduced while the carotid artery can be shown to be normal by using Doppler sonography.

5.3. OODG in temporal arteritis

Also temporal arteritis (Morbus Horton) will result in OODG changes[21] if the ciliary vessels and/or the central retinal artery are involved in the inflammatory and occlusive process. Typical patterns of the spreading of the disease through the vessels are found by combining OODG with orbital dynamography (ODG) and temporal dynamography (TDG). This combined procedure may become of particular importance in therapy control. Corticoid therapy will result in complete normalization of the circulation through recanalization in the regions involved. Any relapses that may occur due to insufficient maintenance dosage can be detected at once by using OODG, ODG and TDG combined and loss of vision can thus be prevented.

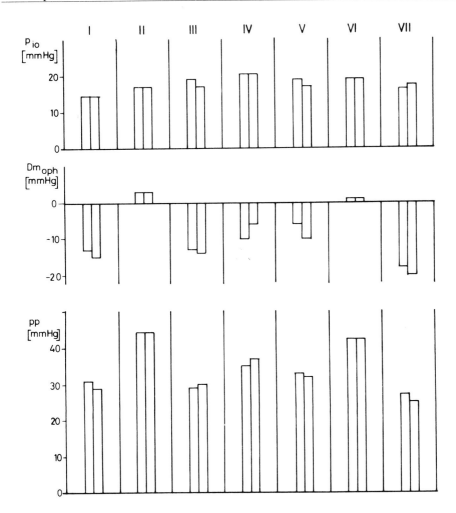

Fig. 11. Evaluated data (IOPs), ciliary perfusion pressures and deviations of ciliary arterial pressures from normal regression) of a 52-year old male patient with low tension glaucoma.
P_{io} IOP, Dm_{oph} deviation of ciliary arterial pressure from normal regression, pp mean ciliary perfusion pressure. The left columns represent data from the right eye, and the right columns those from the left eye.

5.4. OODG and glaucoma

Assuming that glaucoma is a disease involving impairment of ocular and/or optic nerve head circulation, it is desirable to obtain data on ocular perfusion pressures and pulse blood volumes. OODG is a suitable method for obtaining these data without difficulty even in glaucoma patients with narrow pupils.

5.4.1. Ocular perfusion pressure as a criterion in the management of glaucoma: Fig. 11 shows the IOP and the mean effective ciliary perfusion pressure of a male patient aged 52 suffering from progressive low tension glaucoma. Despite normal IOP the deterioration of the visual field progresses continuously. Evidently the ciliary perfusion pressure is insufficient for the blood supply to the optic nerve head as shown by measurements taken at different times (I,III, IV, V, VII). It was only at some times (II, VI) that therapy resulted in improved perfusion pressures. An entirely different situation is shown in Fig. 12. The

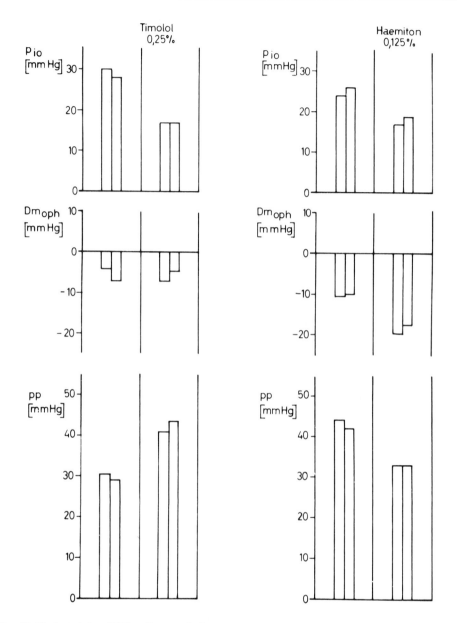

Fig. 12. Evaluated data (IOPs, ciliary perfusion pressures and deviations of ciliary arterial pressures from normal regression) of a 61-year old female patient with primary open angle glaucoma after administration of timolol and haemiton (clonidine), respectively. Abbreviations as in Fig. 11.

IOP is increased and ciliary perfusion pressure is within the normal range. The 61-year old female patient suffers from primary open angle glaucoma with progressing deterioration of the visual field. On administration of haemiton (clonidine, 0.125% solution, 1 drop twice per day) the IOP had decreased, the perfusion pressure, however, had also decreased, indicating that the contrary of the desired improvement of circulation had occurred.

The administration of timolol (0.25% solution, 1 drop per day) instead of clonidine resulted in decreased IOP as well as the desired increase of perfusion pressure.

This confirms that measurements of the IOP alone do not suffice for the diagnosis, functional prognosis and therapy control of glaucoma. It also indicates that ocular (in particular ciliary) perfusion pressure is of higher significance in the diagnosis and management of glaucoma than was assumed in the past.

5.4.2. OODG in primary open angle glaucoma and in low tension glaucoma: In POAG systemic blood pressure tends to rise, and normal or high ocular perfusion pressures are observed. The pulse blood volume is normal or increased in most cases and the pressure difference between retinal and ciliary systems is normal. However, in some cases with rapid deterioration of visual function, very low pulse blood volumes and great retinal–ciliary pressure differences have been observed, *i.e.,* the ciliary perfusion pressure is low relative to the retinal perfusion pressure. In low tension glaucoma, the pulse blood volumes are reduced in the majority of cases and the retinal–ciliary pressure difference is increased.

It can be assumed from these results, provided our interpretation is correct, that in low tension glaucoma the ciliary vascularization pattern deviates from normal in the sense of a more pronounced low tension system.

5.4.3. Ocular perfusion pressures in the assessment of ocular autoregulation: Earlier investigations into the dependence of ocular circulatory parameters on IOP produced results of a wide variability. If, however, circulatory changes in the respective circulatory system (retinal or ciliary) are represented in relation to the perfusion pressure of the system, the variability decreases considerably and the characteristic behavior of the circulation and its autoregulatory mechanism become evident.

Ocular perfusion pressures are thus a basic parameter in the assessment of ocular circulation and its regulation.

References

1. Hayreh SS: The ophthalmic artery, III Br J Ophthalmol 46:212–247, 1962
2. Hayreh SS: Structure and blood supply of the optic nerve. In: Heilmann K, Richardson KT (eds) Glaucoma: Conceptions of a Disease, pp 97–103. Stuttgart: George Thieme 1978
3. Bill A: Physiological aspects of the circulation in the optic nerve. In: Heilmann K, Richardson KT (eds). Glaucoma: Conceptions of a Disease, pp 97–103, Stuttgart: George Thieme 1978
4. Bill A: Ocular circulation In: Moses RA (ed): Adler's Physioklogy of the Eye, pp 184–203. CV Mosby Company 1981
5. Ulrich WD, Ulrich Ch: Einsatz der Okulo–Oszillo–Dynamographie (OODG) für Patientenuntersuchungen. Boucke–Report Tübingen 1984
6. Ulrich WD, Ulrich Ch: Oculo–Oscillo–Dynamography: A diagnostic procedure for recording ocular pulses and measuring retinal and ciliary arterial blood pressures. Ophthalmic Res 17:308–317, 1985
7. Ulrich WD, Ulrich Ch: Okulo–Oszillo–Dynamographie, ein neues Verfahren zur Bestimmung des Ophthalmikablutdruckes und zur okulären Pulskurvenanalyse. Klin Mbl Augenheilk 186:385–388, 1985
8. Ulrich Ch, Ulrich WD: Das Saugnapfverfahren in der okulären Kreislaufdiagnostik. In: Stodtmeister R, Christ Th, Pillunat LE, Ulrich WD (eds): Okuläre Durchblutungsstörungen, pp 80–88. Stuttgart: Ferdinand Enke Verlag 1987
9. Hayatsu H: Measurement of blood pressure in retina, especially on calibration curves for Mikuni's ophthalmodynamometer. I. Calibration curves by Schiötz's standardized tonometer. Acta Soc Ophthalmol Jpn 68:111–119, 1964
10. Hayatsu, H: Measurement of blood pressure in retina especially on calibration curves for Mikuni's ophthalmodynamometer. II. Calibration curves by Goldmann's applanation tonometer. Acta Soc Ophthalmol Jpn 68: 175 – 182, 1964
11. Hayatsu H: Measurement of blood pressure in retina, especially on calibration curves for Mikuni's ophthalmodynamometer. III. Influences of age, refraction and ocular rigidity upon calibration curves. Acta Soc Ophthalmol Jpn 68:1289–1296, 1964
12. Ulrich WD, Ulrich Ch, Schulz Chr. Walther G: Negative pressure to IOP conversion curves for the suction cups of 11, 12 and 13 mm diameter acc. to W.D. Ulrich and Ch. Ulrich, unpublished
13. Ulrich WD: Grundlagen und Methodik der Ophthalmodynamometrie (ODM), Ophthalmodynamographie (ODG) und Temporalisdynamographie (TDG). Abhandlungen aus dem Gebiete der Augenheilkunde. Sammlung von Monographien Bd. 44, Leipzig: VEB Georg Thieme Verlag 1976

14. Strik F: OODG –Ulrich and OPG–Gee: A comparative study. Docum Ophthalmol 69:51–71, 1988
15. Ulrich Ch, Ulrich WD: Okulo–oszillodynamische und dopplersonographische Untersuchungen bei Netzhautarterienverschlüssen. Fortschr Ophthalmol 82:484–487, 1985
16. Ulrich WD, Ulrich Ch, Helm W, Walther G, Sachsenweger M: Perfusionsdruck–Videoangiographie – ein neues Verfahren zur Untersuchung des retinalen und chorioidalen Kreislaufs. Augenspiegel 34:53–57, 1988
17. Hayreh SS: Glaucoma damage. Pathogenesis of optic nerve damage and visual field defects. In: Heilmann K, Richardson KT (eds): Glaucoma: Conceptions of a Disease, pp 78–96. Stuttgart: Georg Thieme 1978
18. Ulrich Ch: Klinik und Praxis der Ophthalmodynamometrie (ODM), Ophthalmodynamographie (ODG), Temporalisdynamographie (TDG). Ein Beitrag zur neuro–ophthalmologischen Kreislaufdiagnostik. Abhandlungen aus dem Gebiete der Augenheilkunde. Sammlung von Monographien Bd 46. Leipzig: VEB Georg Thieme 1980
19. Strik F: Ophthalmodynamography and ophthalmodynamometry in neurological practice. Docum Ophthalmol 49:97, 1980
20. Weigelin E, Lobstein A: Ophthalmodynamometrie. Basel: Karger 1962
21. Ulrich Ch, Ulrich D, Kornotzki M, Ulrich WD: Arteriitis temporalis – Diagnostik und Therapiekontrolle. Z Inn Med 43:526–530, 1988

This paper is discussed together with the other papers on ocular pulse measurements, on page 121 ff.

OCULAR PULSE MEASUREMENTS IN LOW-TENSION GLAUCOMA

George N. Lambrou, Peter Sindhunata, Thomas J.T.P. van den Berg, Caroline H. Geijssen, Pietr Vyborny and Erik L. Greve

Glaucoma Department, Eye Clinic of the University of Amsterdam. Meibergdreef 9, 1105 AZ Amsterdam, The Netherlands.

Introduction

Despite the important advances made in glaucoma research in the last decades, the role of the ocular circulation in the pathogenesis of glaucoma in general and of low-tension glaucoma in particular remains controversial. The so-called vasogenic theory postulates that glaucoma is due to inadequate perfusion of the optic nerve head and/or the retina, resulting from any combination of three mechanisms: decreased perfusion pressure (itself a result of increased IOP), inadequate vascular autoregulation at capillary or precapillary level, or insufficient blood supply to the eye. Of those three mechanisms, the first two would be involved in primary open-angle glaucoma, whereas in "low-tension glaucoma" the third factor would be predominant.

To test this hypothesis, we undertook a pilot study in which we investigated total ocular blood supply in a sample of glaucoma patients and age–matched controls.

Methods

Our study was to be carried out on well-diagnosed and followed-up patients, and was not meant to have any therapeutic implications. It was important, therefore, to use a simple, innocuous and painless method. We chose to measure *ocular pulse amplitudes* (PA) with the help of the Langham Ocular Blood Flow System (Grieshaber, Switzerland). This system uses the Langham pneumatonograph (Alcon Laboratories, USA) whose output is processed by a computer correcting for pressure fluctuations, weight of the probe in supine or sitting position, etc. A pedal-driven scleral suction cup, provided as part of the system, allows artificial IOP elevation.

Prior to the pneumatonographic examination, blood pressure and heart rate were measured for each patient, and Goldmann tonometry performed. The pulse amplitudes from both eyes were then recorded at spontaneous IOP, *i.e.* without suction cup (PA1). Finally, the suction cup was applied and further pulse amplitudes recordings were made, after the IOP had artificially been raised by 10 mmHg (PA2), by 20 mmHg (PA3) and to half the systolic brachial arterial pressure (PA4), first in one eye and then in the other.

From each of these rough ocular pulse measurements we obtained another two ocular perfusion parameters: First, by means of the ocular pressure-volume relationship (Fig.1), we computed the *pulsatile volume*, *i.e.* the rhythmic volume change of the intraocular content, corresponding roughly to the bolus of blood entering the eyeball with every heartbeat[1]. We then multiplied this volume by the heart rate to estimate (pulsatile) minute blood flow, which we divided by an approximation of perfusion pressure to obtain a rough estimate of (pulsatile) *vascular conductance*, in accordance to Ohm's law applied to hydrodynamics:[2]

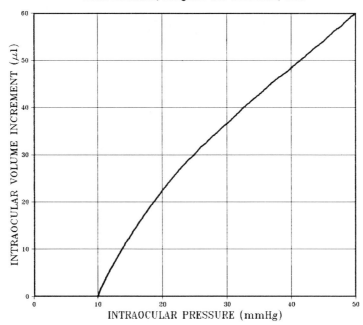

Fig. 1. Graphic representation of the pressure-volume relationship of the human eye, after Langham's data[1]. The curve illustrates the volume of liquid that must be injected into an eye with an initial pressure of 10 mmHg, to reach a given IOP.

$$VC = \frac{PV \cdot h}{(2/3) \cdot BP_{syst} - IOP}$$

where: VC : vascular conductance;
PV : pulsatile volume;
h   : heart rate;
PV · h : estimate of minute blood flow;
BP_{syst} : systolic brachial blood pressure;
IOP : intraocular pressure;
(2/3) · BP_{syst} − IOP : estimate of ocular perfusion pressure[2].

Patients

Sixty-nine patients and sixteen age-matched control subjects were included in the study, irrespective of sex, age or treatment (operated eyes were not subjected to IOP-elevation, though). All patients came from the outpatient consultation of the Glaucoma Department of the University of Amsterdam Eye Clinic. The control subjects were spouses of patients, with no eye problems other than refractive. The purpose of the study and the method of examination were explained, and informed consent obtained from each subject investigated.

The patients were selected so as to fall into two entirely distinct subgroups: "Low-tension glaucomas" (LTG), with pressures below 22 mmHg (although one single IOP peak,

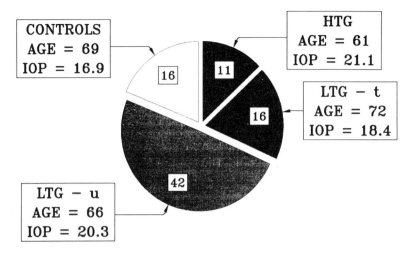

Fig. 2. Distribution into groups and subgroups of the subjects included in the study. The figures inside the pie–chart segments are the numbers of subjects in each subgroup.

not exceeding 26 mmHg, was tolerated in the diurnal curve) and "High–tension glaucomas" (HTG), with pressures above 30 mmHg. LTG patients were further subdivided into untreated (LTG–u) and treated (LTG–t). All patients had visual field loss and disc alterations in both eyes.

Figure 2 shows the number, mean age and mean IOP for each subgroup.

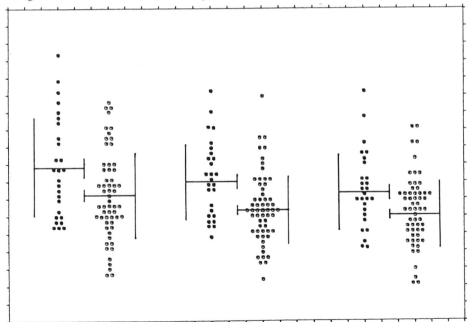

Fig. 3. Dispersion of the values of each of the three blood flow parameters. Each point represents one patient. Pulse amplitudes are depicted in the two leftmost columns, pulsatile volumes in the two center columns, and vascular conductances in the two rightmost columns. Within each pair of columns the left (filled dots) represents the "presumed healthy circulations" group (controls + HTG), and the right the "presumed poor circulations" (LTG). Horizontal lines are means, long vertical lines are standard deviations, short vertical lines are standard errors of the mean. Mean values of all three parameters are significantly lower in the LTG group, but the overlap is considerable. (Vertical scaling of pulse amplitudes is expanded by two, for clarity).

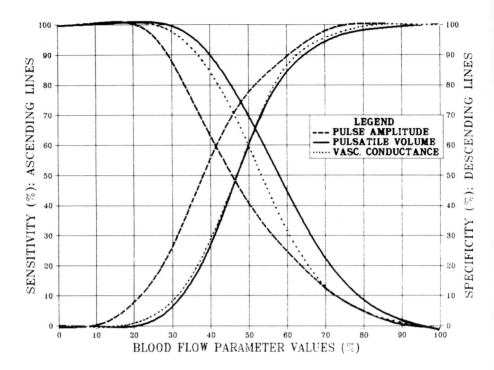

Fig. 4. Sensitivity (decreasing from left to right) and specificity (rising from left to right) curves for each of the three blood flow parameters, illustrating the poor diagnostic value of the technique.

Results

1. It became very soon obvious that there was a very important variability of the results, making any statistic interpretation hazardous. To remove part of the variability, we decided to average the values of the two eyes for every patient, as if they were a single organ. We felt justified in doing so as (a) all patients had bilateral and, in most cases, symmetrical disease and (b) the values from the two eyes were very highly correlated ($r=0.76$, $p<0.0001$). In the case of operated eyes, where no suction–cup was applied, the reading of the non–operated eye alone was taken into account.
2. The mean pulse amplitudes for each subgroup and IOP–level are summarized in Table 1. The inter-subgroup differences in pulse amplitudes were not significant and decreased as IOP increased. We decided therefore to discard the measurements performed under artificially raised IOP, and carry the subsequent analysis only on the parameters calculated from measurements at spontaneous IOP.
3. Similar to the PA, neither of the two calculated parameters was significantly

Table 1 Mean pulse amplitudes in the four subgroups (control, HTG, untreated and treated LTG), at spontaneous and artificially increased IOP. See text for details.

	PA_1	PA_2	PA_3	PA_4
CON	1.4 ± 0.5	1.1 ± 0.4	1.0 ± 0.3	0.5 ± 0.1
LTG u	1.3 ± 0.4	1.0 ± 0.4	0.9 ± 0.3	0.5 ± 0.2
LTG t	1.1 ± 0.4	0.8 ± 0.4	0.8 ± 0.3	0.5 ± 0.1
HTG	1.6 ± 0.4	1.1 ± 0.4	0.9 ± 0.4	0.5 ± 0.1

Table 2 Mean pulse amplitudes (PA), pulsatile volumes (PV), and vascular conductances (VC) at spontaneous IOP, in each of the four subgroups and in the two merged groups, "presumed healthy circulations" (CNT+HTG) and "presumed poor circulations" (LTG u+t).

Groups	Parameters		
	P.A.	P.V.	V.C.
CNT	1.36 ± 0.46	2.65 ± 0.80	2.34 ± 0.76
HTG	1.63 ± 0.49	2.73 ± 0.70	2.60 ± 0.68
CNT + HTG	1.47 ± 0.47	2.68 ± 0.73	2.45 ± 0.72
LTG–u	1.24 ± 0.42	2.12 ± 0.70	2.05 ± 0.68
LTG–t	1.15 ± 0.41	2.05 ± 0.60	1.99 ± 0.60
LTG (u+t)	1.22 ± 0.41	2.10 ± 0.66	2.03 ± 0.64

different between the groups. All three parameters, however, were lower in LTG (and even more so in the treated subgroup) and slightly higher in HTG than in the control group (Table 2). We merged, therefore, our subgroups into "presumed healthy circulations" (controls + HTG) and "presumed poor circulations" (LTG–t + LTG–u). The ensuing increase of the number of subjects per group caused the differences to cross the significance threshold (Table 3). Figure 3 shows the distribution of values for each of the three parameters.

Table 3 Comparison of the three parameter means among subgroups with a two-sided t-test. Only the pulsatile volume is significantly different between control subjects and untreated LTG patients. Merging of the (statistically and conceptually similar) subgroups into "presumed healthy circulations" (CNT+HTG) and "presumed poor circulations" (LTG u+t), reveals more significant differences, in favor of a vascular component in the pathogenesis of low-tension glaucoma.

	P.A.	P.Vol.	Vasc. Cond
CNT – HTG	NS	NS	NS
LTG: u – t	NS	NS	NS
CNT – LTG u	NS	S++	NS
(CNT + HTG) – LTG u	NS	S+++	S++
(CNT + HTG) – (LTG u + t)	S+	S+++	S+++

NS: Not Significant ($p > 5\%$)
S: Significant   +   : $p \leq 5\%$
               ++ : $p \leq 1\%$
              +++ : $p \leq 0.1\%$

Comments

The above results corroborate the hypothesis that ocular blood supply is deficient in low–tension glaucoma as compared to normal eyes or to "high-tension" glaucoma. There is, however, a very high interindividual variability in the perfusion parameters calculated from ocular pulse measurements. This variability is not altogether unexpected. Indeed, pulse amplitudes are relevant for the assessment of ocular blood flow only to the extent that they relate to (pulsatile) blood flow. This relationship, expressed by the curve of Fig. 1, depends upon many other factors, such as volume of the eyeball, scleral rigidity, thickness of the choroid, etc., themselves subject to a more or less important interindividual variability. Moreover, those measurements reflect the perfusion of the entire choroidal bed, of which an extremely reduced part may have some role to play in the pathogenesis of glaucoma.

It is evident, from Fig. 3, that the diagnostic value of such measurements is small. This

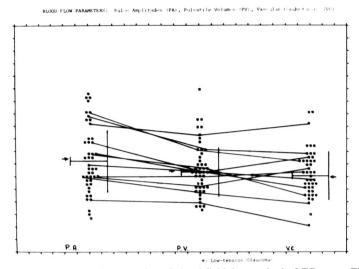

Fig. 5. Blood flow parameters and progression of visual field damage in the LTG group. The layout is the same as in Fig. 3, except that the "presumed healthy circulations" group has been omitted for clarity. When available (40 cases out of 58), the visual fields of LTG patients over two years prior to the examination were clinically assessed. A clear-cut deterioration was found in 11 patients, whose individual values have been linked with oblique lines. The arrows show the mean values of this 11-patient subgroup, situated within the confidence interval of the group mean for all three parameters.

is confirmed by the sensitivity and specificity curves of the three parameters (Fig. 4), especially if one keeps in mind the low incidence of LTG.

At best, therefore, one might use those parameters to diagnose a very deficient circulation as a potential risk factor in a low-tension glaucoma patient or in an ocular hypertensive. However, this use of ocular pulse measurements has to be confirmed by prospective studies. As a possible encouragement to future such studies, we attempted a retrospective assessment of the prognostic value of our three perfusion parameters: we identified the patients whose visual field had undergone undeniable deterioration during the two last years before the measurement (irrespective of visual field stage: indeed, it is not so much the stage of the visual field, highly dependent on the length of the disease, as its rate of deterioration that is relevant as a prognostic factor). The parameter values corresponding to each of those patients have been linked by continuous lines in Fig. 5. As can be seen, the "progressive" damage subgroup is in no way different from the stabilized patients.

References

1. Langham M.E., Eisenlohr J., Maumenee A.E.: Manometric studies of the pressure–volume relationships in living and enucleated eyes of individual human subjects. Br J Ophthalmol 46: 536 – 548.
2. Langham M.C.: Personnal communication.

DISCUSSION

Erik L. Greve : It was decided, since the three papers in this session dealt with very similar methods, to discuss them all in the end of the session. Before we start, let me remind you of the conclusions drawn by each author. Dr Ulrich claims to be able to measure separately the arterial and the ciliary perfusion pressures, and that the latter is reduced in glaucoma, especially of the low-tension type. Dr Langham described his system for ocular pulse amplitude measurements and a method by which he claims to derive blood flow. Dr Lambrou presented the results of the study we undertook in Amsterdam with Langham's method hoping that we would be able to use it for the individual low-tension-glaucoma patient. It turned out that it can't be used for diagnosis so far, because of the high overlap between groups. These were the main points of the three presentations; the discussion is now open.

Richard Stodtmeister : Dr Langham, how did you measure the ophthalmic artery pressure ?

Maurice E. Langham : We plotted the curve of pulse amplitude against IOP. The IOP for which the pulse is extinguished is the ophthalmic artery pressure.

Bernard Schwartz : How large was your population, Maurice ?

Maurice E. Langham : The results I have shown in the table were from a small group of eight healthy adults. But we have done hundreds by now for confirmation.

Erik L. Greve : Dr Ulrich, how can you be so sure that the first pulse that you measure corresponds to the retinal circulation only and that you can later pick up the first pulses of the ciliary circulation ?

Wulff D. Ulrich : We are absolutely sure of that. We confirmed it by doing simultaneous video fluorescein angiography and OODG: the first small pulse of the OODG was recorded at the very moment that fluorescein appeared in the central retinal artery. Similarly, the choroid started filling at the moment we recorded the first ciliary pulse.

Richard Stodtmeister : We have also been using this method and we have seen a number of cases that are relevant for this issue. We had, for instance, a patient with disseminated choroiditis, and his retinal pulsations were normal while the choroidal were very diminished. And in some patients with carotid obstruction, both pulsations were absent until the IOP was very low. Also, as Dr Ulrich showed, the retinal pulsations are abolished in central retinal artery occlusion. Moreover, we compared the retinal and ciliary systolic pressures, as measured by OODG, to the systemic blood pressure and found very good correlations within the limits of biological variation. So I think that we can indeed accept this claim of Dr Ulrich.

Wulff D. Ulrich : Since you mentioned central retinal artery occlusion, we did simultaneous video-angiography and OODG in a few such cases, and it seems that there are two sorts of occlusion, real and functional. In functional occlusion, there is a residual flow in the central retinal artery, but with very low perfusion pressures.

Yves C.A. Robert : There are two remarks I would like to make. The first concerns the pressure-lowering effect in therapeutic trials. If the pulse amplitude is about 2 mmHg, this means that the measurement error when reading an IOP of 20 mmHg is 10%. So if in a therapeutic trial we demonstrate a pressure-lowering effect of less than 4 mmHg, this result is useless, because it is within the error interval of the two measurements, before and after therapy. My second remark is that there seem to be very many patients, in Switzerland, at least, where you can't see any pulsations at all when you do Goldmann tonometry. What is the explanation for these people, who seem to be pulseless and are yet in an absolutely normal ocular condition ?

Maurice E. Langham : I am rather surprised at what you say. We have measured about 4000 patients by now, and the only ones with low pulse have either carotid disease or very important posterior segment disease, like retinal detachment.

Harry A. Quigley : About your first remark, Dr Robert, the mean error is only 1 mmHg if you make an attempt to average the pressure values where the rings clear each other and where they overlap, in the Goldmann tonometer. And I don't think that this 1 mmHg is so crucial to our therapeutic trials.

Yves C.A. Robert : Yes, but do we always try to take the average? Or do we just take the value we happen to read at a given instant? You have to be very careful if you want to measure always in the same way, and I am not sure that everyone is, especially since this is seldom specified in the protocol of the trials.

Maurice E. Langham : I would like to go back to George's study. I think it is very encouraging, George, that you found those differences between groups even by making a coarse approximation of the perfusion pressure. I believe that differences will come out even more strongly if you put all the parameters together, including the correction for rate of pulsatile flow. And as for the implications of a low value for the individual patient, I would say that if a given patient has very low flow values then he is at a high risk.

Erik L. Greve : This may be so, Maurice, but the variability is so important that we can draw this conclusion only in the very extreme cases.

Harry A. Quigley : I want to understand better Dr Lambrou's study. Did you say that for you a low tension glaucoma is someone with pressures not exceeding 26 mmHg? Is 26 the dividing line ?

George N. Lambrou : Not exactly. We used for this study the low tension glaucoma population of the glaucoma department of the University of Amsterdam. Patients in this population have all had IOP day-curves. Mean IOP is below 22mmHg, usually around 19, but we allow one peak above 22, not exceeding 26 mmHg.

Harry A. Quigley : And were the mean ages and age distributions the same in your low-tension glaucoma and normal groups ?

George N. Lambrou : Yes, they were.

Harry A. Quigley : Were your different glaucoma subgroups stage-matched with respect to visual field damage ?

George N. Lambrou : No, they were not.

Harry A. Quigley : I ask these questions because I think it is very important, especially if you are looking at a prognostic feature, to know how much damage there is, because it may indicate which patients are in fact more susceptible to injury; that is, those who have more field loss. I understand that it is very laborious to get such a group together, but it is important not to compare people who are in the early phase of the disease to those who are more advanced, because then you have an uncontrolled variable.

George L. Spaeth : I think that what Harry says is very important, because one would assume that with advancing glaucoma one would have a reduction in the number of blood vessels. And Harry has shown that to be the case, in the optic nerve head at least.

Erik L. Greve : Yes, but you wouldn't expect anything similar in the choroid.

George L. Spaeth : Perhaps also there. Well, I am speculating, of course, but if you stage-match your patients, then your point becomes very convincing.

George N. Lambrou : It is true that one should take into account the progression of the disease. However, more than the stage of loss, it is rather the rate of progression that one should consider. And that was the idea behind the last figure: we picked out of all our population those patients who had shown visual field deterioration during the last two years, and it turned out that their flow parameters were distributed exactly like the rest of the patients, whose visual fields – whatever their stage – had remained unaltered during that period.

Erik L. Greve : There is one more question, Dr Ulrich, I would like to ask. The fact that the pulse volume is lower in low-tension glaucoma is confirmed by many studies. However, there seems to be an important variability in the results. What was the variability in your study? Do you think that you can draw conclusions from your measurements for the individual patient?

Wulff D. Ulrich : We found, as you said, a decrease of both the pulse volume and the ciliary perfusion pressure in low-tension glaucoma, but the variability was indeed very high. It is only by taking mean values from the whole low-tension glaucoma group that you can find this decrease. But then the difference is highly significant, contrary to the primary open-angle glaucoma, the ocular hypertensive and the normal groups, where no significant difference is to be found. Now as far as the individual patient is concerned, there are some patients with very low pulsatile volume. What exactly pulsatile volume means is difficult to say, but I think that it does reflect blood flow, and therefore we can say that in those patients choroidal blood flow is indeed reduced.

George N. Lambrou : I think that the extrapolation from pulse amplitudes, because that's what we are measuring, to pulsatile volume and, one step further, to pulsatile blood flow is a little hazardous, since the pulse amplitude depends on a number of things. It depends on the pulsatile volume of course, and that is what we are trying to get to. But it also depends on the volume of the choroid relative to the total volume of the eyeball – and in normal persons there is a 10% variation in the anteroposterior ocular diameter, which makes a 30% variation in ocular volume. Then of course scleral rigidity will also influence the pulse amplitude and add some more variability to the measurements. And this is what makes the technique tantalizing: it seems that there is something in it, but we can't reach it yet. The day we can control all these parameters, we might have a simple and elegant way to evaluate global ocular blood flow. Now about optic nerve head blood flow in particular, we should keep in mind that the pulse comes from the entire choroidal vascular bed, while only a tiny fraction of the choroid is in some way involved in the vascularization of the optic nerve head. So even if we manage to solve all the other problems of the technique and to measure global blood flow accurately, we will still not have the key to the role of the circulation in the pathogenesis of glaucoma – supposing of course the damage to occur primarily in the optic nerve head.

Maurice E. Langham : Speaking of variability, George, there is one more source adding to it if you use Oculo-Oscillo-Dynamography, due to the fact that the IOP is not measured directly but is derived from the suction pressure with the help of a statistic curve, whereas pneumatonography measures IOP directly.

George N. Lambrou : That's right, yes.

Sohan S. Hayreh : One of the most important factors to keep in mind with ocular pulse measurements is, I think, that they reflect global choroidal perfusion while, as Dr Lambrou rightly pointed out, the blood supply to the disc depends only on the peripapillary choroid. You can have disturbances there with a massive impairment of the optic nerve head circulation while the rest of the choroid remains normally perfused. A negative finding is therefore meaningless.

Erik L. Greve : This is entirely correct, and I think that the point is well made.

Douglas R. Anderson : I am a bit puzzled by what it all means. We assume that the problem in glaucoma is localized in the optic nerve head. Yet, it seems that on the average the values are lower for the whole choroid. Why would the choroidal circulation be abnormal in those people ?

George N. Lambrou : This could be due to either of a number of things: the circulation from heart to eye might be impaired; or there could be an increased vascular resistance in the posterior ciliary arteries; anything, as a matter of fact, that would reduce the amount of blood reaching the eye would cause the pulse amplitude to drop. These factors might not be clinically important under normal circumstances – which, incidentally, would explain why many normal eyes have low pulse amplitudes – but in case of a drop of systemic pressure they could result in a major disturbance, especially in the more vulnerable parts such as the watershed zones or the optic nerve head. Now if you have such a combination of circumstances, decreased blood supply plus low systemic pressure plus a vulnerable optic nerve head, then some nerve fiber damage will occur which you will diagnose as glaucoma. Whereas if you happen to have just one vulnerable area, watershed or whatever, somewhere in the mid-periphery, then the damage which will occur over there will probably remain unnoticed forever.

Yves C.A. Robert : Some years ago, Perkins modified a Goldmann tonometer to measure the ocular pulse and he found that it was increased in glaucoma. This is not very easy to explain, either.

George N. Lambrou : What he found in low-tension glaucoma was a wider spreading of the pulse values as if there were two LTG-subpopulations. But he didn't try to interpret this any further*.

Yves C.A. Robert : Yes, that's right.

Harry A. Quigley : I would like to draw attention to the fact that we are using here terms like "pulsatile volume" and "ocular blood flow" for the results of computations based on measurements that can be influenced by quite a number of factors, so that we do not know whether the "blood flow" we are talking about really reflects ocular blood flow. I think it would be reassuring if some studies were done on animals, together with some actual quantitative measurements of blood flow, like those presented in the first part of this meeting, so that we can be sure that the parameters we are computing correspond indeed to real blood flow parameters.

Richard Stodtmeister : With regard to the sources of interindividual variability, there is obviously too much scatter in the results to be used for the individual patient. However, Dr. Pillunat has studied simultaneously the retinal and ciliary perfusion pressures in low tension glaucoma and the observed differences with normals are clear-cut and with very low scatter. This is because the measurements are done in the same eye and the sources of variation cancel out.
And one final remark about the relation between the suction pressure and the IOP increase: It is a statistical relation with some variability in it, so that if you calculate IOP from the suction pressure there is some uncertainty in your result. This uncertainty, however, is of the same order of magnitude as the uncertainty in the relation between the pressure in the cuff and the blood pressure in the brachial artery. So if in everyday medicine we rely with confidence on a method with such accuracy (or inaccuracy), then I think that we can just as well rely on the suction-pressure-to-IOP-increase relation.

Erik L. Greve : Thank you very much for this last piece of information. We have heard some interesting remarks and suggestions for future research concerning pulse measurements. I think that we can close the discussion at this point and move to the next session.

---

* *Editors' note* : Perkins ES, Phelps CD: Die okuläre Pulskurve beim Glaukom ohne Hochdruck. Klin Monatsbl Augenheilk 184: 303-304, 1984

III. LASER DOPPLER VELOCIMETRY
BLUE FIELD ENTOPTOMETRY
REFLECTOMETRY OF THE OPTIC DISC

NONINVASIVE MEASUREMENT OF THE OPTIC NERVE HEAD CIRCULATION*

Charles E. Riva, R. D. Shonat, B. L. Petrig, Constantin J. Pournaras[1] and J. B. Barnes[2]

University of Pennsylvania, Department of Ophthalmology and Scheie Eye Institute, Philadelphia, PA, USA, [1]University of Geneva, Switzerland and [2]Alcon Laboratories, Inc. Fort Worth, TX, USA

Introduction

The role of the circulation of the optic nerve head (ONH) in the pathogenesis of glaucoma is still controversial, mainly because of the lack of a clinical method capable of measuring blood flow in this region of the eye fundus.

Among the various techniques developed so far to investigate the ONH circulation in human subjects, laser Doppler velocimetry (LDV) appears to be the most promising[1]. It is noninvasive and can provide results in a matter of seconds. In this technique, a weak laser

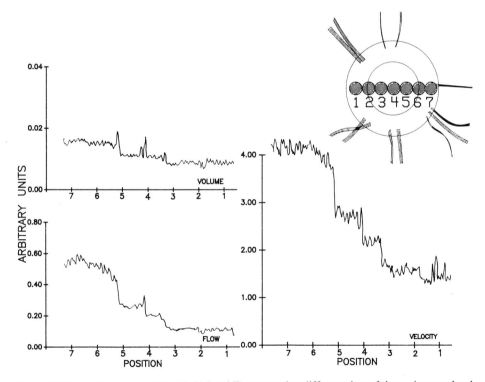

Fig. 1. LDV blood flow parameters (V, Vol and F) measured at different sites of the optic nerve head (ONH) tissue of an anesthetized cat.

*Supported by NIH Grant EYO-3242, Alcon Research Institute Award (to CER), Swiss National Science Foundation for Research # 3965087 and The Vivian Simskins Lasko Research Fund.

Correspondence to: Dr. Charles Riva, Scheie Eye Institute, 51 N, 39th Street, Philadelphia, PA 19104, USA.

beam (usually from a HeNe laser or more recently from a near-infrared diode laser) is focused on a small region of the ONH tissue. Care is taken to avoid regions traversed by visible blood vessels. This laser light is scattered by the tissue and the moving RBCs. The frequency of the light scattered by the RBCs is Doppler shifted by an amount that is proportional to the velocity of the RBCs. When a range of RBCs speeds is present in the region of measurement, a range of frequency shifts (the so-called Doppler shift power spectrum, DSPS) is measured.

Previous LDV investigations in monkeys and human subjects have demonstrated the capability of the ONH circulation to autoregulate.[1,2] Sebag et al.,[3,4] combining LDV and fundus reflectometry were able to document blood flow changes caused by atrophy of the ONH. In all these investigations, a parameter α, which can be associated with the width of the DSPS was determined. Based on a simple model for the scattering of the laser light by the tissue and the RBCs as well as for the distribution of RBCs velocities in the capillaries of the ONH, α was shown to vary linearly with RBC velocity[5].

Application of 3-wavelength reflectometry has allowed Sebag et al.[3,4] to measure, in addition to α, a parameter γ that was shown to vary, under certain conditions, in proportion to the volume of blood within the region of measurement and to use as an index of blood flow the product $\alpha \cdot \gamma$. Analysis of the properties of the LDV signal reveals, however, that reflectometry may not be needed to determine blood flow since, theoretically, changes in blood volume can be extracted directly from the LDV signal.

LDV signals contain indeed three components: (a) a constant term which gives rise to the dc (zero frequency) component of the DSPS. The value of this constant depends linearly on the intensity of the incident laser light; (b) a shot noise term and (c) a fluctuating component generated by the Doppler shifted light that has been scattered by the RBCs moving within the illuminated volume.

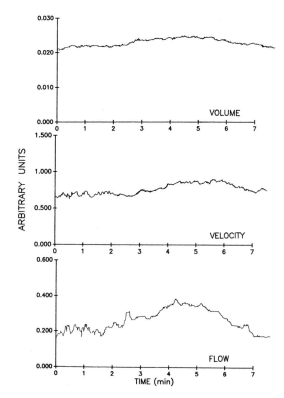

Fig. 2. Effect of an increase of PCO_2 in the arterial blood of a cat on the LDV blood flow parameters in the cat ONH tissue.

Measurement of optic nerve head circulation

The LASERFLO blood perfusion monitor (TSI, Inc., BPM 403) is an instrument that extracts three parameters from the Doppler signal obtained from a microcirculatory bed such as that of the skin: (1) the velocity, V, (2) the volume, Vol, and (3) the flow, F, of blood. These three parameters, given in relative units, are divided by the dc term and are, therefore, independent from the intensity of the incident light. We have built an electronic interface that links our LDV fundus camera detection system[6] to the LASERFLO instrument so that the signal processing unit of this device can be used to obtain V, Vol and F from the tissue of the ONH. In addition, we have adopted an illumination/detection system that is different from the one previously described,[1,2] where the light collecting optical fiber was placed on top of the illumination spot. We now detect the scattered light from a region of the ONH adjacent to the site of illumination. In this manner, direct reflection of the incident light at the surface of the ONH tissue is avoided. This was found to provide a much more stable signal and it also enables us to better filter out the Doppler shift signal caused by eye motion from the signal produced by the moving RBCs.

Experimental part

Anesthetized cats and minipigs were used to test this new approach. Calculated diameter of the incident beam at the ONH was approximately 50 μm and the diameter of the detecting optical fiber aperture was about 150 μm.

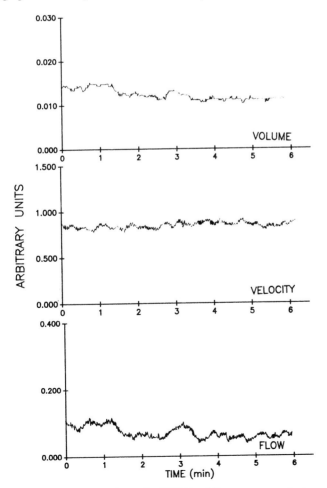

Fig. 3. Effect of breathing 100% O_2 on the LDV blood flow parameters in the cat ONH tissue.

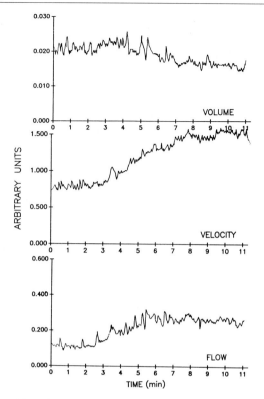

Fig. 4. Effect of breathing 10% O_2, 90% N_2 on the LDV blood flow parameters in the cat ONH tissue.

a. Effect of varying the site of illumination on V, Vol and F

Fig. 1 shows how these parameters vary when the illumination site is moved horizontally across the ONH of the cat, while the position of the detecting fiber aperture relative to the illumination site was left unchanged. There was a marked decrease in F caused by a change in both V and Vol as the site of measurement approached the center of the ONH. Also F is notably smaller in the nasal than in the temporal region of the ONH.

b. Effect of changing the breathing conditions

Increasing the arterial blood PCO_2 from 34 to 48 mm Hg in the arterial blood of the cat resulted in marked increases of Vol and F but little change of V (Fig. 2). Fig. 3 shows the effect of the animal breathing 100% O_2 and Fig. 4 that of breathing 10% O_2, 90% N_2. With hypoxia, most of the change in F resulted from a change in V.

c. Effect of bilateral carotid occlusion

Both carotid arteries in the cat were transiently closed by ligation. As expected, blood flow did not decrease to zero (Fig. 5) due to the contribution of the vertebral circulation. For comparison, we also show the change in centerline velocity of the RBCs measured under identical conditions from a main artery located in front of the pigmented area of the retina.

d. Rhythmical variations in ONH blood flow parameters

Continuous recordings of V, Vol and F in the optic nerve head of minipigs using a

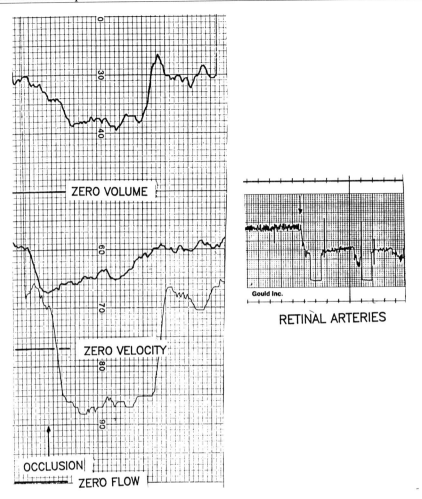

Fig. 5. Effect of transiently ligating the carotid arteries on the LDV blood flow parameters in the cat ONH tissue. Graph at right represents the change in centerline velocity in a retinal artery.

near-infrared diode laser at 795 nm showed rhythmical variations of these parameters at a frequency of approximately 3 cycles/min (Fig. 6). Interestingly, the variations in V and Vol were always out of phase, with a phase difference that was not significantly different from 180°. As a result, the variations of F were comparatively strongly attenuated. These oscillatory variations are most certainly associated with the active, rhythmical vasomotion reported previously by others in different tissues.[8,9] These recordings demonstrate that the LDV technique has the potential to become a useful tool for the study of vasomotion in the microcirculation of the central nervous system.

In all measurements presented in this report, the irradiance of the laser beam at the ONH was about 0.75 W/cm^2. The Ansi 136.1 standards for the maximum permissible level of irradiance for extended sources[9] indicate that such an irradiance would be allowed in man for about 1 sec, a period of time too short from a practical point of view. Assuming conservatively that measurement times of a few minutes will be needed, two options are available for clinical measurements: a reduction of the irradiance by about 100 times, resulting in a dramatic and undesirable decrease of signal-to-noise ratio of the Doppler signal or the use of a laser emitting in the near-infrared. This second alternative was now chosen for future work with this technique.

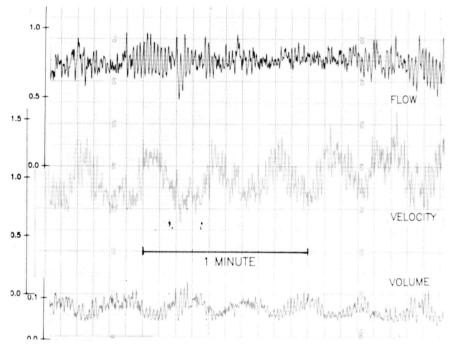

Fig. 6. Rhythmic variations of the blood flow parameters measured from the ONH tissue of an anesthetized minipig during normal air breathing.

Acknowledgements

The authors wish to thank Tom McLaughlin for technical help.

References

1. Riva CE, Feke GT, Loebl M: Proceedings of the 5th Congress of the European Society of Ophthalmology, François J, (ed) Hamburg 1976, pp 414–416. Stuttgart:Ferdinand Enke Verlag, 1978
2. Riva CE, Grunwald JE, Sinclair SH: Laser Doppler measurement of relative blood velocity in the human optic nerve head. Invest Ophthalmol Vis Sci 22:241-248, 1982
3. Sebag I, Feke GT, Delori FC et al.: Anterior optic nerve blood flow in experimental optic atrophy. Invest Ophthalmol Vis Sci 26:1415-1422, 1985
4. Sebag I, Delori FC, Feke GT et al: Anterior optic nerve blood flow decrease in clinical neurogenic optic atrophy. Ophthalmology 93:858-865, 1986
5. Stern MD, Lappe DL: Method and apparatus for measurement of blood flow using coherent light. U.S. Patent No. 4, 109, 647, 1978
6. Riva CE, Grunwald JE, Sinclair SH et al: Fundus camera based retinal laser Doppler velocimeter. Appl Optics 20:117-120, 1981
7. Salerud EG, Tenland GT, Nilsson GE et al: Rhythmical variations in the human skin blood flow. Int J Microcirc Clin Exp 2:91-102, 1983
8. Colantuoni A, Bertuglia S, Intaglietta M: Quantitation of rhythmic diameter changes in arterial microcirculation. Am J Physiol 246 (Heart Circ Physiol 15): H508-517, 1984
9. Delori FC, Parker JS, Mainster MA: Light levels in fundus photography and fluorescein angiography. Vision Res 20:1099-1104, 1980

DISCUSSION

Sohan S. Hayreh : When you do measurements on the disc, Dr Riva, which layer are you measuring? The surface layer, which is part of the retinal circulation, or the prelaminar layer, which comes from the choroidal circulation ?

Charles E. Riva : This point is not clear yet. We are sure that we do measure the superficial layer. But we don't really know how deep our measurements go. In the skin it has been shown that if you want to do a deeper reading you must put your detection probe a little further from your laser source, because in that way you have more chances of picking up light backscattered from the depth. This is something that we intend to try in the optic nerve head, taking the readings and then comparing them with measurements of the retinal and choroidal blood flow, the latter measured with infrared laser with which you can see the choroidal vessels.

Harry A. Quigley : I would suspect that you can indeed go deeper into the tissue if you use longer wavelengths. We have done some work on the penetration of light into connective tissue (in relation to transscleral laser cyclodialysis) and we realized that red light penetrates quite well, in contrast to the blue or green-yellow light used in fluorescein angiography. So if your reflected light isn't too much shifted towards the yellow, then you have very good chances of illuminating the red blood cells inside capillaries surrounded by connective tissue and of detecting the backscattered light.

Charles E. Riva : The shift is really very small, around 500 Hz* and therefore the incident and reflected light penetrate the tissues in the same way. But we also plan to do measurements using blue and green lasers to see whether we can selectively measure different layers.

Harry A. Quigley : Are you not worried about shining blue laser light on the retina ?

Charles E. Riva : No, the intensities involved are really very low: detectors are much more sensitive in the blue than in the red.

Harry A. Quigley : Still, when you apply the method to glaucoma patients you are likely to encounter some problems because of their cataracts.

Charles E. Riva : That could well be, yes.

Douglas R. Anderson : I am wondering if you aren't really measuring the blood flow over quite a large area of the disc put together. Most of the light that you send in does not hit a red blood cell but reaches the lamina cribrosa, then is scattered to all directions through the optic nerve head tissue, and eventually comes back to be detected. So the light that you detect from a certain part of the disc is really a summation of light scattered from the whole area, no matter where you place the illuminating probe.

---

* *Editors' note*: At visible light energies this frequency shift corresponds to a wavelength shift of less than a billionth of a nanometer.

Charles E. Riva : That is possible. But if such were the case, you wouldn't see any details on the disc: the reading would be more or less the same, wherever you place the illuminating spot. With green light however, which is less scattering, you still see a lot of detail. With red light there is some loss of detail but the reading is still not uniform.

François Delori : I am not sure that there is so much scattering either within the optic nerve head tissue or at its surface. I think that the light penetration is fairly easy up to the lamina cribrosa level, otherwise how could we explain the appearance of the cup? The main "scatterer" is the lamina cribrosa itself. There is another thing however that I am wondering about. Are your measurements absolute or relative? I mean, if the ocular media aren't completely clear and they cause a lot of scattering or absorption, will that affect your reading ?

Charles E. Riva : No, it will not: the values read are divided by the shot noise. So the instrument is self-calibrated, in a way. This is one of the nice things about the method.

Harry A. Quigley : Do the scattering properties of the tissue influence laser Doppler velocimetry spectra or not ?

Charles E. Riva : Not directly, no. But they do interfere with the interpretation of the results, because – depending on the transmission properties – you measure velocities of red blood cells that are nearer to or further from your illuminating spot. So we need to understand better their influence.

Harry A. Quigley : The reason I am asking that question is this: If you measure a glaucoma patient, there is a very important loss of nerve fibers but also the reflectance characteristics of the remaining tissue have changed, because there are much more astrocytes with respect to axons and capillaries. Can this interfere with the interpretation of the results ?

Charles E. Riva : Only if you make your measurements right on the spot that you are illuminating. Because then, if there are a few red blood cells most of the light you will collect will come from a single scattering; while if there are much more cells moving at the same speed you will collect light after multiple scattering, which will broaden the spectrum and give you the impression that the speed is higher. But if you measure systematically at some distance from the point you are illuminating, you always collect multi-scattered light, whatever the number of red blood cells present.

Douglas R. Anderson : But won't the multiple reflections cancel each the effects of the other? I mean if the first reflection is on a red blood cell moving in one direction and the second on another moving in a different direction, do you still know where you are ?

Charles E. Riva : Yes, the overall effect will be to broaden the spectrum, and that is what we are measuring.

Douglas R. Anderson : And don't you need to know how many reflections there have been ?

Charles E. Riva : No: each new reflection adds less than the preceding ones, so that after a while more reflections do not add anything significant.

LASER DOPPLER VELOCIMETRY AND BLOOD RHEOLOGY; PRELIMINARY TRIALS

H. Hamard[1], A. Parent de Curzon[1], J. Dufaux[2] and P. Hamard[1]

[1]*Service d'Ophtalmologie II, Hôpital des Quinze–Vingts, 28 rue de Charenton, 75571 Paris Cédex 12;* [2]*Laboratoire de Biorhéologie et d'Hydrodynamique physicochimique, UA CNRS 343, 2, Place Jussieu 75005 Paris; France*

Abstract

The blood flow characteristics in the microcirculatory network of the optic nerve are not well known because they are practically inaccessible. However, the utilization of Laser Doppler Velocimetry recently enabled us to obtain data on red blood cell (RBC) velocity in that area[1,2]. We have therefore set up a system that simultaneously uses a fundus camera and a laser Doppler velocimeter. With this device, the retina can be illuminated in the peripapillary area by a laser beam of low intensity. The light penetrates superficially into the tissues and is backscattered by the moving RBCs. The frequency of the light is shifted proportionally to the RBC velocity.

Our system is being tested on RBC suspensions flowing in glass capillaries (100 µm in diameter) and on the rabbit eye. At the same time, the rheological properties of the RBC suspension or of the blood are being measured with a Couette viscometer and an aggregameter. The reversible RBC aggregation is also studied.

Animal models allow us to study, by means of injections of specific products (such as Dextran solutions), the consequences of the modifications of aggregation. Our practice with rats has shown us that the blood flow velocity can slow down considerably during a long period (approximately two hours) after the injection.

Our purpose is to demonstrate such modifications in the peripapillary area of the rabbit eye. Our system will be used on man if this study succeeds.

Introduction

Blood flow in microcirculatory networks is a complex phenomenon affected by a great number of factors, such as network topography, blood rheology and blood cell to vessel wall interactions. These microcirculatory networks are the sites of exchange of oxygen, carbon dioxide, nutritional elements and wastes.

Every disturbance of blood flow – be it a slowing down or a stop – is a risk to its good functioning. Many studies have clearly proved this in various medical fields: hypertension[1], cardiology[2], angiology[3], diabetology[4] and more recently in ophthalmology[5].

We have, for our part, worked on demonstrating the importance of the rheological properties of the red blood cells. Their importance is not only due to their number but also to two characteristics of their membrane:

- membrane deformability: during their course in the microcirculation, the RBCs must pass through capillaries that have a diameter inferior to that of the RBCs and the flow rate can slow down;
- their aggregability: if the flow rate is slow enough, the RBCs can form a reversible structure, *i.e.*, an aggregate. These aggregates will be destroyed if the flow velocity, or rather the shear stress, increases. The stress needed will be greater since the concentration of the suspending medium in protein and fibrinogen will be high.

Blood is a non newtonian fluid. The aggregation level and the deformation rate can be appreciated or measured thanks to a more or less sophisticated apparatus. We will briefly describe some of them before discussing laser Doppler velocimetry.

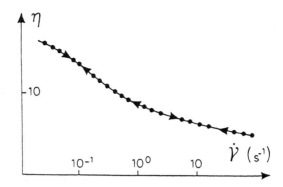

Fig. 1. Viscosity against shear rate in a Couette viscometer for normal human blood (hematocrit H = 46, T + 37°C).

Couette viscometer[6]

This viscometer enables us to measure the viscosity coefficient of a given blood sample in different flow conditions (Fig. 1). The Couette system consists of two concentric cylinders with an annular gap of 0.5 mm or 1 mm. The shear rate

$$\dot{\gamma} = \frac{\Delta v}{e} = \frac{V_o}{e}$$

is generated across the gap by rotating the outer cylinder; the inner cylinder remains stationary. The shear rate can vary from $0.017 s^{-1}$ to $128 s^{-1}$ in 30 discrete steps. The amount of blood needed is approximately 0.5 cm^3. The temperature of the system is regulated.

Aggregameter[7]

This apparatus uses a modified Couette viscometer; the two cylinders are transparent and the suspension placed between them is illuminated by a laser beam. The backscattered

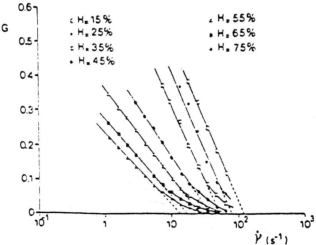

Fig. 2. Reflectometric index G against the shear rate in a Couette flow for normal red blood cells suspended at various hematocrit in PBS 1.2g%, Dextran T 80 (T = 20°C) (from[2]).

light is collected on a photodiod. The reflectivity signal is directly related to the mean RBC bridging area per unit volume of the suspension, the shear stress required to disperse the RBC suspension can be easily measured (Fig. 2).

Capillary viscometer[6]

This device is closer to the micro–circulation flow conditions than the Couette system. The tube (50 µm ≤ inner diameter ≤ 200 µm) is in a horizontal observation chamber filled with a liquid, the refractive index of which is matched to the index of the glass.

Flow is observed through a microscope, with natural light, with a long working distance objective. The image is photographed or shown on a video screen and can be recorded on videotape.

The flow is driven by the variation of air pressure in the tank and is very regular. This set–up allows pressure drops as low as 0.5 mm H$_2$O. The flow rates are very low (Q = 10^{-6}cm/s) and are measured by means of a double–slit velocimeter.

RBC aggregation is always very close to normal in order to avoid the problems due to RBC sedimentation.

To determine the viscosity coefficient η, we used the Poiseuille law

$$\eta = \frac{\Pi R^4}{8} \frac{\Delta p}{L} \frac{1}{Q}$$

where R = tube radius, L = tube length, Δp = pressure drop in the tube, Q = flow rate.

Fig. 3 gives an example of the results we have obtained. It can be shown that at low flow rate, the viscosity coefficient can be multiplied by a factor 10 because of the aggregation of the RBCs. The existence of a yield stress is also clearly demonstrated.

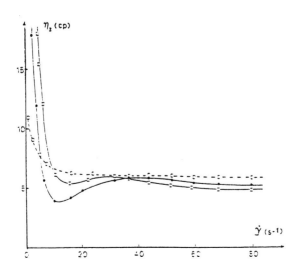

Fig. 3. Viscosity against shear rate in a capillary viscometer for different RBC suspensions. RBCs in a saline solution (no aggregation). RBCs in a D$_x$ 70 solution c = 3%. RBCs in a D$_x$ solution c = 3.5%.

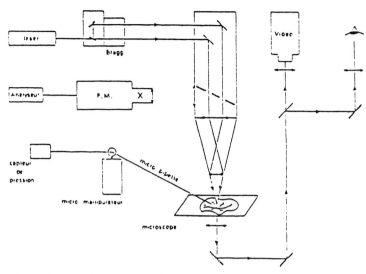

Fig. 4. Experimental set-up of the laser Doppler velocimeter, adapted to microscopic measurements.

In vivo experiments

We have also carried out *in vivo* experiments[3] on the rat cremaster or mesentery, where the vessel walls are nearly transparent. Different techniques have been set up:
- video visualization of the RBC flow
- measurements of the vessel diameter;
- pressure drop measurements ΔP with micropipettes in vessels down to 25 µm;
- velocity measurements with laser Doppler velocimetry (double beam system)(Fig. 4).

Thanks to these techniques many characteristic parameters can be measured, such as:
- the flow rate Q
- the hydraulic resistance $R_H = \dfrac{\Delta P}{Q}$

The evolution of these parameters can be followed when rheological properties of the RBCs are modified (Fig. 5). At the same time, we have recorded the variations of some important parameters in order to point out the importance of blood supply:
- electrocardiogram (Fig. 6)
- systemic pressure
- heart frequency

Drug effects can be easily studied with this animal model.

Study of the irrigation of the optic nerve head

The blood flow characteristics in the microcirculatory network of the optic nerve are not well known because they are practically inaccessible. However, the utilization of the Laser Doppler Velocimetry recently enabled us[9] to obtain data on red blood cell (RBC) velocity in that area. Therefore, we have realized a system simultaneously using a fundus camera and a laser Doppler velocimeter. With this device, the retina can be illuminated in the peripapillary area by a laser beam of low intensity (Fig. 7).

The laser light illuminates the superficial layers of the optic nerve head and is backscattered by the moving RBCs. The frequency of the light is shifted proportionally to

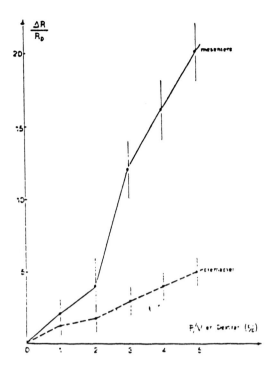

Fig. 5. Relative variations of the hydraulic resistance versus dextran 500 concentration in the rat circulation (cremaster and mesentery).

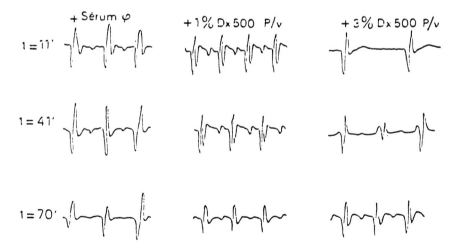

Fig. 6. Rat electrocardiograms versus dextran 500 concentration in: blood.

RBC velocity.

In our case, the illuminated region is relatively large in comparison with the dimension of the capillary network we wish to study.

Backscattered light comes from RBCs moving at different velocities in different directions, so the frequency spectrum is very broad. Thanks to a frequency analysis, the maximum velocity V_{max} in the illuminated region can be determined[10].

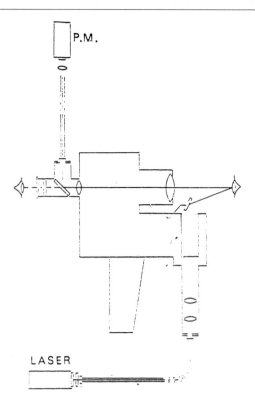

Fig. 7. Fundus camera adapted to laser Doppler measurements.

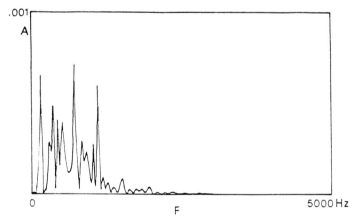

Fig. 8. Power spectrum of the light scattered from a capillary tube ($V_{max} = 0.8$ mm/s)

$$\alpha = \frac{V_{max}}{\lambda}$$

where α = maximum frequency detected in the spectrum and λ = light wavelength.

First the system has been tested on the capillary system, at different flow rates, with different RBC suspensions (Fig. 8).

Then, similar measurements have been made on an albino rabbit's eye in the peripapillary area. The rabbit was anesthetized and the pupil was dilated. It was placed on a platform

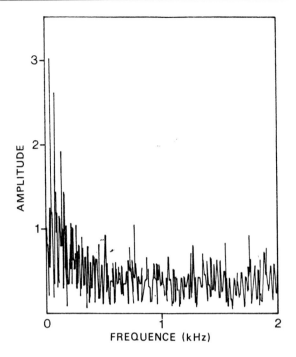

Fig. 9. Power spectrum of the LDV signal obtained in the peripapillary area of the rabbit eye.

and its head was restrained. Fig. 9 shows preliminary results. Observation of the rabbit's fundus immediately after the experiment and the following days did not show damage after an exposure of one minute with a beam of 0.3 mW intensity.

Conclusion

We are preparing a series of more accurate experiments. The RBC aggregation will be artificially modified by means of injections of dextran, at different concentrations. Viscosity coefficients and disaggregation shear stress will be determined with the techniques described above. At the same time, the blood velocity on the head of the optic nerve will be recorded.

A rheological study of the circulating blood seems particularly appropriate for glaucoma patients, as most of the experimental studies or clinical angiographies show localized signs of ischemia.

Any rheological change is indeed a factor of ischemia, and whether being due to reduced blood inflow, or to stasis, or to anoxia, or responding to Ditzel's classification, this ischemia induces the local formation of oxygen free radicals. In neurology, the latter have a well–known action on various parameters, such as capillary permeability, mitochondrial metabolism, calcium metabolism and glial tissue proliferation. Oxygen free radicals are thus inducing a slower axonal transport and appear as the common denominator of all types of optic neuropathy, among which the glaucomatous neuropathy.

References

1. Chien S: Blood rheology in myocardial infarction and hypertension. Sixth International Congress of Biorheology Plenary lecture. Biorheology 23:633–653, 1986
2. Dufaux J, Lardoux H, Othmane A, Bregevin A: Evolution of ergometric and hemorheological parameters for healthy non smoker and smoker volunteers. 5ème Congrès d'Hémorhéologie Clinique, Bordeaux 1987
3. Le Devehat C, Lemoine A, Bertrand A, Vellay P: Hémorhéologie et insuffisance veineuse: facteurs de risque thrombotique. In: Phlébologie 85. Negus D, Jantet G (eds), pp 812–814. John Libbey et Co Ltd 1986
4. Othmane A, Bitbol M, Snabre P, Mills P, Grimaldi A, Bosquet F: Red cell aggregation in insulin dependent diabetics. Clin Hemorheol (to be published)
5. Wolf S, Bertram B, Kiesewetter H, Jung F, Reim M: Iso and hypervolumic hemodilution in central retinal vein occlusion. 5ème Congrès d'Hémorhéologie Clinique, Bordeaux 1987
6. Dufaux J: Couette viscometry. Capillary viscometry in standardization in clinical haemorheology, pp 60–72: March 13th–14th 1987
7. Snabre P, Bitbol M, Mills P: Cell disaggregation behavior in shear flow. Biophys J 51:795–807, 1987
8. Dufaux J, Durussel JJ: Physiologie de la microcirculation. In: Innovation et Technologie en Biologie et en Médicine, Vol 7, No 2, 153–163, 1986
9. Riva C, Ross B, Benedex GB: Laser Doppler measurements of blood flow in capillary tubes and retinal arteries, Invest Ophthalmol 3/11:936–944, 1972
10. Stern MD: Laser Doppler velocimetry in blood and multiply scattering fluids; theory. App Opt 23/31:1068–1986, 1985
11. Feke GT, Riva CE: Laser Doppler measurements of blood velocity in human retinal vessels. J Opt Soc Am 68:526, 1978
12. Riva CE, Grunwald JE, sinclair SH: Laser Doppler measurement of relative blood velocity in the human optic nerve head. Invest Ophthalmol Vis Sci 22:241–248, 1982
13. Sebag J, Feke GT, Delori FC, Weiter JJ: Anterior optic nerve blood flow in experimental optic atrophy. Invest Ophthalmol Vis Sci 26:1415–1422, 1985
14. Sebag J, Delori FC, Feke GT, Gogger D, Fitch K, Tagawa H, Deupree D, Weiter JJ, McMeel JW: Anterior optic nerve blood flow decreases in clinical neurogenic optic atrophy. Ophthalmology 93:858–865, 1986
15. Sebag J, Feke GT, Delori FC: Letter to the editor. Ophthalmology 94:88–89, 1987

DISCUSSION

Henry Hamard : Before the discussion of our paper is open, I would like to outline the rationale that led to this investigation. Blood viscosity and aggregability are parameters of paramount importance in cardiology and neurology, perhaps even more than flow rate itself. It is a well established fact that increased blood viscosity induces stasis anoxia which leads to the production of oxygen free radicals which in turn are known to increase the permeability of the vessels, to reduce the metabolism of mitochondria, to block calcium exchange and to stimulate glial proliferation. All these phenomena are known to occur in optic neuropathy of any kind. So we decided to start a preliminary study on the subject, which may open new perspectives for research in the future.

Albert Alm : Dr Dufaux, which vessels are you measuring in the fundus ?

Jacques Dufaux : We are measuring in the papillary area. We are not sure, however, if our measurements come from the optic nerve head exclusively or from some of the retinal vessels as well.

Douglas R. Anderson : Why did you have to develop a totally new technique for measuring blood viscosity in the capillaries? Would you not get the same results if you drew some blood from an artery and measured its viscosity in the traditional way ?

Jacques Dufaux : Our purpose was not so much to develop a new technique for blood viscosity measurements as to correlate the rheologic parameters of the blood with the flow rate.

Charles E. Riva : Moreover, the rheologic properties, and especially their effect on flow rate are very much dependent on vessel size, and that is one of the difficult problems in microcirculation studies. Viscosity in the capillaries, and whole blood viscosity which you measure with the traditional techniques, aren't necessarily the same.

RETINAL HEMODYNAMICS IN OPEN-ANGLE GLAUCOMA

Juan E. Grunwald

Scheie Eye Institute, Department of Ophthalmology, University of Pennsylvania

Introduction

Abnormalities of blood flow supply and its regulation have been implicated in the development of glaucomatous damage[1]. The loss of ganglion cells due to glaucomatous pathology is most evident at the optic nerve head. This is most probably the reason why most of the interest has been focused so far on the circulation of the optic nerve head and very little is known about the retinal circulation in this disease. It is important to remember, however, that the bodies of these ganglion cells are located in the inner retina and receive their blood supply from the retinal circulation. It is possible, therefore, that the abnormalities of the retinal circulation may have some role in the etiology of glaucomatous pathology.

Previous investigations have suggested alterations of the retinal circulation in glaucoma. Baurmann et al.[2] reported a decrease in number of leukocytes perceived entoptically by glaucoma patients. Increased intraretinal transit time[3] and a prolonged dye appearance rate in the ocular fundus[4] have been described in fluorescein angiographic studies of glaucomatous eyes. In patients with glaucoma, the intraretinal fluorescein transit time appears to increase with an increase in intraocular pressure, whereas in patients with ocular hypertension the fluorescein angiography is usually normal even at IOPs high enough to cause collapse of retinal blood vessels[3]. These findings suggest an impairment in the autoregulation of the retinal blood flow in glaucoma. In other words, at elevated IOPs in glaucoma retinal blood flow may not be maintained as well as in ocular hypertension.

We have studied the retinal blood flow autoregulation in open-angle glaucoma and glaucoma suspects using the blue field entoptic phenomenon which enables the perception of one's own leukocytes moving in the macular retinal capillaries.

Subjects and methods

This technique has been described in detail previously[5-7]. Subjects are asked to look alternately into two blue field entoptoscopes (Mira, BFE-l00), one in front of each eye. By means of a scleral suction cup, the IOP in one eye is first raised and then lowered while subjects are asked to compare the speed of the entoptic particles in the eye with the suction cup with the speed observed in the other eye at resting IOP. The highest acutely raised IOP for which macular blood flow can be maintained constant by autoregulation (*i.e.*, equal to the speed in the fellow eye) is considered as IOP_{max}. IOP is monitored throughout the experiment by pneumatonometry (Digilab, Model 30R). When the suction cup is removed, the patients are again asked to compare leukocyte speeds between eyes. An immediate perception of a faster speed in the eye which had the suction cup is considered as indicative of a hyperemic response.

Because of the design of the experimental protocol, we had to select glaucoma patients who observed equal speeds in both eyes at resting IOP. Of 49 primary open-angle

Portions of this chapter were published previously and appear courtesy of Ophthalmology (1984; 91, 1690-4)

glaucoma patients screened, 16 observed the same speed in both eyes. Out of the 16 patients, five were excluded because of history of systemic hypertension and systemic drug therapy.

Results of the autoregulation experiments in the 11 glaucoma patients were compared with those obtained in nine glaucoma suspects who had elevated IOPs and no visual field damage and 13 normal subjects. All subjects were matched with regard to age and systemic blood pressure. The examiner was unaware of the patients' diagnosis at the time of the study.

Results and discussion

Among the 49 glaucoma patients, 33 described a difference in the baseline leukocyte speed between eyes; 28 of the 33 patients reported slower speed in the eye with more advanced glaucoma. Compared to the 33 glaucoma patients who observed asymmetric speeds, those who observed the same speed in both eyes were younger (two tailed student's t-test, $p < 0.001$), had a disease of shorter duration ($p < 0.05$) and had a smaller difference in the highest recorded IOP ($p < 0.01$); their disease was probably less advanced and more symmetric in nature.

Average IOP_{max} in the 11 glaucoma patients studied (24.9 ± 1.5 mmHg, ± 1 SD) was significantly lower than that in the 13 normals (29.9 ± 3.6 mmHg, $p < 0.001$). In the eight glaucoma suspects studied average IOPmax (30.8 ± 4.6) was not significantly different from normal. The average difference between resting IOP and IOP_{max} was 14.3 ± 3.1 mmHg in normals, 4.7 ± 3.3 mmHg in glaucoma suspects (significantly different from normal, $p < 0.01$) and 3.7 ± 4.3 mmHg ($p < 0.001$) in glaucoma patients.

Perception of a hyperemic response following the removal of the suction cup was present in 94% of the normals, 71% of glaucoma suspects and only 47% of glaucoma patients.

These results suggest an abnormality of the retinal autoregulation in glaucoma. Average IOP_{max} is significantly reduced in glaucoma patients. This is probably not an effect of antiglaucomatous therapy since the average IOP_{max} in three eyes that were not receiving any topical medication was very close to that of the other eyes that were under different antiglaucomatous medications.

The range of increased IOPs above rest for which the macular circulation could maintain a constant blood flow was also significantly decreased in glaucomatous eyes. Moreover, the absence of hyperemia in most of these glaucomatous eyes supports our contention that autoregulation is abnormal in glaucoma. This effect results most probably from the lack of autoregulatory vasodilatation that normally occurs when IOP is acutely increased[8].

Quantitative determinations of leukocyte velocity during acutely increased IOP in normal eyes have been previously obtained using the blue field simulation technique[9,10]. In this technique, subjects compared and matched the speed of simulated leukocytes displayed by a computer on a screen to that of their own entoptically perceived leukocytes. Leukocyte velocity remained fairly constant at or near baseline up to IOPs around 30 mmHg. Above this pressure, a linear decrease in leukocyte velocity was observed. Average IOP_{max} determined by this technique in six healthy volunteers was 29.2 ± 2.5 mmHg, a value which closely matches the IOP_{max} obtained in our study.

The effect of acutely increased IOP on normal retinal blood flow has also been investigated by Riva et al. using laser Doppler velocimetry and monochromatic fundus photography[11]. Blood velocity was not statistically significantly different from normal for elevations of IOP up to a range between 23 and 26 mmHg. Only at IOPs in a range between 27-30 and above were blood velocities significantly reduced from normal.

These results are again within the range of what we have found, demonstrating that the normal retinal circulation can be maintained by autoregulation for acutely elevated IOPs up to 27-30 mmHg. For pressures above this range retinal blood flows are reduced.

Abnormal autoregulation of the retinal circulation in glaucoma could lead to impairment of flow when the IOP is raised above $10P_{max}$. Although our measurements have been obtained during an acute rise in IOP caused by suction pressure and the effect of a more chronic and spontaneous elevation such as that present in glaucoma is not known, it must be considered that retinal blood flow may be impaired under such conditions leading to damage of the retinal ganglion cells and progression of the glaucomatous optic nerve disease.

References

1. Harrington DO: The pathogenesis of the glaucoma field; clinical evidence that circulatory insufficiency in the optic nerve is the primary cause of visual field loss in glaucoma. Am J Ophthalmol 47 (2):177-185, 1959
2. Baurmann H, Fink H, Cornelius P: Entoptische Zirkulationsmessungen an den Augen Glaukomkranker. Klin Mbl Augenheilk 165:477-482, 1974
3. Spaeth GL: Fluorescein angiography: its contribution towards understanding the mechanisms of visual loss in glaucoma. Trans Am Ophthalmol Soc 491-553, 1975
4. Moses RA: Intraocular blood flow from analysis of angiograms. Invest Ophthalmol Vis Sci 24:354-360, 1983
5. Riva CE, Sinclair SH, Grunwald, JE: Autoregulation of retinal circulation in response to decrease of perfusion pressure. Invest Ophthalmol Vis Sci 21:34-38, 1981
6. Grunwald JE, Sinclair SH, Riva CE: Autoregulation of the retinal circulation in response to decrease of intraocular pressure below normal. Invest Ophthalmol Vis Sci 23:124-127, 1982
7. Grunwald JE, Riva CE, Stone RA, Keates EV, Petrig BL: Retinal autoregulation in open angle glaucoma. Ophthalmology 91: 1690–1694, 1984
8. Wilson TM, Constable IJ, Cooper RL, Alder VA: Image splitting - a technique for measuring retinal vascular reactivity. Br J Ophthalmol 65:291-293, 1981
9. Petrig BL, Werner EB, Riva CE, Grunwald JE: Response of macular capillary blood flow to changes in intraocular pressure as measured by the blue field simulation technique. In: Proceedings of the 6th International Vision Field Symposium, pp 447–451. Heijl A, Greve EL (eds). Dordrecht: W. Junk 1985
10. Riva CE, Petrig B: Blue field entoptic phenomenon and blood velocity in the retinal capillaries. J Opt Soc Am 70:1234-1238, 1980
11. Riva CE, Grunwald JE, Petrig BL: Autoregulation of human retinal blood flow. Invest Ophthalmol Vis Sci 27:1706-1712, 1986

DISCUSSION

Richard Stodtmeister : How exactly do you measure the velocities of leukocytes in the retinal capillaries, Dr Grunwald?

Juan E. Grunwald : We did not measure the actual velocities in the first set of patients. We only compared them to the velocities in the fellow eye, which had not been submitted to artificial IOP changes.

Harry A. Quigley : Did you ask the patients to tell you if their leukocytes seemed to be moving twice as fast or three-quarters as fast as in the fellow eye?

Juan E. Grunwald : No, we only asked them to say if they seemed to be moving faster or slower in the eye with altered IOP. To quantitate the velocities we used a computer simulation of the leukocyte movement, presented to the fellow eye, and asked the patient to say which was faster. By speeding up or slowing down the simulation until the two speeds matched we could make an estimation of the blood velocity.

Richard Stodtmeister : How long does it take to make a measurement at each IOP step?

Juan E. Grunwald : It takes some minutes because there are a number of adjustments to be made, about a couple of minutes I would say. But we do multiple measurements for each subject: we first raise the pressure, wait for the autoregulation to take place and then we make the actual measurement.

Douglas R. Anderson : Are your IOP increments in random sequence? I mean do you first make a measurement at IOP+25mmHg, then at IOP+15, then at +30 and so on?

Juan E. Grunwald : Yes, the subjects had no idea of what the sequence of IOP increments was. And the experiments were done in different sessions on the same subject.

Harry A. Quigley : I do not doubt that the patient can't tell the difference between IOP increments of 40 and of 45 mmHg. But with a suction cup on my eye, I can assure you that I do know the difference between a +20 and a +50!

Juan E. Grunwald : Of course you do; I did not say that it was completely masked, only that the subject didn't know beforehand what the pressure would be, neither if it was higher or lower than the previous times.

Erik L. Greve : You mentioned, Juan, that for pressures between 23 and 26 mmHg there is no significant difference from normals in blood velocity. Is that due to statistical variation, or to autoregulation, or to what?

Juan E. Grunwald : I think that we ought to be very careful when we interpret our results in terms of autoregulation. Suppose that by using a given technique you measure some blood flow parameters at different IOP levels, and you find constant flow up to, say, 50 mmHg and then a sudden drop. It is very unlikely that you are looking at a system which is perfectly autoregulated up to a given point, after which the autoregulation suddenly breaks down; your results are probably due to the sensitivity of your technique, which can only detect a decrease if it is important enough, above a certain threshold, that is. It is very probable that as the IOP increases blood flow decreases, but this decrease is very small up to 27 or 30 mmHg due, precisely, to autoregulation. From that point on, the decrease becomes more and more important until, eventually, blood flow drops to zero. Now what you will measure depends entirely on the sensitivity of your technique. If it is sensitive enough you will be able to pick up even small decreases in blood flow, in the 27 to 30 mmHg IOP-range. If it is less sensitive, the first changes you will detect will occur at around 35 mmHg. And if it is not sensitive at al, then you will not be able to detect any decrease in blood flow, even at zero perfusion pressure when the flow has dropped to zero! It is very important to know what the sensitivity of the technique, is before you speak of autoregulation.

Albert Alm : What Dr Grunwald just said is right. Blood flow decreases even in the presence of an efficient autoregulation, because you need a metabolic drive to get your regulatory mechanisms to work. If flow kept on being absolutely normal, there would be no accumulation of metabolites, and hence no vasomotive response.

Charles E. Riva : Of course, otherwise you would have a system with infinite gain and there can be no such system in the body.

Wulff D. Ulrich : With respect to the autoregulatory capacity, which seems to be around 15 mmHg in the normals and more or less diminished in glaucoma patients, our results basically agree with yours. But we think that the first site of glaucoma pathogenesis is the ciliary system, while you are measuring the retinal circulation. Could it be that when the ciliary system is impaired the retinal arterioles are at the limit of their capabilities so that the two systems show similar behavior?

Juan E. Grunwald : I don't think that I can answer your question. The way I see it, it could be that there is a problem in the ciliary circulation at the same time as well.

Gisbert Richard : Dr Grunwald, let me mention that our results with video-angiography led to the same conclusions as yours, before I ask you two questions: Did you try the opposite experiment, lowering the IOP that is? And how well do you think that your results on the macular capillaries apply to the optic nerve head?

Juan E. Grunwald : We did not do any experiments involving exclusive lowering of the IOP. But we did make flow measurements after taking the suction cup off, when the IOP was below its resting level and we found as a rule a reactive hyperemia, although it was absent in some glaucoma patients. As far as your second question is concerned, I tend to think that the problem is in the retina. I imagine that optic nerve head and retina behave in a very similar way and laser Doppler velocimetry measurements tend to confirm that.

Harry A. Quigley : Retinal and optic nerve head capillaries are indeed very similar, structurally. But whether they also behave in the same way, I am not that sure. They certainly have different sorts of input: a single input to each retinal capillary through a very elongated arteriole versus multiple inputs through a number of more or less short arterioles of various origins, retinal, choroidal or retrolaminar, for the optic nerve head. Still, they might behave in similar ways and there is only one way to find out: measure them.

Another point that I want to mention is that the group which showed a clearly different behavior in your experiment was the glaucoma group with well established cup and disc changes. This means that they had already lost half their optic nerve fibers – and probably much more if they had cup/disc ratios of 0.9 or so – and therefore also half or more of their retinal fiber layer so that the capillaries supplying that layer would also have decreased in proportion. So the reason these patients perceive fewer leukocytes moving is that there are fewer capillaries with leukocytes moving inside them to be seen. Now whether that would change the autoregulatory response and how, I can't speculate but you should also take that into account.

Juan E. Grunwald : It is a fact that most of the patients with an asymmetry in behavior between the two eyes showed the smaller velocities and the smaller number of leukocytes in the eye with more advanced visual field defects. This seems to corroborate your hypothesis, but it might also mean that there is something more wrong in those eyes than in the others. That was one of the reasons why we tried to pick patients with disease as symmetric as possible.

Douglas R. Anderson : Being accustomed to thinking that the site of the damage is the optic nerve head, I am a bit confused by what you are telling us, that there is a problem with retinal autoregulation. So I am thinking of what Harry just said, that the variation of speed you measure in the retina might be due to capillary dropout secondary to the loss of optic nerve fibers. You could put that to test if you had a patient with a dense field defect causing him a split fixation, provided he was astute enough to compare the leukocyte velocities above and below fixation.

Juan E. Grunwald : The problem is that he wouldn't be able to see the leukocytes in the part of the field with the scotoma.

Sohan S. Hayreh : I think that there is some contradiction in these last speculations. To be able to participate in your experiment, patients must have a good central vision. So how can one say that there is an important nerve fiber loss when the central vision is perfectly normal? Or isn't it?

Juan E. Grunwald : Visual acuity was better than 0.6 or 0.75 and there were no central visual field defects as far as we could test with Goldmann perimetry and Amsler grids, although there were some more peripheral defects, sometimes even as near as the corners of the Amsler grid which is about 10 degrees away from fixation.

Sohan S. Hayreh : Then you can't invoke the nerve fiber loss to account for capillary dropout!

Harry A. Quigley : Sohan, I heard in the ARVO meeting, last year, that in the central 12 degrees you have to lose at least 40% of the ganglion cells to have a 10 dB defect on the Octopus or on the Humphrey. So, although in principle you are correct, it may well be that each one of those glaucoma patients had indeed ganglion cell and nerve fiber loss even though they could still see 20/20 with their central half degree or one degree which is anyway not measured here, since it is completely capillary-free.

Erik L. Greve : But Harry, aren't you stretching your hypotheses too far, speculating that (1) there is nerve fiber loss, even if undetected, (2) as a result of that there is a capillary dropout, then (3) as a result of that the speed in the capillaries is different ?

Harry A. Quigley : I didn't take that last step. I didn't speculate at all about the speed in the capillaries.

Erik L. Greve : But it's speed that Juan is measuring, isn't it? And it's speed differences that seem to indicate a poor autoregulation in glaucoma patients.

Juan E. Grunwald : I think we need to sort things out a bit. There is literature data that glaucoma patients see less leukocytes, but that is not my work. I couldn't compare one subject to another in my experiment, I only compared one eye to the other. And the patients where a difference was found between the two eyes, usually saw slower speeds and less leukocytes in the eye with more advanced glaucoma.

Harry A. Quigley : Now what I find hardest to accept in the implications of your hypothesis, Juan, is that if indeed the autoregulation in the retina is deficient and if this results in anoxia and atrophy of parts of the retina, then much more than nerve fibers and ganglion cells ought to die! Histologically this should look like central retinal artery occlusion, with the middle layers of the retina severed or gone. But there is no histologic evidence in the literature of damage extending deeper than the ganglion cell layer. Now if your results are very well documented and other interpretations discarded, maybe we ought to reevaluate our histology, but you must admit that it flies in the face of our notions so far.

George L. Spaeth : I think, Harry, that you could consider another possibility. It can well be that if you have some mechanical damage occurring at optic nerve head level due to high IOP or to a kink at the lamina or to whatever, then the fibers become much more susceptible to other toxic effects, such as anoxia, whether those act at optic nerve head or at ganglion cell level.

Harry A. Quigley : That is a good hypothesis; it could be tested in the laboratory, I guess.

Bernard Schwartz : I have a question about methodology. I am a little concerned about using a suction cup to increase the IOP. There are more ways to achieve the same result. The suction cup technique, even if artifacts due to the cup itself are eliminated, may well cause all sorts of changes in the eye, due to the fact that it is acute and completely anti-physiological. One could use steroids or even pick up cross-sections of the population with different IOP-levels. I wonder if our tendency to use suction-cups so easily doesn't lead us to conclusions that do not apply to the natural course of the disease.

Erik L. Greve : You may be right, Bernie, but I do not think that at this point we can answer your question, no more than the one George has brought up just before. So I think that we can close the discussion of Juan's paper and move to the next speaker.

REFLECTOMETRY MEASUREMENTS OF OPTIC DISC BLOOD VOLUME

François C. Delori

Eye Research Institute of Retina Foundation. 20 Staniford Street, Boston, MA 02114, USA

Introduction

The condition of the optic disc tissues is often clinically assessed by the degree of its pale-red color which results from the presence of capillaries in the disc tissues. A decrease in redness of the disc, clinically called "pallor", is generally associated with a decrease in the amount of blood in the disc tissues. Spectral reflectometry of the optic disc is used here to document the reflectance properties of the disc, to provide an objective measure for disc "color", and to study the optical properties of the disc tissues. A simple empirical model for disc reflectance is then reviewed and a method for blood volume determination based on that model is used to assess blood volume in normal and diseased conditions. Finally, another more complete model for light propagation in the disc tissues is proposed and used to derive tissue thickness, blood volume, O_2 saturation of the capillary blood, and information on the ocular media from the measured spectra. The limitations of both models, and of disc reflectometry in general, in providing quantitative information on the vascularization of the disc tissues are discussed.

Reflectance characteristics of the optic disc

The reflectance characteristics of the optic disc were measured with an experimental fundus reflectometer[1]. The disc is illuminated with white light over a circular area of 2.1° in angular diameter. The light reflected by the disc is imaged by the camera optics onto a diaphragm which defines a circular area of 1.4 to 1.6° in angular diameter. The detected light is analyzed by a system containing a grating monochromator, a Vidicon camera, and a multichannel analyzer. This system provides the spectrum of the reflected light intensities in 512 wavelength channels from 400 to 912 nm (effective spectral resolution: 7.5 nm). A reference spectrum is obtained from a standard diffuse reflector, using the same flash power, illumination and sampling apertures as used for the disc measurement. The reflectance of the fundus is computed at all wavelengths by comparing the disc and reference signals. The measured reflectances are "equivalent reflectances" since they include ocular media transmission and are based on an ocular focal length of 22 mm.

Reflectance spectra were obtained from the optic disc of 15 normal subjects (age: 22-64 years). The pupil of one eye was dilated to a diameter of at least 6 mm. Reflectance spectra were recorded from the temporal and nasal disc in all subjects, and from the physiological cup in some subjects.

Fig. 1 shows reflectance spectra obtained from the cup (C), the temporal (T) and nasal (N) side of the disc of a young individual (age: 27 years) and from the temporal (T') and nasal (N') side of the disc in an older subject (age: 60 years). All spectra reveal the absorption characteristics of oxyhemoglobin[2] by distinct reflectance minima at 540 and 575 nm (absorption maxima) and by high reflectance in red light (low absorption). Table 1 gives, for selected wavelengths, the average reflectances for the temporal and nasal side of the disc and for the physiological cup. The reflectance of the temporal side is signifi-

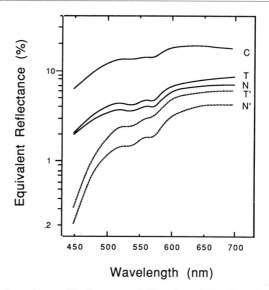

Fig. 1. Reflectance spectra from the cup (C), the temporal (T) and nasal (N) sides of the disc of a young individual (age: 27 years) and from the temporal (T') and nasal (N') sides of the disc in an older subject (age:60 years).

cantly higher than that of the nasal side at all wavelengths between 480 and 700 nm ($p<0.01$). The ratio of temporal to nasal reflectance is highest around 575 nm (average 1.4, SD = 0.4). The ratio R(675)/R(575) is on the average 2.3 (SD = 0.5) nasally and 1.9 (SD = 0.3) temporally. This ratio is significantly higher nasally than temporally ($p = 0.02$) indicating that the hemoglobin absorption bands are more pronounced nasally. This corresponds with the redder (less pale) appearance of the nasal disc compared to the temporal disc.

Table 1. Average disc reflectance in % (coefficient of variation in %)

λ(nm)	Temporal (n=15)	Nasal (n=15)	Cup (n=4)
455	1.2 (43)	1.2 (54)	6.4 (64)
480	2.3 (38)	1.9 (43)	10.1 (55)
522	3.3 (32)	2.5 (33)	13.6 (44)
540	3.0 (32)	2.3 (33)	13.3 (42)
559	3.4 (32)	2.5 (34)	14.2 (39)
565	3.5 (32)	2.6 (32)	14.1 (38)
569	3.4 (32)	2.6 (31)	14.4 (38)
575	3.4 (32)	2.5 (32)	14.4 (38)
585	4.2 (32)	3.1 (31)	15.6 (35)
610	5.9 (26)	4.8 (30)	17.9 (31)
675	6.5 (24)	5.5 (29)	18.0 (28)

The amplitude and shape of the disc reflectance spectra (and hence the color of the disc) are substantially affected by the dimension of the illumination aperture. Fig. 2 shows a comparison of spectrum T*, obtained with an illumination area of 7.7° (entire disc illuminated as in fundus photography), with spectrum T, obtained from the same site with an illumination area of 2.1°. The reflectances with large field illumination are higher at all wavelengths and the absorption bands are more distinct. This effect occurs because light incident outside the sampling area is scattered by the disc tissues and diffuses towards the sampling area, thereby increasing to focally reflected light. The longer effective path length through tissues (capillaries) and the eventual contribution of light transmission

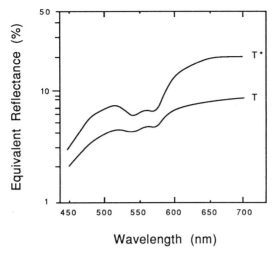

Fig. 2. Reflectance spectra from the temporal side of a disc using different areas of illumination. T: illumination area of 2.1° in diameter, and T*: illumination area of 7.7° in diameter. The detection area was 1.4° in diameter in both cases.

through large retinal vessels on the disc cause the hemoglobin absorption bands of the T* spectrum to be more pronounced than those of the T spectrum. Thus, disc tissues observed with a focal illumination would appear paler (less red) and less reflective than with full-disc illumination.

The equivalent reflectance of the disc decreases with increasing age, significantly so for wavelengths shorter than 540 nm ($p<0.0007$ at 455 nm). The reflectance spectra also become steeper with age (Fig. 1). This results from the age-related increase (most marked at short wavelengths) in the density of the ocular media and of the crystalline lens in particular[3]. The steepening of the spectra is illustrated in Fig. 3 by the variation with age of the slope M of the line through the 540 and 575 nm points of each spectrum (see inset

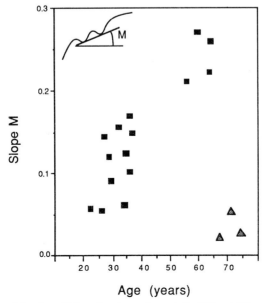

Fig. 3. Inset: Definition of the slope M for a line drawn through the 540 and 575 nm points of a spectrum. Variation of slope M, expressed in log. reflectance units per 100 nm, with age of subject.

in Fig. 3). The slope M (square symbols) correlates significantly with age ($r=0.8$, $p=0.0005$), and therefore M could be used as an index for ocular media density. Reflectance spectra were also obtained from three aphakic subjects; the corresponding slopes (triangles) are smaller than those of the youngest phakic subjects, indicating a very flat spectrum in these eyes. This demonstrates that the crystalline lens is the major contributor to ocular media absorption and scattering, and that any quantitative analysis of disc reflectometry must account for the ocular media transmission characteristics.

Semi-empirical model for disc reflectance

A relatively simple disc reflectometry method was developed to assess anterior optic disc blood volume. The reflectometry method was used in conjunction with blood speed measurements by the laser Doppler method, to assess blood flow in the capillaries of the anterior optic nerve in experimental and clinical optic atrophy[4,5]. The discussion here will be limited to the reflectometry technique; more details can be found in the original reports of the study[4,5].

The reflectometry method is based on a semi-empirical model for disc reflectance. Because the volume fraction of blood in the disc tissue is small, 2 to 4%[6], it is reasonable to assume that the reflectance R_λ at a wavelength λ is given by:

$$R_\lambda = R_{bl,\lambda} (1 - \gamma \cdot K_\lambda) \tag{1}$$

where $R_{bl,\lambda}$ is the equivalent reflectance of the bloodless disc (as measured through the ocular media), γ is a measure for the amount of blood in the tissues (in cm), and K_λ is the known absorption coefficient of hemoglobin (in cm^{-1}). Equation (1) must be considered as a first-degree approximation valid when γ is small. A similar relationship can be derived from the Kubelka-Monk theory[7] in the assumption that the blood volume fraction v_{Hb} is very small: the quantity Y is then proportional to v_{Hb} and inversely proportional to the scattering coefficient of the tissue. Thus, the measurement of λ does not permit a differentiation between changes in blood volume and changes in scattering properties of the tissues.

The equivalent reflectance of the bloodless disc cannot *a priori* be considered to be wavelength independent. Transmission characteristics of the ocular media and scattering properties of the disc tissues are responsible, as shown above, for an increase in reflectance with increasing wavelength. For a narrow spectral range we assume that the following first degree approximation is valid:

$$R_{bl,\lambda} = R_{bl,\lambda_0} \cdot [1 + \beta (\lambda - \lambda_0)] \tag{2}$$

where β is an unknown factor (in nm^{-1}), λ_0 is a reference wavelength (in nm), and R_{bl,λ_0} the bloodless disc reflectance at λ_0.

Equations (1) and (2) contain three unknowns: γ, β, and R_{bl,λ_0}. Thus disc reflectance measurements at three wavelengths are needed to determine γ and eliminate β and R_{bl,λ_0}. We selected $\lambda_0 = 569$ nm, $\lambda_1 = 559$ nm, and $\lambda_2 = 585$ nm because interference filters (halfwidth 7.5 nm) corresponding to these wavelengths existed in the retinal vessel oximeter instrument[8] and because these wavelengths were also an appropriate choice for solving Equations (1) and (2). Elimination of the unwanted unknowns gives the measure γ for blood volume as:

$$\gamma = \frac{\omega\,(r_1 - 1) - r_2 + 1}{K_{569}\,(\omega \cdot r_1 - r_2) - K_{559}\,\omega + K_{585}} \quad (3)$$

where $r_1 = R(559)/R(569)$ and $r_2 = R(585)/R(569)$. The reflectances $R(559)$, $R(569)$ and $R(585)$ are the three measured disc reflectances. Because ratios of reflectances (r_1 and r_2) are used, the method does not require absolute reflectance measurements. The parameter W is given by $(585-569)/(559-569) = -1.6$, and K_{569}, K_{559}, and K_{585} are the absorption coefficients of hemoglobin at the three wavelengths. Assuming that hemoglobin concentration is 15 g/100 ml and that the oxygen saturation of the blood in the disc capillaries is 80%, then $K_{569} = 237$ cm^{-1}, $K_{559} = 202$ cm^{-1}, and $K_{585} = 153$ cm^{-1} [2].

Applying these algorithms to the above-described spectral data of 15 normal subjects, we found on average $\gamma = 12.5$ µm (SD = 2.7 µm) for the temporal sites, and 13.3 µm (SD = 3.9 µm) for the nasal sites. The difference between the γ's for the two sites of the disc was not statistically significant.

The method of measuring γ was also applied using a three-wavelength fundus reflectometer to study blood volume in the disc tissue of nine patients with unilateral neurogenic optic atrophy. The instrument was the Retinal Vessel Oximeter operated in its reflectometry mode[8]. Blood volume index γ was measured from the disc of the affected eye and from that of the normal fellow eye. The blood volume index γ for the normal discs was found to be on average 12.7 µm (SD = 2.0 µm) and 14.3 µm (SD = 2.7 µm) for the temporal and nasal sites, respectively. The value of γ for the atrophic optic nerve was on average 6.6 µm (SD = 2.3 µm) and 12.0 µm (SD 2.3 µm) for the temporal and nasal sites, respectively. The difference between the affected and unaffected eyes was statistically significant for the temporal sites ($p<0.0001$, paired t-test) but not for the nasal sites ($p=0.06$).

Interpretation of the results for the blood volume index λ depends upon the magnitude of tissue scattering in the anterior optic nerve. For high tissue scattering, γ is proportional to the fractional blood volume (and inversely proportional to the scattering coefficient). For low tissue scattering, γ is proportional to the total amount of blood in the layer of disc tissue (the product of fractional blood volume and layer thickness). It is known from ophthalmoscopy that the reflectance by the disc tissues increases as the thickness of the tissue layer anterior to the highly reflecting lamina cribrosa decreases. The physiological cup (thin layer of glial tissue) reflects more light than the disc rims, even for red wavelengths where blood absorption is minimal (Fig. 1, Table 1). Backscattering of light by the disc tissues cannot therefore be a dominant factor because reflectance would then increase with layer thickness (see Fig. 4). Reflectance by the lamina cribrosa must play a role in the overall disc reflectance. The index γ would therefore correspond more to a measure of total blood volume than of blood volume fraction. This is an important distinction, as was pointed out by Quigley[9] and further discussed by Sebag[10], since a decrease in total blood volume in optic atrophy would correspond to a decrease in tissue thickness, whereas a decrease in fractional blood volume would correspond to a decrease in vascularization per unit volume (nutrition). To obtain a more quantitative analysis of the effect of light scattering, we have investigated a more physical model of light reflectance by the disc tissues.

Optical model for disc reflectance

The model for disc reflectance consists of an absorbing layer (simulating absorption and scattering in the ocular media), a homogeneous scattering-absorbing layer with uniformly distributed hemoglobin and neutral absorber (simulating the disc tissues), and a reflecting surface (simulating the lamina cribrosa). Mathematical solutions describing light reflectance by such layers were derived by Kubelka and Munk[7]. The reflectance R of the optic disc, at any wavelength, is then given by:

$$R = 10^{-2(K_{om}+\rho) D_m} \cdot \frac{1-R_{lc}(A-B \coth B S d)}{A + B \coth B S d - R_{lc}} \qquad (4)$$

where R_{lc} is the reflectance of the lamina cribrosa, K_{om} is the density spectrum of the ocular media normalized at 420 nm[11], P is an ocular media scattering term, and D_{om} is the density of the media at 420 nm. The parameter $B = (A^2-1)^{1/2}$, and A is given by:

$$B = (A^2-1)^{1/2}$$
$$A = \frac{K_{total}}{S} = \frac{[K_0 OS + K_r (1-OS)] v_{Hb} + N}{S} \qquad (5)$$

where K_o and K_r are the absorption coefficients of oxygenated and de-oxygenated hemoglobin, respectively[2]; OS is the O_2 saturation of capillary blood; d is the thickness of the disc tissue layer; v_{Hb} is the fractional blood volume in the disc tissue; N is the neutral absorption coefficient; and S is the scattering coefficient of the disc tissue.

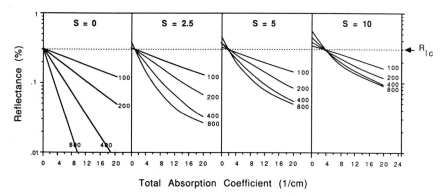

Fig. 4. Relationship between disc reflectance and total absorption for four different values of the scattering coefficient S (0, 2.5, 5.0, and 10 cm^{-1}) and four different layer thicknesses (100, 200, 400 and 800 μm).

Fig. 4 illustrates, for four different values of the scattering coefficient S (0, 2.5, 5.0, and 10 cm^{-1}) and four different layer thicknesses (100, 200, 400, and 800 μm), how the disc reflectance varies as a function of the total absorption coefficient K_{total} of the tissue. For high tissue scattering (S large), reflectance is less affected by changes in layer thickness and total absorption than for low tissue scattering. When S is large and the total absorption low, reflectance increases with layer thickness. This phenomenon is reversed as total absorption decreases. To account for the observation that reflectance of the disc decreases with increasing layer thickness, one must introduce a light loss in the form of the neutral absorber coefficient N. This absorption represents light losses by absorption in the disc tissues themselves (other than absorption by blood in the disc capillaries) and/or by scattering of light outside the sampling aperture.

Fig. 5 demonstrates the relationship between the absorption spectrum of blood and the reflectance spectrum of the disc. A reduction of the fractional blood volume (v_{Hb} decreases) will cause the reflectance spectrum to flatten and the disc to appear more pale. However, pallor would also result from any flattening of the reflectance-total absorption curve, either due to an increase in scattering (S increases) or to decrese in layer thickness

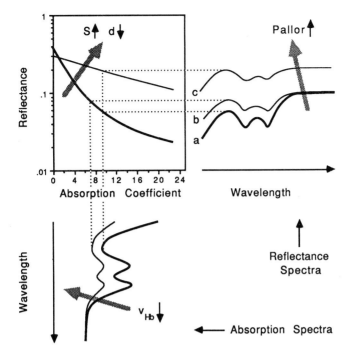

Fig. 5. Relation between the absorption spectra of hemoglobin and reflectance spectra of the optic disc. Starting from a normal disc (spectrum a), an increase in pallor (decrease in redness) can result from a decrease in the fractional blood volume v_{Hb} (spectrum b), from an increase in the tissue scattering coefficient S (spectrum c) or from a decrease in the disc tissue layer thickness d (spectrum c).

(d decreases). These changes are also seen in Fig. 4. Thus disc pallor can result from three possible causes: a decrease in V_{Hb} (caused, for example, by an acute elevation of the IOP), an increase in S (secondary to astrocyte proliferation), and a decrease in d (thinning of the disc tissue layer). This conclusion corresponds with observations made by Quigley[12].

The 34 spectra from the group of 15 normal subjects were fitted to the model (Equations 4 and 5), using the curve-fitting procedure "Curfit" described by Bevington[13]. The measured reflectance at 13 wavelengths between 505 and 700 nm were used (weights = 1/measured reflectance). Four parameters were calculated from the regressions for each individual spectrum: d, d_{Hb}, D_m, and OS. The blood layer thickness d_{Hb} is equal to the product $v_{Hb} \cdot d$. The other parameters were kept equal for all spectra, but were varied for the entire group of spectra to optimize the regressions and to bring the layer thickness d in the range 500-800 μm, corresponding to anatomical data for normal, uncupped discs. After an evaluation of the overall and individual quality of the regressions, the following common values were selected for all subjects and sites: R_{lc}=35%, S=1.5 cm^{-1}, N=6.0 cm^{-1}, and p = 0.095 D.U.

All the regressions were highly significant ($p<0.0001$) and the standard deviations of regression were smaller than 0.5% reflectance in all cases. Table 2 gives the average results of the curve fitting calculations for the four unknown parameters (d, d_{Hb}, OS, and D_m). The fractional blood volume v_{Hb} was calculated from the individual regression results ($v_{Hb} = d_{Hb}/d$) and the average v_{Hb}'s are also shown in Table 2.

The disc tissue is thicker nasally than temporally, by an average of 24% (SD = 27%). The thickness d of the temporal side correlates significantly with that of the nasal side ($p<0.001$). The total blood volume d_{Hb}, at each site, correlates significantly with d ($p<0.0004$). The blood volume d_{Hb} is larger nasally than temporally, but the fractional blood volume v_{Hb} is not statistically different for the different sites. The average value for v_{Hb}, 3.1%, is somewhat higher than the 2.35% found by Quigley[6] for the nerve head of

Table 2. Mean results of curve fitting to the model (coefficient of variation in %)

Parameters		Temporal (n=15)	Nasal (n=15)	Cup (n=4)
d	[μ]	565 (31)	688 (31)*	89 (63)*
d_{Hb}	[μ]	15 (51)	24 (71)*	3 (27)*
OS	[%]	62 (12)	57 (13)	73 (10)*
D_m	[D.U.]	0.61 (36)+	0.61 (41)+	0.50 (67)+
v_{Hb}	[%]	2.6 (28)	3.4 (52)	4.2 (36)
F(575)[%]		55 (34)	69 (29)*	9 (60)*
F(675)[%]		46 (33)	56 (30)*	10 (46)*

* Parameter significantly different from temporal value ($p<0.05$).
+ Significant correlation with age.

monkeys (*Macaca fascicularis*). The larger variability of the nasal values for d_{Hb} and v_{Hb} compared with the temporal values may be associated with the more variable geometry of the nasal disc sites. The O_2 saturations OS are not statistically different for the temporal and nasal sites, but OS for the cup capillaries is significantly higher than those of the disc rims. The standard errors of regression for OS are large, especially when d_{Hb} is small. The ocular media densities D_m determined independently for the different sites are not statistically different from each other, and the temporal D_m's correlate significantly with the nasal ones ($p<0.0001$). The density D_m at all sites correlates significantly with age ($p<0.0007$), and the mean values agree well with the standard observed value of 0.58[11].

The contribution of the reflectance of the disc tissues anterior to the lamina to the total reflectance was calculated from the fitted and fixed parameters. Table 2 gives, for $\lambda= 575$ and 675 nm, the mean ratio F(λ) of disc tissue reflectance to total reflectance. The tissues at the disc rim are thus moderately scattering, reflecting on average 40 to 70% of the total reflected light. This contribution increases significantly with the thickness of the tissue layer anterior to the lamina ($p<0.0001$, temporal and nasal sites).

The model for disc reflectance is a first step toward a better understanding of the optical properties of the disc tissue. Because several parameters were fixed for all spectra (R_{lc}, S, N, and P), the results of Table 2 do not represent a unique solution, but rather an average solution valid for the group of normal optic discs investigated in this study. Furthermore, the model does not account for variations in the size of the illumination and detection areas. A more complex optical model of light propagation in the disc needs to be developed to include illumination and detection geometries, and more *in vivo* and *in vitro* measurements are required to better characterize some of the optical parameters.

Conclusions

Reflectance spectra of the optic disc of normal subjects are influenced by the ocular media transmission (age), disc tissue layer thickness, tissue scattering, and amount of blood in the tissues. An enhanced understanding of light propagation by the disc tissue improves our interpretation of disease-related changes of the nerve head, and optical modelling allows quantification of clinically important parameters such as thickness of the disc tissue layer, degree of vascularization of the tissue, and O_2 saturation.

References

1. Delori F, Pflibsen K: Spectral reflectance of the human ocular fundus, Applied Optics (in press)
2. Van Assendelft OW: Spectroscopy of Hemoglobin Derivatives. Springfield, Illinois: CC Thomas, 1970
3. Boetner EA, Wolter JR: Transmission of the ocular media, Invest Ophthalmol 1:776, 1962
4. Sebag J, Feke GT, Delori FC, Weiter JJ: Anterior optic nerve blood flow in experimental optic atrophy. Invest Ophthalmol Vis Sci 26:1415, 1985
5. Sebag J, Delori FC, Feke GT, Goger D, Fitch K, Tagawa H, Deupree D, Weiter JJ, McMeel JW: Anterior optic nerve blood flow decreases in clinical neurogenic optic atrophy. Ophthalmology 93:858, 1986
6. Quigley HR, Hohman RM, Addicks EM, Quantitative study of optic nerve head capillaries in experimental optic disc pallor, Am J Ophthalmol 93:689, 1982
7. Kortum G: Reflectance Spectroscopy, p 116. New York: Springer-Verlag 1969
8. Delori FC: Noninvasive technique for oximetry of blood in retinal vessels. Applied Opt 27:1113 1988
9. Quigley HA, Letter to the Editor. Ophthalmology 94:87, 1987
10. Sebag J, Feke GT, Delori FC: Letter to the Editor, Ophthalmology 94:88,1987
11. Van Norren D, Vos JJ: Spectral transmission of the human ocular media, Vision Res 14:1237,1974
12. Quigley HA, Anderson DR: The histologic basis of disc pallor in experimental optic atrophy, Am J Ophthalmol 83:709, 1977
13. Bevington PR: Data Reduction and Error Analysis for the Physical Sciences, p 235. New York: McGraw-Hill Book Company, 1969

DISCUSSION

Sohan S. Hayreh : Obviously, Dr Delori, your measurements reflect to some extent the color and more specifically the redness of the disc. About twenty years ago we studied the significance of disc color by doing fluorescein angiography in normal eyes as well as in eyes with optic atrophy of various origins. And we found that the color of the disc didn't reflect its vascularity at all. So I have some difficulty in understanding what your test shows.

François Delori : I didn't really study the correlation between our measurements and disc color, though I believe that the calculated amount of blood will be related to the redness of the disc.

Sohan S. Hayreh : Then your measurements would suggest that there is more blood on the nasal than on the temporal side?

François Delori : Not necessarily: there was no statistically significant difference between nasal and temporal side as far as fractional volume of blood is concerned. The total amount of blood was higher temporally, but so was the thickness of the disc tissue.

Sohan S. Hayreh : The reason why I raised this point is that it is often somehow taken for granted that a pale disc is less vascular, but this isn't necessarily the case. Dr Schwartz's studies have confirmed that.

Richard Stodtmeister : Dr Delori, I would like to ask you a few questions as a clinician. How can reflectometry be used for glaucoma diagnosis? Is it possible to detect slight changes in vascularization? And is the technique easily applicable in clinical practice?

François Delori : I must admit that I can't myself explain all the data that we collected. I do not think that actual blood volume can be measured with accuracy, because we have to make certain assumptions about some parameters. I believe that the method can be used to improve our understanding of disc reflectance properties and maybe to measure clinically important parameters, such as oxygen saturation or degree of vascularization. But the major problem is that we can't very well differentiate between a change in scattering with no change in disc tissue thickness, and a change in disc tissue thickness with no change in scattering.

Harry A. Quigley : I have seen the original data, Dr Stodtmeister, and have discussed them extensively. From a clinician's point of view, there is no doubt that the method can detect optic atrophy and, which is more, yield a reading that is proportional to nerve fiber loss judged clinically. We don't know yet if the method measures actual blood flow or blood flow per gram of nerve tissue, but either way the information is valuable. True, the measurements are done in the anterior part of the optic nerve head and not in the lamina cribrosa where we suspect the pathogenic mechanism to act, but I think that it is a very promising method, even if it is rather unlikely that we will be able to use it very soon in routine practice.

François Delori : Since you mentioned the optic atrophy study, Dr Quigley, I think that its one weak point was the blood volume estimation. We hadn't yet worked everything out then, as we have now. But the other part of it, the laser Doppler velocimetry measurement is simple, elegant and very promising.

George N. Lambrou : Speaking of that optic atrophy study, Dr Delori, you had measured two parameters: alpha, reflecting blood velocities, and gamma, reflecting the amount of blood present. After optic nerve transection had caused optic atrophy, both parameters were reduced as anticipated. However, if you look at the degree of reduction, it is almost exactly the same for the two parameters in every single one of the five experimental eyes. That made me wonder at the time whether the two techniques, reflectometry and laser Doppler velocimetry, aren't measuring two aspects of the same phenomenon, the optic nerve fiber loss, say, or if they aren't critically dependent on some other factor.

François Delori : That is a good point. You are suggesting that changes in scattering properties, for example, might be the predominant parameter. I don't think that I can give you an answer now, but I will think about it.

PHOTOMETRY OF THE OPTIC DISC

Yves C. A. Robert and Phillip H. Hendrickson

Universitätsspital, Augenklinik, CH 8091 Zürich, Switzerland

In any consideration of the papillary perfusion, we have to bear in mind that it cannot be measured simply. At best we can estimate individual perfusion-related parameters. Among these, we should mention the mean blood pressure of the afferent artery (calculated from the systolic and diastolic upper-arm arterial blood-pressure), the velocity of erythrocytes, the number and cross-section of the capillaries, and the vascular resistance. Of these five quantities mentioned, none can been measured without problems. In the following, we want to show that vascular resistance can, under certain circumstances, become a measure of the papillary perfusion which can provide information about the vitality of the organ. As you know, vascular resistance in the case of laminar flow can be described by Hagen and Poiseuille's law. It is, for the most part, dependent on the cross–section of the vessels.

What can we actually determine at the papilla? When we illuminate it with white light, we can measure the redness of the rim. Fortunately, this redness is the result of the summation of the entire prelaminar vital tissue of the papilla, and not – as in the case of illumination with monochromatic light – only representative of one particular tissue depth. The redness is directly dependent on the amount of hemoglobin and, therefore, on the amount of whole blood present in the vessels at the time of the measurement. When measuring the redness of the rim, we are determining its blood-volume. The blood-content of the papilla is, itself, inversely proportional to the vascular resistance. It is high when the vascular resistance is low and *vice versa*. Therefore, one can evaluate the vascular resistance by observing/measuring the blood-content or redness of the papilla. The vascular rigidity is, in itself, an extremely important circulatory parameter, because it reacts to systemic as well as local provocation. Therefore, the regulation of the papillary vascular bed is multifactorial and subject to autoregulatory influence. Looking simply at the redness of the papilla at any one moment does not yield much information, even when it is altered by atrophy or glaucoma. Only when the disease has progressed so far that the regulatory mechanisms can no longer compensate for deficiencies, are we able to see excavation and increased paleness. However, the disease is by then already in its late stages. What then must we do to detect the early stages of the disease? We have to provoke the system, which means that we have to force it artificially out–of–balance and, therefore, test its ability to react. For this purpose, a test of the vascular rigidity is highly appropriate.

The basis for our method of examination of the optic disc is a phenomenon, well known to those who perform ophthalmodynamometry and easy to observe, the change of the brightness of the vital rim following an acute intraocular pressure increase. An increase in papillary brightness is its only specific response to a pressure provocation. No other structure of the eye responds so obviously as does the rim. It is true that at the same time the papilla and the lamina cribrosa are shifted posteriorly, but this is not generally measurable today.

Is the pressure provocation sensible?
It is a physiological stimulus, since, normally, the IOP shows strong variations.
It is specific for the disease under consideration, glaucoma.
It is simply and quickly performed, even at the slit–lamp.
It involves no discomfort to the patient.

What, then, are we able to determine when the intraocular pressure is abruptly elevated and the brightness of the papilla is simultaneously measured? By using our Photopapillometer we establish a Dynamic Provoked Circulatory Response (DPCR) curve[1], showing the course of the papillary brightness before, during, and after the intraocular pressure provocation. First we measure the brightness of a particular location on the papilla rim under normal pressure conditions; we call this the "baseline brightness", B_o. Thereafter, the intraocular pressure is abruptly elevated. Following a certain period of time, which we call the "latency time, T_L, an increase in brightness is detected, eventually leading to a brightness maximum, B_M, the level of which depends in part on the extent of the pressure elevation. When the provocation is ended, the brightness returns to baseline, sometimes even deepening to a brightness minimum, B_m. Our attention should be directed to the latency time, the time between the onset of the pressure provocation and the initial reduction of capillary blood volume (increase in rim brightness).

This reduction of blood volume in the capillaries is effected through the narrowing of their diameters. This, in turn, is directly dependent on the vascular resistance or rigidity. Obviously, this is a measure of the vascular resistance directly at the papilla! One might argue that the vascular resistance is only one of at least five parameters involved in perfusion. However, we should note here that (1) this parameter is exactly and thoroughly determined and (2) although only indirectly measured, it may be nonetheless considered representative of the perfusion.

The following experiment shows in what manner the latency time can be altered according to the vascular resistance:

In young subjects requiring general anesthesia for surgery, we performed the DPCR-examination alternatively on both eyes immediately before the operation began, with their informed consent. In the first eye, the DPCR-examination was performed during normal, laughing–gas/oxygen anesthesia. With this anesthetic gas the cerebral circulation remains uninfluenced. The resulting latency times averaged about 2.5 seconds, now considered normal. During the subsequent ten minutes, the patient was given Halothane^R, an anesthetic gas which strongly reduces cerebral vascular resistance. Then the DPCR-examination was performed on the contralateral eye. But, from a physiological point of view, the situation was different, since the vascular resistance of the cerebral circulation had been drastically reduced. Whereas, thanks to the stabilizing influence of anesthesia, no discernible brightness changes prior to provocation could be noticed, all these patients showed a shortening of the latency time to a uniform 0.5 seconds! The change of the vascular rigidity expressed itself directly as a difference in latency time specific to the papilla! This obviously shows that, by measuring the latency time, we are determining the vascular resistance and, therefore, describing the vascular condition of the organ in question. This result becomes even more interesting, since the same effect was documented in ambulatory glaucoma patients. These were compared with a group of ten normal subjects of similar age. As reported earlier[1], we found shortened latency times for the glaucoma patients which, interestingly, are the same as those for the Halothane patients. Larger subject populations will determine whether the coincidence of these values is due to different causes or whether they are both expressions of the same vascular resistance. What we can say today is that stronger evidence is now available that glaucoma is related to changes of the vascular condition of the papilla.

References

1. Robert Y: Understanding the dynamic provoked response of the papilla. Int Ophthalmol 13:15-19, 1989

DISCUSSION

Erik L. Greve : To what level did you raise the IOP, Dr Robert ?

Yves C.A. Robert : To about 40 mmHg. But the actual level is not very critical for the experiment, since it is only the latency times that we are interested in.

Juan E. Grunwald : By what means did you achieve that increase ?

Yves C.A. Robert : We do it with a very fast suction cup; it is the same device that is used in oculo-oscillo-dynamography. You don't have to raise the pressure very high, really, but the increase must be very fast, almost instant.

George L. Spaeth : You said that the latency time was reduced in your glaucoma group. What was the actual value ?

Yves C.A. Robert : It was the same as in normals under Halothane, 0.5 seconds, while in normal eyes under normal circumstances it is 2.5 seconds.

Harry A. Quigley : Dr Robert, your technique, as I understand it, consists in illuminating the disc with white light and then measuring the light reflected back. But I did not understand what wavelengths you are measuring. Is it the whole spectrum?

Yves C.A. Robert : That's what we did in the beginning, indeed. But nowadays we only record the short wavelengths, 500 nanometers and below, which correspond to blue and green. When the IOP increases the papillary rim seems to grow paler, as if the redness was decreasing. What happens in fact, is that at some moment after the increase of IOP there is a reduction of the amount of blood present in the disc capillaries and therefore less absorption of the green and blue wavelengths: the reflectance in the red remains the same but it increases in the blue and green. That is the reason why we now restrict our measurements to the short wavelengths.

Sohan S. Hayreh : I think that the issue of the redness of the disc is a very important one. We are not absolutely sure as to what redness represents. We did some experiments to investigate the question and we found that sectioning the posterior ciliary arteries doesn't affect the color of the disc, whereas sectioning the central retinal artery causes immediate pallor. So if you are measuring redness, I think that you are studying the superficial, retinal circulation - which is probably not relevant in glaucoma pathogenesis - and that you are not collecting any data about the deeper layers of capillaries at laminar and prelaminar level.

Yves C.A. Robert : Thank you for bringing up what I think is indeed an important question. As you said, the cause and the meaning of disc redness aren't straightforward and we studied them for years before starting our actual investigation. Maybe you remember the studies of Sørensen in Denmark* and of Gloster in

---

* *Editors' note*: Sørensen PN: The color of the optic disc. Variation with illumination. Acta Ophthalmol 58 : 1005-1016, 1980.

London*, who also tried to investigate the question. Imagine that you are examining the fundus at the slit-lamp using a very fine slit. While you are sweeping it over the retina and choroid, all you see is the slit itself, with darkness on either side of it. But as soon as it reaches the rim of the optic nerve head, then the entire disc lights up until the slit has moved away from it. This indicates that the light coming from the disc is, to a great extent, backscattered light. Interestingly, the retinal nerve fiber layer does not backscatter light in the same way.

Another interesting point is the position of the central vessels. If they are in the center of the disc, then it will light up in the same way, whether you approach your slit from the nasal or from the temporal side. But if they are shifted nasally, then you will have much less light backscattered from the temporal half than from the nasal half of the disc. And it is my personal opinion that temporal pallor of the disc is due to a shift of the central vessels.

Now to come back to the significance of the redness of the disc, I admit I do not know for sure what it is due to. But it is certainly a sign of vitality: a red disc is a disc in good shape, while a pale disc is either damaged or in danger. And I think there can be no doubt that by bleaching it we test its vitality.

Harry A. Quigley : Another question, Dr Robert: were the cup-to-disc ratios in the glaucoma group much higher than in the normals ?

Yves C.A. Robert : Not really; we tried to match glaucomas to normals with respect to cup-to-disc ratios, IOP values, etc. So the cup-to-disc ratios of glaucoma patients were either similar or very slghtly higher than those of the normals.

Harry A. Quigley : But still the glaucoma patients did have visual field loss, didn't they?

Yves C.A. Robert : Yes, although very slight.

Harry A. Quigley : It is rather surprising, then, that they didn't have higher cup-to-disc ratios. I believe that what you are somehow measuring is similar to what Dr Delori measures, and that is the amount of red blood cells in a part of the disc. Now the rapidity with which it will turn white under pressure, in other words the rapidity with which red blood cells will be pushed out of it, is proportional to the volume of tissue present. In the glaucomatous disc there is less tissue and therefore it will be easier for you to push the red blood cells out of it faster. It may well be, then, that you are indeed measuring something which is characteristic of the glaucomatous disc, but which is only related to the amount of tissue present and not to the vascular resistance. And I would also like to ask about the elevated IOP: was it raised to the same level in glaucoma and normal eyes ?

Yves C.A. Robert : Yes, it was the same. As I told you, we matched glaucoma patients and normal subjects also with respect to baseline IOP and then raised the IOP to the same level.

Eric L. Greve : Harry, what you were saying about differences in amount of tissue present doesn't explain the effect of Halothane.

---

* *Editors' note*: Gloster J: The colour of the optic disc. Doc Ophthalmol 26: 155-163, 1969

Discussion

Harry A. Quigley : I am just guessing, but Halothane lowers the IOP, so that you have a very different baseline measurement in normal patients with Halothane as compared to glaucoma patients. Did you measure the IOP after Halothane was given?

Yves C.A. Robert : Yes, it was somewhat lower, but very slightly so. It was not a complete Halothane anesthesia. We just added to the routine anesthesia the minimum active dose of Halothane in order to influence the cerebral and, hopefully, the ocular blood flow.

Richard Stodtmeister : It is true that the mechanisms subtending disc redness are not well understood, and neither is its clinical meaning. But I think that this is slightly beyond the point, here. What is most important is that you are measuring a time delay, which seems to be different in normal and glaucomatous eyes. Now if this time delay turns out to be of of diagnostic value and if it can be measured reliably, then we can consider these results to be very promising and apply the technique further, even without understanding everything about it for the time being.

Harry A. Quigley : Of course it would be absolutely vital if one could demonstrate that the glaucoma suspects with a behavior different from normals, according to some technique, were the ones to develop visual field loss. But if you want to have a large group of patients, such a study would take at least five or six years. So you want to be certain before you start that the parameters you are measuring are the correct ones. That's why you need to understand the phenomenon you are studying, in this case the reason why the disc's reflectance characteristics change. For instance, the baseline must certainly be different from one subject to the other, so that you make relative measurements of the ratio between maximum brightness and baseline brightness. Is there any difference in that ratio between normals and glaucoma patients ?

Yves C.A. Robert : The baseline is different for each subject, as you said, and the maximum brightness depends on the final IOP, which in turn depends on the baseline IOP and on scleral rigidity. We collect all this data, of course, but we restrict our analysis to the latency time, which seems to be particularly promising, so far.

Bernard Schwartz : I think that to understand this test better and to interpret its results, a lot of data is indeed required. Harry just mentioned a few of the most important parameters, such as the initial amount of pallor. But also the demographic characteristics of the groups and the general condition of the patients are important: were they vascular hypertensives? Did they have any systemic medication? I am sure you thought of such things.

Yves C.A. Robert : Yes, our exclusion criteria were very strict, because in the beginning we didn't believe too much in the usefulness of the test ourselves.

Gisbert Richard : Dr Robert, I think that your method is very interesting, but I have one question which also applies to Dr Riva's technique. When you are trying to measure a spot in the fundus over some time, you have the problem of eye movements. Not only the large movements, for which you can more or less correct, but also the micromovements can be very important if you want to be analyzing the same spot all the time. We faced this problem when we started doing image processing, and we only could solve it through a rather complicated and expensive tracking system. How do you deal with this problem ?

Yves C.A. Robert : What we do is use the suction cup to hold the eye stable and of course there is a fixation light for the other eye and we only do it with well-cooperating subjects. I think that for us the problem wasn't so crucial, since we do not do image analysis; we only measure over a few seconds the light reflected from a small spot, about 500 microns in diameter. If there is a micromovement, the spot will move slightly but it will not leave the rim. If it did, of course, we would get an artificial result, but that would require a much wider movement.

Charles E. Riva : Since you also addressed the question to me, Dr Richard, this is how we proceed: we put the suction cup on the eye with just enough suction pressure to hold it there, raising the IOP by only 5 mmHg or so. Then we align everything, get ready to measure, raise the IOP to about 40 mmHg, correct the alignment if need be, and then make the measurement. And up to now we have only been using staff members like us, who understand what it is all about, or selected patients who can cooperate.

IV. ELECTRODIAGNOSTIC TESTS AND OCULAR BLOOD FLOW

PRESSURE TOLERANCE TEST:
I. Clinical technique and specificity*

Richard Stodtmeister and Lutz E. Pillunat

University Eye Clinic (Director: Prof. Dr. R. Marquardt), Prittwitzstr. 43, 7900 Ulm, FRG

Introduction

The damage of the optic nerve head is not strictly connected with the elevation of the intraocular pressure[1]. It has to be assumed that there are additional mechanisms which play a role as damaging factors. Undoubtedly the intraocular pressure plays an important role in the pathomechanism of optic nerve fiber damage, but it can no longer be assumed that this force is the only cause for this damage.

According to the knowledge presently available the optic nerve fiber damage occurs in the prelaminar layer of the optic nerve head which is nourished by the ciliary circulation[2].

In this region the vessels are a "backwater" (Hayreh, personal communication) of the ciliary circulation system which itself has a lower blood pressure than the retinal system. Thus the optic nerve head circulation has to be assumed to be very susceptible to disturbances.

According to our experience the systolic ciliary blood pressure measured by oculo-oscillodynamography according to Ulrich and Ulrich[3] does not differ in glaucoma patients and in healthy volunteers. However, the site of measurement is in the ciliary arteries just after leaving the ophthalmic artery[3]. Thus the ciliary systolic blood pressure is not

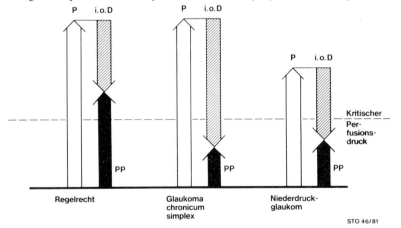

Fig. 1. Interdependency of blood pressure in the vessels of the eye (open arrows), intraocular pressure (hatched arrows) and perfusion pressure (black arrows). Kritischer Perfusionsdruck = Critical perfusion pressure: perfusion pressure below which damage occurs. Regelrecht = healthy subject. Glaukoma chronicum simplex = primary open angle glaucoma. Niederdruckglaukom = low tension glaucoma.

---

*Supported by Deutsche Forschungsgemeinschaft Grant Sto–180/1–2 and Dr. Helmut und Margarete Meyer–Schwarting Stiftung

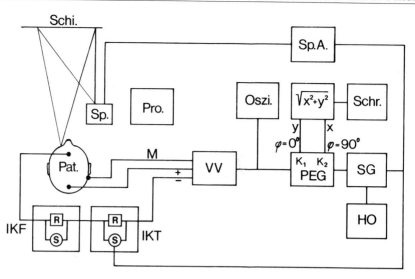

Fig. 2. Block diagram of the experimental set–up for the pressure tolerance test by recording steady state visually evoked cortical potentials. Abbreviations: HO = master oscillator. IKF = integral calibration (free running). IKT = integral calibration (triggered). K1 = channel 1. K2 = channel 2. M = symmetry electrode. Oszi = oscilloscope. Pat. = patient. PEG = phase sensitive detector. Pro. = slide projector. R = resistor 10 Ω. SG = signal generator. S = signal source for calibration. Schi. = projection screen. Schr. = strip chart recorder. Sp = moving mirror. Sp.A. = driving unit for the mirror. VV = preamplifier. x^2+y^2 = vector calculator. φ = phase. (From: Stodtmeister *et al.*, 1987b[14]).

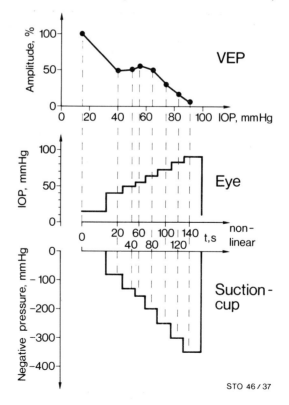

Fig. 3. Diagrammatic demonstration of the pressure tolerance test. Ordinate: pressure scale is linear. Time scale is non linear.

measured at the site of the optic nerve fiber damage. One reason for this observation may be seen in the wide scatter of measured values[4,5].

It has to be kept in mind that the crucial parameter for the pressure head in the tissue is not the blood pressure itself but the perfusion pressure. This value results from the blood pressure minus the intraocular pressure. It can be concluded that this parameter is one of the most determining characteristics for the circulation in the optic nerve head (Fig. 1). A damage to the optic nerve fibers can be assumed when the perfusion pressure is falling short of a critical value. That can be the case at high intraocular pressure or at low blood pressure.

Glaucoma can be regarded as the disease in which the perfusion pressure is temporarily or permanently too low to maintain a sufficient circulation. Until now there is no method available, according to the literature accessible to us, by which this pressure can be measured in the optic nerve head.

In physics and in biology it is a general principle to test the susceptibility to damage by stress tests. One widely used method in medicine is the exercise electrocardiogram.

This principle has been applied by Benedikt et al.[6], by Bartl et al.[7,8] and by Bartl[9] to the glaucoma problem. These authors have registered visually evoked cortical potentials at artificially increased intraocular pressure in a few volunteers and in a few glaucoma patients. The artificial pressure rise was done by impression dynamometry[10]. Ulrich[11] has shown one single experiment in a healthy volunteer slightly modifying the method of Benedikt et al.[6] by using the suction cup[13] for the artificial pressure rise.

We have designed an examination set-up which enables us to perform this test more quickly and easily[13,14]. By this improvement the test could be introduced into the clinical diagnostics[15-18]. Benedikt et al.[6], Bartl et al.[7,8], Ulrich[11] and Bartl[9] used the averaging technique for the recording of the visually evoked cortical potentials. We applied phase sensitive detection[19-21], a method which is more effective to separate the evoked potentials from the spontaneous electrical brain activity than the averaging technique[22]. Our first set-up was based on analog technique (Fig. 2). Presently we are using a digital instrument which also performs the formerly quite time consuming evaluation of the strip chart

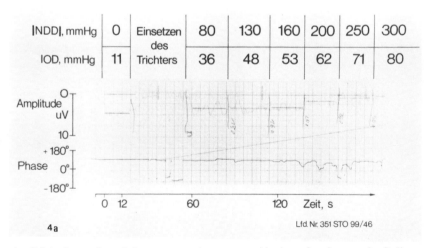

Fig. 4a. Original recording of the pressure tolerance test. Abscissa: time in seconds. Ordinate upper trace: amplitude of the steady state visually evoked cortical potential at the output of the vector voltmeter. Ordinate lower trace: phase angle at the output of the vector voltmeter. The straight ascending line is an auxiliary line. (NDD) = absolute value of the negative pressure difference in the suction cup. IOD = intraocular pressure. Einsetzen des Trichters = insertion of the suction cup. (From Stodtmeister et al., 1988b)[5].

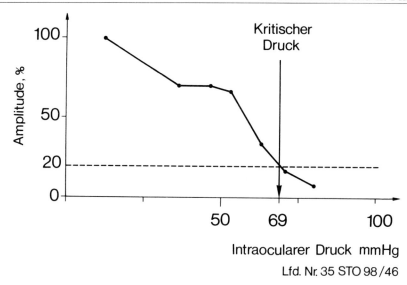

Fig. 4b. Amplitude/pressure curve plotted according to the values of the recording in Fig. 4a. Ordinate: amplitude of the visually evoked cortical potentials in percent of the initial value at uninfluenced intraocular pressure. Abscissa: intraocular pressure. Kritischer Druck: intraocular pressure at which the 20% level is reached. This amplitude/pressure curve shows a weakly monotone behavior. (From: Stodtmeister *et al.*, 1988b)[5].

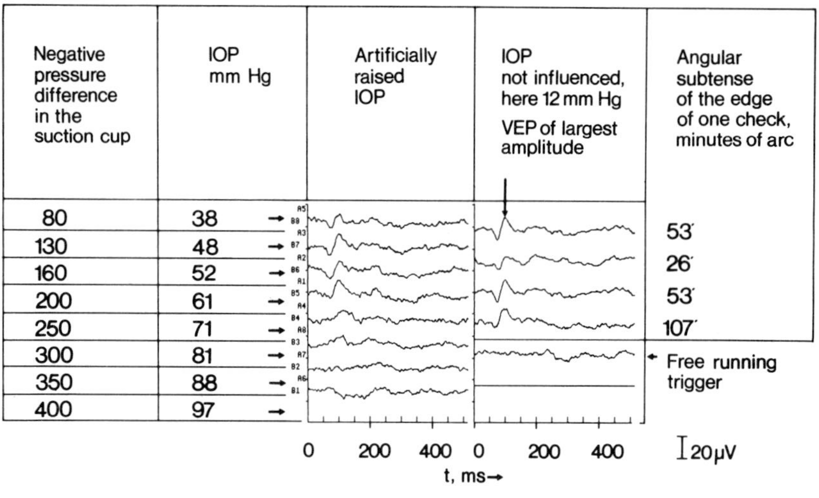

Fig. 5. Arrangement of the transient visually evoked cortical potentials obtained by the program used by us. Ordinate: amplitude. Abscissa: time. The pattern reversal occurs at 0.

recordings. An additional new feature of this set-up is the computer controlled pressure rise. This characteristic is important for the standardization of the test procedure.

Methods

The test procedure is as follows and diagrammatically shown in Fig. 3.

The intraocular pressure is measured. Visually evoked cortical potentials are elicited by checkerboard reversal stimuli and that pattern is determined at which the highest amplitude is recorded. Monocular stimulation is used. The pupil is not dilated. Then the suction cup is applied and recordings are carried out at predetermined values of negative pressure

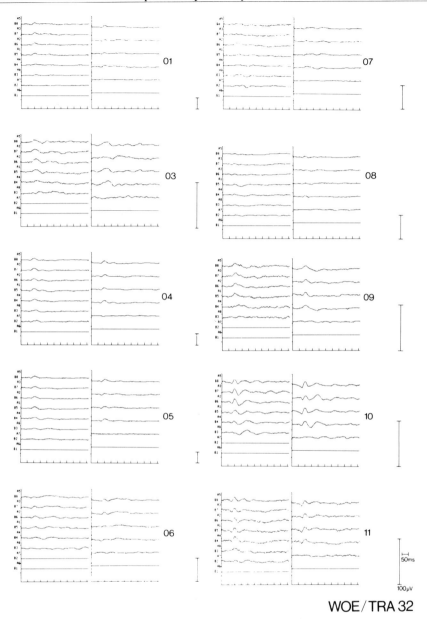

WOE/TRA 32

Fig. 6a. Pressure tolerance test. Visually evoked cortical potentials at 1.9 Hz r/s, 50 sweeps per average, of ten subjects. Ordinate: the bars of different length on the right of the systems represent 100 µV. Further information in Fig. 5.

difference in the suction cup. The recordings are stopped when a potential seems not to be recordable. With our first set-up the recording time at one pressure step was about 15–20 seconds. Thus the recordings at elevated intraocular pressure were done in about two to three minutes. During the major part of this time the perfusion pressure can be assumed to be above zero.

The value of the artificially elevated intraocular pressure has been calculated by using the regressions of Hayatsu[23,24]. We have determined these regressions in a large sample of healthy subjects using the standardized suction cup (Taberna pro medicum, Lünenburg) which is mandatory in the Federal Republic of Germany. Our regressions do not differ widely from these of Hayatsu. We are using our regressions: According to our data we can

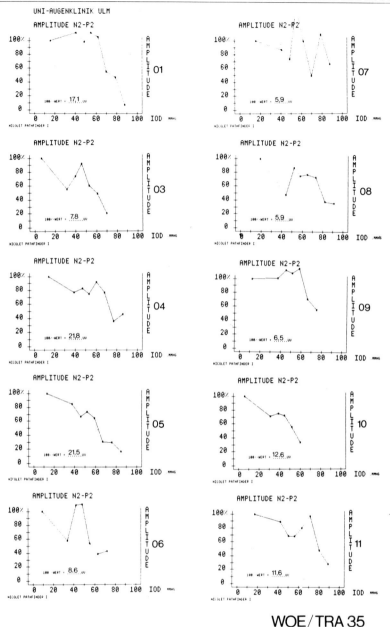

Fig. 6b. Amplitude/pressure curves plotted according to the values measured in Fig. 6a.

quite easily calculate by computer the actual intraocular pressure.

The amplitude of the visually evoked cortical potential at uninfluenced intraocular pressure is set to 100% and the amplitudes at artificially increased intraocular pressure are plotted as percent values versus the intraocular pressure. These curves are called amplitude/pressure curves.

Generally it is advisable to calculate differences of measured values. In the case of the pressure tolerance test described here the use of percentages is more appropriate: It is generally known that the amplitudes of the visually evoked cortical potentials show a wide interindividual variability. By using differences the comparison of the results of the pressure tolerance tests of different subjects would be practically impossible. Because

Pressure tolerance test: Technique and specificity

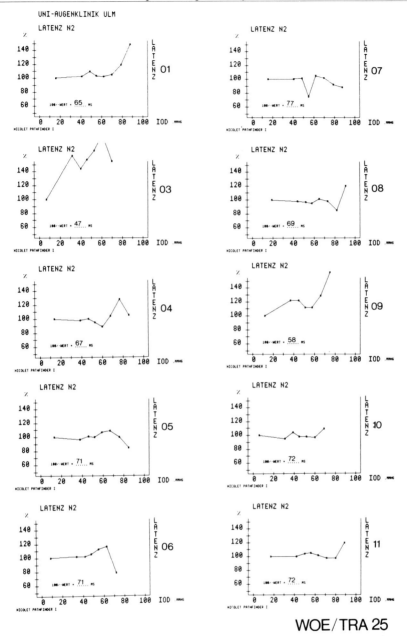

Fig. 6c. Latency N2/pressure curves plotted according to the values measured in Fig. 6a.

the amplitude values at uninfluenced and artificially increased intraocular pressures are dependent from each other it is admissible to use percentages from the practical as well as from the theoretical point of view[25].

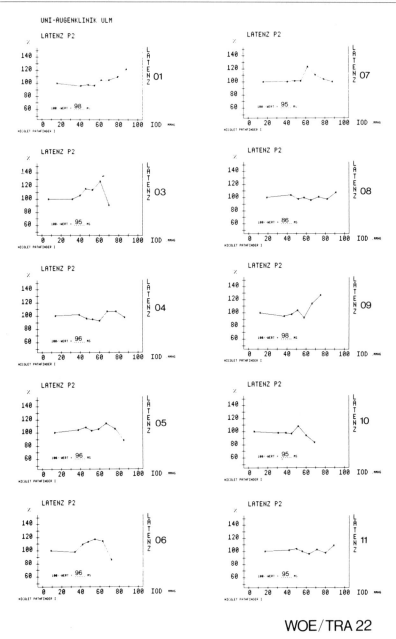

Fig. 6d. Latency P2/pressure curves plotted according to the values measured in Fig. 6a.

Results

Analog technique

Fig. 4a shows an original recording of a pressure tolerance test with the method described. The poor quality of reproduction is taken into account for the sake of the originality as recommended by Van der Tweel et al[26]. The recording of the phase gives information on the reliability of the amplitude recording. As seen at intraocular pressures

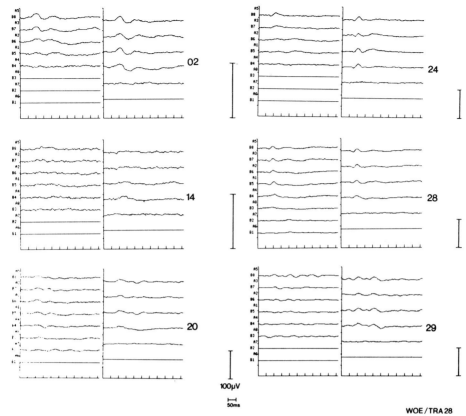

Fig. 7a. Pressure tolerance test. visually evoked cortical potentials at 1.9 Hz r/s, 50 sweeps per average of ten subjects. Ordinate: the bars of different length on the right of the systems represent 100 μV. Further information in Fig. 5 (From: Stodtmeister et al., 1988a)[4].

of 36, 48 and 53 mm Hg the phase is quite steady. At 62 mm Hg there are phase instabilities which are hinting at influence of interfering activity from outside the visual cortex. Fig. 4b shows the amplitude/pressure curve plotted from the records in Fig. 4a.

Averaging transients technique

We have also carried out the pressure tolerance test by using transient visually evoked cortical potentials at a pattern reversal rate of 1.9 Hz[4,5,13,14]. Because the autoregulatory phenomenon of optic nerve head circulation as supposedly recorded by the pressure tolerance test has a time constant in the order of magnitude of 40 seconds, the recordings have to be made in a very rapid sequence. For this purpose a larger examination unit is needed for quick recording, storing and handling of visually evoked cortical potentials. We used a Pathfinder I (Nicolet Instruments). The sequence of the test was controlled by a program written by us. Thus the interruptions between the single recordings were only due to the time required for the increase of the intraocular pressure. Fig. 5 shows the arrangement of the recordings of a pressure tolerance test obtained by this method.

In Fig. 6a the recordings of ten out of 30 healthy subjects are shown and the amplitude/pressure curves plotted from these recordings are seen in Fig. 6b. In all of the amplitude/pressure curves a non–monotone behavior can be seen. In subject 07 the amplitude does not go down to the noise level. It can be explained by a high noise level. According to the definitions used the peaks N2 and P2 have to be determined. It does not seem to be advisable to allow too much influence of subjective judgement. It would introduce too much of observer bias to the evaluation. The latencies of N2 and P2 (Fig.

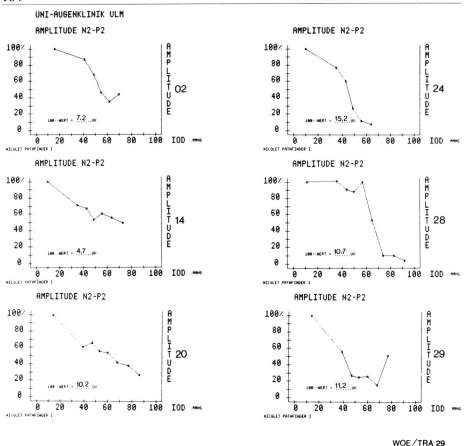

Fig. 7b. Amplitude/pressure curves plotted according to the values measured in Fig. 7a. (From: Stodtmeister *et al.*, 1988a)[4].

6d) do not show a pattern which can be brought in connection with the pressure rise.

In Fig. 7a the recordings of six further cases of the series are shown and in Fig. 7b the amplitude/pressure curves derived from these recordings. Case 24 clearly shows a monotone behavior. The behavior of case 02 has to be classified also as monotone because the final rise of the amplitude has clearly to be attributed to the influence of noise. In cases 14 and 20 the classification depends on the definitions used because it has to be kept in mind that smaller deviations from the monotone behavior can also be due to noise.

The latencies of N2 and P2 (Fig. 7d) do not show a clear influence of the artificial pressure rise.

We have done these experiments also by averaging 25 single responses at 1.9 Hz. In Fig. 8a ten out of 30 recordings are shown and in Fig. 8b the amplitude/pressure curves derived from these recordings.

It is seen that the recordings are of reasonable quality. The peaks in the averages of 25 responses could as easily be identified as the peaks in the averages of 50 responses. By averaging 25 single responses the recording time is nearly halved and the signal to noise ratio is reduced from 7 to 5 only. According to our experience this reduction in signal to noise ratio can be taken into account.

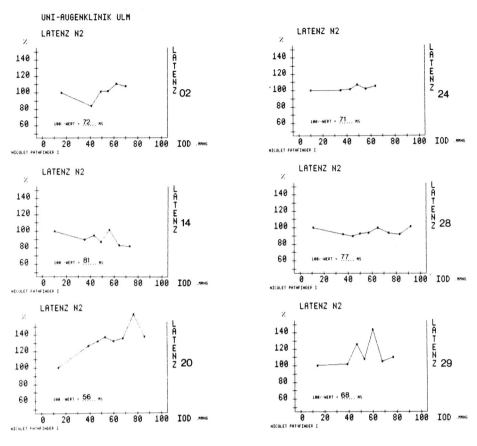

Fig. 7c. Latency N2/pressure curves plotted according to the values measured in Fig. 7a.

Discussion

It had been assumed that there is no autoregulation of the circulation in the optic nerve head until 1984[27]. We were the first who could demonstrate by a clinically applicable method using visually evoked potentials that there are signs of an autoregulatory process in the optic nerve head[15].

Comparison of the two techniques

We are regarding a non monotone or weakly monotone behavior of the amplitude/pressure curves as sign of autoregulation in the circulation of the optic nerve head and a monotone behavior as sign of lack of this autoregulation which can be observed in patients with primary open angle glaucoma[15] and in patients with low tension glaucoma[17,18].

The monotone behavior can therefore be regarded as pathognomonic for primary open angle glaucoma and low tension glaucoma.

The specificity (the fraction of true negative test results in a sample of healthy subjects) is for the analog method 0.8. For the averaging methods shown here (1.9 Hz, 25 sweeps or 50) the specificity is also 0.8. Thus averaging seems to be suitable for pressure tolerance testing. However, pressure tolerance testing as done by us has to be carried out quite fast which results in the necessity of handling a relatively large amount of data in a limited time[13,14]. This should be regarded in planning experiments and in judging results.

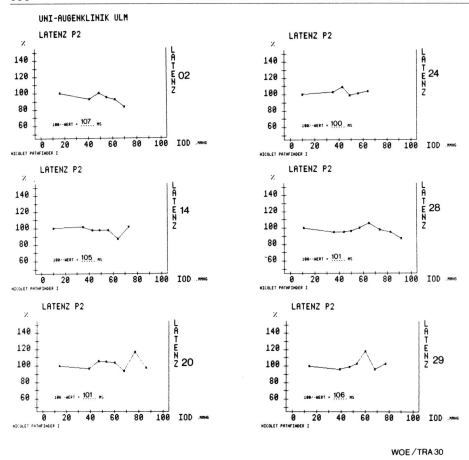

Fig. 7d. Latency P2/pressure curves plotted according to the values measured in Fig. 7a.

According to the experiments done until now the phase information given by the vector voltmeter seems to give no additional information with regard to the influence of the artificial pressure rise. It is however useful in judging the quality of the potentials.

Information in the time domain is of great importance in the diagnosis of diseases of the optic nerve, *e.g.*, optic neuritis[28]. Our hope that the measurements of latencies could improve the pressure tolerance testing by averaged transient potentials has not been fulfilled according to experiments done by us until now[4,5,13,14]. Thus it seems feasible to carry out the pressure tolerance test by using a vector voltmeter either analog or digital.

The fact that in averaging the potentials can be inspected is not as advantageous as it seems to be because the potentials themselves give only a limited amount of information on the influences of unwanted signals. The seeming drawback of the vector voltmeter not showing the signals can be overcome by an appropriate test method devised by two of us[29] and recommended by Van der Tweel *et al.*[26].

For the assessment of the autoregulatory phenomenon the time course of the experiment should be fixed. Artifacts however are disturbing the recording of the visually evoked cortical potentials. With the vector voltmeter these artifacts can be easily recognized and taken into account in the evaluation process. In the averaging technique it is advisable to use an artifact rejection which prevents too large artifacts to be included in the average. This fact may influence the time course and has to be regarded in the evaluation.

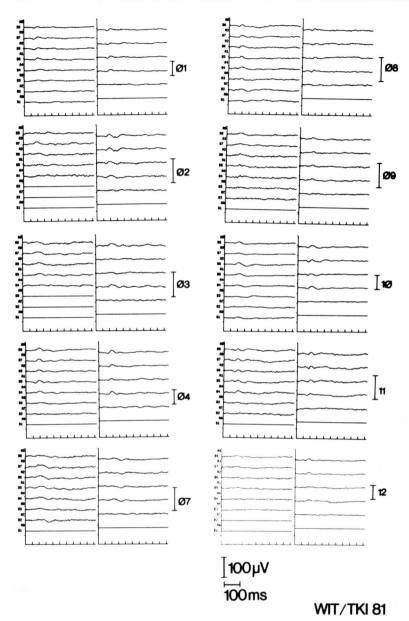

Fig. 8a. Pressure tolerance test. Visually evoked cortical potentials at 1.9 Hz r/s, 25 sweeps per average of ten subjects. Ordinate: the bars of different length on the right of the systems represent 100 µV. Further information in Fig. 5.

General aspects

In pressure tolerance testing we are regarding the eye as a "black box" and are recording the function – monitored by visually evoked cortical potentials – during stepwise artificially increased intraocular pressure. The method applied shows in the amplitude/pressure curves differences which can be interpreted as a sign of the presence or absence of an autoregulatory phenomenon. That this autoregulation is due to processes in the circulation of the optic nerve head is hypothesized by us. The site of origin and the underlying

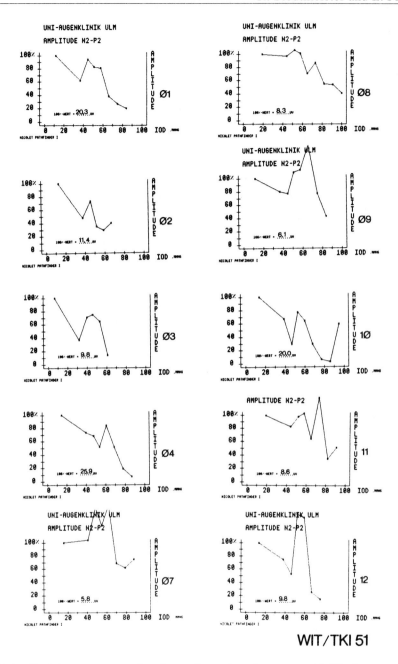

Fig. 8b. Amplitude/pressure curves plotted according to the values measured in Fig. 8a.

mechanism may be different. The specificity of 0.8 is of an order of magnitude which is sufficient to consider this test for early diagnosis of glaucoma.

References

1. Graham P: Epidemiology of chronic glaucoma. In: Heilmann K, Richardson K (eds): Glaucoma – Conceptions of a Disease, pp 7–17. Stuttgart: Thieme 1978
2. Hayreh SS: Structure and blood supply of the optic nerve. In: Richardson K, Hielmann K (eds): Glaucoma – Conceptions of Disease, pp 78–96. Stuttgart/New York: Thieme 1978
3. Ulrich WD, Ulrich Ch: Okulooszillodynamographie, ein neues Verfahren zur Bestimmung des Ophthalmikablutdruckes und zur okulären Pulskurvenanalyse. Klin Mbl Augenheilk 186:385–388, 1985
4. Stodtmeister R, Hornberger M, Hoefer M, Gaus W, Pillunat L, Swobodnik W, Bischof G: Okulo–Oszillo–Dynamographie nach Ulrich und Ulrich: Ergebnisse bei Augengesunden. Klin Mbl Augenheilk 192:219–233, 1988a
5. Stodtmeister R, Pillunat L, Wilmanns I: Drucktoleranzprüfung des Sehnerven mit gemittelten transienten visuell evozierten kortikalen Potentialen. Fortschr Ophthalmol 85:402–406, 1988b
6. Benedikt O, Bartl G, Hiti H, Mandl H: Die Änderung der elektrophysiologischen Antwort am menschlichen Auge bei kurzzeitiger Erhöhung des intraokularen Druckes. Graefes Arch Clin Exp Ophthalmol 192:57–64, 1974
7. Bartl G, Benedikt O, Hiti H, Mandl H: Das elektrophysiologische Verhalten gesunder und glaukomkranker menschlicher Augen bei kurzzeitiger intraoculärer Druckbelastung. Graefes Arch Clin Exp Ophthalmol 195:201–206, 1975
8. Bartl G, Benedikt O, Hiti H: The effect of elevated intraocular pressure on the human ERG and VER. Docum Ophthalmol 275–279, 1976
9. Bartl G: Das Elektroretinogramm und das evozierte Sehrindenpotential bei normalen und an Glaukom erkrankten Augen. Graefes Arch Clin Exp Ophthalmol 207:243–269, 1978
10. Müller A, Brühning HK, Sohr H: Ein Dynamometer. Ber Dtsch Ophthalmol Ges 52:434–438, 1938
11. Ulrich WD: Grundlagen und Methodik der Ophthalmodynamometrie (ODM), Ophthalmodynamographie (ODG), Temporalisdynamographie (TDG), pp 1–147. Berlin/Leipzig: Georg Thieme 1976
12. Kukan F: Weitere Angaben zur experimentellen Hypotonie und Hypertonie. Klin Mbl Augenheilk 89:553, 1931
13. Stodtmeister R, Pillunat L, Wilmanns I: Drucktoleranztestung des Sehnervs mit Hilfe gemittelter, visuell evozierter kortikaler Potentiale. Spektrum Augenheilk 1:311–314, 1987a
14. Stodtmeister R, Wilmanns I, Pillunat L: Methodik okulärer Kreislaufdiagnostik beim Glaukom. In: Stodtmeister (ed): Okuläre Durchblutungsstörungen, pp 95–101. Stuttgart: Enke Verlag 1987b
15. Pillunat L, Stodtmeister R, Wilmanns I, Christ Th: Autoregulation of ocular blood flow during changes of intraocular pressure. Graefes Arch Clin Exp Ophthalmol 223:219–223, 1985
16. Pillunat L, Stodtmeister R, Wilmanns I, Christ Th: Oculäre Kreislaufdiagnostik beim Niederdruckglaucom. Klin Mbl Augenheilk 188:526–529, 1986
17. Pillunat L, Stodtmeister R: Oculäre Kreislaufdiagnostik bei verschiedenen Glaukomformen. In: Stodtmeister R, Christ Th, Pillunat LE, Ulrich WD (eds): Okuläre Durchblutungsstörungen. Grundlagen–Diagnostik–Therapie, pp 102–107. Stuttgart: Enke Verlag 1987a
18. Pillunat L, Stodtmeister R, Wilmanns I: Pressure compliance of the optic nerve head in low tension glaucoma. Br J Ophthalmol 71:181–187, 1986b
19. Fricker SJ: Application of synchronous detector techniques for electroretinographic studies in patients with retinitis pigmentosa. Invest Ophthalmol Vis Sci 10/5:329–339, 1971
20. Fricker SJ: Numerical measurements of retinal and occipital function. Arch Ophthalmol 76:37–46, 1974
21. Padmos P, Norren D van: The vector voltmeter as a tool to measure electroretinogram spectral sensitivity and dark adaption. Invest Ophthalmol Vis Sci 11/9:783–788, 1972
22. Regan D: Comparison of transient and steady state methods. Ann NY Acad Sci 338:45–71, 1982
23. Hayatsu H: Measurement of blood pressure in retina, especially on calibration curves for Mikuni's ophthalmodynamometer. 1. Calibration curves by Schiötz's standardized tonometer. Acta Soc Ophthalmol Jpn 68:119–119. 1964a
24. Hayatsu H: Measurement of blood pressure in retina, especially on calibration curves for Mikuni's ophthalmodynamometer. 2. Calibration curves by Goldmann's applanation tonometer. Acta Soc. Ophthalmol Jpn 68:175–180, 1964b
25. Batschelet E: Introduction to mathematics for life scientists. Berlin: Springer 1971
26. Van der Tweel H, Carr R, Hellner K: Report of the committee on instrumentation and procedures in visual electrophysiology at the request of the Concilium Ophthalmologicum Universale. Docum Ophthalmol 1–13, 1981
27. Ulrich WD, Ulrich Ch: An electrophysiological approach to the diagnosis and treatment of glaucoma. Dev Ophthalmol 9:140–146, 1984
28. Halliday AM, McDonald WI, Mushin J: Visual evoked potentials in patients with demyelinating disease. In: Desmedt (ed): Visual Evoked Potentials in Man: New Developments, pp 438–449. Oxford:Clarendon 1977
29. Wilmanns I, Stodtmeister R: Ein neues Verfahren zur Kalibrierung elektrophysiologischer Untersuchungseinheiten. Graefes Arch Ophthalmol 205:33–39, 1977
30. Stodtmeister R, Pillunat L, Mattern A, Polly E: Die Beziehung zwischen negativer Druckdifferenz und künstlich erhöhtem Augeninnendruck bei der Saugnapfmethode. Klin Mbl Augenheilk: in press

DISCUSSION

Erik L. Greve : Are the IOP values on your graphs actual measurements or are they estimates from the suction pressure?

Richard Stodtmeister : They are estimates from the suction pressure. However, as it was pointed out earlier, this estimation is as accurate as the estimation of the arterial blood pressure from the pressure in the sphygmomanometer cuff. We feel, therefore, that it is reliable enough for our purpose.

Harry A. Quigley : How long did the IOP elevation last at each point measured ?

Richard Stodtmeister : The time was not fixed. We switched each step to the next, only after we had had a reliable recording. This takes usually about 10 to 20 seconds.

Harry A. Quigley : Do you know approximately how many pattern reversals you had at each point ?

Richard Stodtmeister : The number of pattern reversals is of some importance when the averaging technique is used. Our preference goes to the analog, or steady-state potentials, where you have a continuous recording and you only read the amplitude of the potentials, as on a voltmeter. Of course there is a time constant which you have to fix on your equipment, and it plays some role in the quality of your recordings, but I don't think that we should go into such complicated details. We used a time constant of 4 seconds and it gave reliable recordings in 60 patients. The quality can be poor at very low amplitudes, so it is advisable to consider as critical pressure the IOP where the amplitude drops to 20% of the baseline, instead of extrapolating to zero.

Harry A. Quigley : What are the sizes of the test field and of the checks, and the reversal rates that you think give the best quality recordings ?

Richard Stodtmeister : We have used reversal rates of 7 and 15 Hz. The field size was 12 to 16 degrees wide and the individual checks between 26 and 100 minutes of arc. You have to determine for each patient which check size gives you the best results.

Harry A. Quigley : It seems, from your graphs, that in glaucoma patients the response is better maintained to higher intraocular pressures. Is this true ?

Richard Stodtmeister : No, there is no real difference: the amplitudes are of the same order in glaucoma patients and in normals.

Harry A. Quigley : Well, at intraocular pressures of 50 mmHg, or slightly less, there seems to be quite a difference in amplitude values, with the glaucoma patients doing better than the normals.

Richard Stodtmeister : Yes, the normal eyes have somewhat lower amplitudes at intermediate pressure levels. This is because it is a well regulated system that can react with some decrease, while in glaucoma the system is working at full power. It is as if you had an overheated house in one case, and in the other a normally heated house which will counteract the drop in temperature brought about by the opening of a door.

Douglas R. Anderson : We should also keep in mind that these amplitudes are expressed as percentages of the baseline. And if in the glaucoma patients the baseline amplitude is already diminished then you will have higher percentages in the course of your experiment.

Harry A. Quigley : I rather doubt that the baseline amplitude will have decreased from normal, Doug, unless of course there are just a few percent of the nerve fibers left! What we seem to have here, is a set of glaucoma eyes that appear to maintain a normal function under abnormal conditions longer than the normals. They seem to be over-regulating, if anything, but maybe that's just a question of terminology.

Juan E. Grunwald : Maybe the explanation is in the time-course of the experiment. The normal curve seems straightforward to me: the dip in amplitude occurs at the first point with raised IOP, that is at about 20 seconds of suction, because at that time there is no regulation yet. But by the time you have reached an IOP of 50 or so, one or one-and-a-half minutes have elapsed and the autoregulation is working. It is a bit more difficult for me to understand the glaucoma curves which lack the dip. Is it possible that the measurements took longer in glaucoma patients, so that the autoregulation was already active at lower intraocular pressures ?

Richard Stodtmeister : No, there was no difference. The time course was the same as in normals.

Lutz E. Pillunat : I think that the amplitude/pressure curves are not the best way to judge the time course of the autoregulation because the amplitude is plotted against pressure, which is dependent on the timing of the experiment, so that the effects of time and pressure are mixed. But if you take a normal subject and increase his IOP to a certain level and then wait for two minutes or so before increasing it further, you see that the amplitude goes down at the onset of pressure, then rises again after one minute or so, to remain stable until the next pressure increase. We haven't done this yet in glaucoma patients, though.

Harry A. Quigley : But can't that be due to a tonographic effect that may have reduced your baseline IOP to, say, 7 instead of your original 15 mmHg ?

Lutz E. Pillunat : We cannot exclude that, of course, but we believe that it is rather the circulation that has adapted to the IOP increase.

Maurice E. Langham : But you can't expect any dramatic tonographic effect in the one or two minutes that each step takes!

Harry A. Quigley : Maybe not, Maurice, but at that rate the whole series of steps will take something like 15 minutes, and that's surely long enough for important tonographic changes.

Juan E. Grunwald : That would be easy to find out: you would have to repeat your experiment with the same pressure steps and measure the IOP instead of the cortical evoked potentials. You would then know exactly what your IOP is at each moment.

Discussion

Lutz E. Pillunat : Yes, that is a possibility.

Erik L. Greve : But, finally, what is the answer to the original question: do the glaucoma patients seem to preserve their function better than the normals or don't they?

Richard Stodtmeister : They do; in this range of pressures, their amplitudes seem to decrease more slowly. As I said before, I think that this is because they have a disturbed autoregulation and their initial flow is higher. But even if this interpretation isn't correct, the important thing to look at is whether the technique can be used to separate normals from glaucoma patients with good predictive performance, that is with high sensitivity and specificity. If it does, then we can start using it without understanding everything from the beginning.

Tom van den Berg : I have one question about the monotone, weakly monotone and non-monotone behaviors that you described. Is it possible that they just reflect variability and that all behaviors would turn out to be the same if the signal-to-noise ratio was better ?

Richard Stodtmeister : Maybe. In some cases the recordings are rather noisy, especially with the transient averaging technique, which can't separate very efficiently visually evoked potentials from brain activity. Still, as it is the most widely used technique, we are trying to evaluate if it is reliable enough to be used for this test, even if it isn't the best choice.

Erik L. Greve : But do you think that there is an essential difference in behavior or that it is just due to the technique ?

Richard Stodtmeister : No, there is an essential difference in behavior, only it isn't always correctly brought out by the transient averaging technique: its specificity is about 80%, which means that it will show a monotone, glaucoma-like behavior in 20% of the normals. This is a quite good performance for a diagnostic technique, equivalent to the performance of X-ray in lung disease. We think, therefore, that we can recommend its use with the figures given in the paper (1.9 Hz, 25 or 50 pattern reversals).

Harry A. Quigley : What is the reproducibility of the method? If you tested the same person ten times, would you always get the same values ?

Richard Stodtmeister : We haven't tested that yet, but it is planned as one of our next steps.

Douglas R. Anderson : But do you know if your patients would show the same behavior, monotone or non-monotone, if tested on two separate occasions ?

Richard Stodtmeister : Glaucoma patients will, yes. But in normals we haven't found out yet. We plan to do it shortly, as I told you.

PRESSURE TOLERANCE TEST:
II. Clinical results and sensitivity

Lutz E. Pillunat and Richard Stodtmeister

*University Eye Clinic (Dir: Prof. Dr. R. Marquardt),
Prittwitzstr. 43, 7900 Ulm, FRG*

Introduction

Since many years the blood flow of the eye and especially optic nerve blood flow was investigated with different methods and by various investigations[1,11,20,28]. One major question in this field concerns the regulation of ocular blood flow. The retina, unlike the choroid, has an efficient autoregulation so that blood is mainly unaffected by intraocular pressure.

As shown by Hayreh[14-16] the peripapillary choroid is the primary source of blood supply to the prelaminar part and retrolaminar regions of the optic nerve head while the lamina cribrosa is usually supplied by branches of the short posterior ciliary arteries. The surface nerve fiber layer is supplied by branches from the retinal arteries. In spite of the fact that the main blood supply of the optic nerve head has the same source as the choroid, many hints were given[9,10] that an efficient vascular autoregulation controls the blood flow in the optic nerve head. Geijer and Bill[13] and Sossi and Anderson[29] showed that a quite efficient autoregulation of optic disc blood flow exists – meaning that there is practically no reduction in blood flow in the optic nerve head or at the region of the lamina cribrosa until the intraocular pressure approaches the arterial pressure, reducing the blood flow in all intraocular structures more or less simultaneously.

Also, during the last few years, experiments in man suggest that a vascular autoregulation in the human optic nerve head exists. As previously shown[23,24] autoregulation of optic nerve circulation can be assessed by recording visually evoked responses under artificial intraocular pressure increase. By this test method, *i.e.*, pressure tolerance testing of the optic nerve head[33,25] it seems possible to describe such a physiological behavior as well as to differentiate different types of glaucoma.

Reproducibility

Beside the interindividual differences in using a test method and beside the methodology-dependent variability, the reproducibility, *i.e.* the intraindividual differences, has to be regarded as a major important fact.

To judge the reproducibility of the results in pressure tolerance testing of the optic nerve head, seven healthy subjects were examined. The pressure tolerance test was carried out by using steady state evoked (15 Hz) potentials. The signals were processed by a two-channel phase sensitive detector, which works rather like a vector-voltmeter. Projected checkerboard-reversals were used for stimulation (for exact methods and technical data see refs[23,24,33].). Seven healthy subjects were examined under the same conditions between two and five times. In all healthy subjects the intraindividual variability of an individual amplitude/pressure curve (a/p-curve) ranged in an acceptable order of magnitude. As described earlier[23] a weakly monotonous or not monotonous slope of the a/p-curve (see

*Supported by the Deutsche Forschungsgemeinschaft

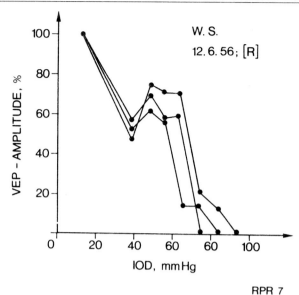

Fig. 1. Amplitude/pressure-curves of the right eye of a 32-year-old male healthy subject. The test was repeated on three different days under the same conditions.

Fig. 1) has to be regarded as normal, *i.e.*, as a physiological behavior in "pressure tolerance testing". This behavior was found to be highly specific[30] in healthy subjects, also when using different test methods.

In seven subjects in which the reproducibility of an individual a/p-curve was tested only a change from weakly monotonous to not monotonous and *vice versa* could be observed. A drift to a monotonous behavior was not found in the subjects examined. Therefore, the main criterion for judging an a/p-curve remained unchanged when the test was repeated up to five times.

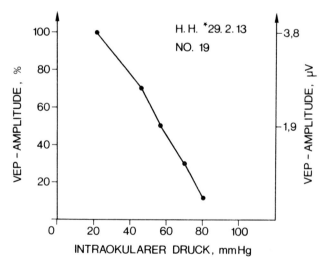

Fig. 2. Amplitude/pressure-curve of a 76-year-old male subject suffering from advanced primary open angle glaucoma with visual field loss and severe cupping of the optic disc. The absolute values of the VER–amplitudes are given on the right ordinate, the relative values of the VER–amplitudes in percent are given on the left ordinate.

Table 1. Behavior of the amplitude pressure curves in 37 randomly chosen eyes of 37 glaucoma patients. The sensitivity of the monotonous criterion amounts to 81%.

Classification	n	n	S
Weakly monotonous	4	8	19%
Not monotonous	4		
Monotonous	29	29	81%
	37	37	100%

Primary open angle glaucoma (POAG)
Low tension glaucoma (LTG)

As described in previous papers[23,25,26] the results of pressure tolerance testing in patients with confirmed primary open angle glaucoma are quite different compared to those of healthy subjects. The slope of the a/p-curve shows no intermittent plateau or intermittent increase (defined as weakly monotonous or not monotonous behavior) but a monotonous decrease to the noise level, *i.e.*, in patients with confirmed primary open angle glaucoma, the VER-amplitudes drop continuously under artificial intraocular pressure increase (Fig. 2).

Thirty-seven consecutive, confirmed POAG-patients (advanced visual field loss in automated computer perimetry; c/d–ratio>0.5; decreased outflow facility and IOP exceeding 25 mmHg without therapy) were examined. In patients who suffered from POAG in both eyes one eye was randomly chosen for evaluation. In 29 patients the VER-amplitude dropped under artificial intraocular pressure increase monotonously down to the noise level, four patients showed a weakly monotonous a/p-curve and in four patients a not monotonous behavior was observed (Table 1).

Using the criteria mentioned that an intermittent plateau or increase in the a/p-curve represents the physiological behavior, a sensitivity of 81% was found in 37 consecutive, confirmed glaucoma patients.

In 19 consecutive, confirmed low tension glaucoma patients the VER amplitude dropped in all cases under minor artificial intraocular pressure increases down to the noise level. In none of the patients examined was a weakly monotonous or not monotonous a/p-curve found. This means a sensitivity of 100% in patients suffering from low tension glaucoma. The critical pressure (see [30]), *i.e.*, that IOP which corresponds to the 20% VER-amplitude (noise level), was reached at 58 mmHg. This value proved to be statistically significantly lower than in POAG patients (Table 2).

The pressure tolerance test was also carried out by using transient visually evoked potentials at a pattern reversal rate of 1.9 Hz. As Stodtmeister[30] showed, the monotonous curve characteristic in patients with primary open angle glaucoma and in patients with low tension glaucoma can also be assessed by using this method. In Fig. 4 a,b,c, the original recordings and the a/p-curve of a young patient suffering from advanced low tension

Table 2. The mean value of the critical pressure in patients suffering from low tension glaucoma set as a border value (58 mmHg). Using a 4 chart board and by statistical analysis using the Fisher test (comparable to the chi–square test) the difference between low tension glaucoma and high tension glaucoma is statistically significant on the $p=0.01$ level

	≥ 58 mmHg	<58 mmHg
Low tension glaucoma	7	12
High tension glaucoma	36	1
	43	13

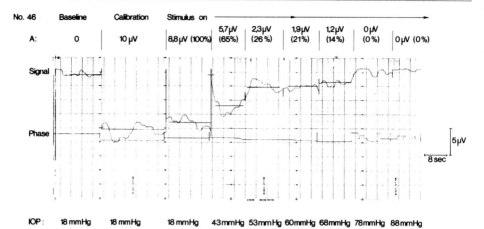

Fig. 3A. Original continuous registration of the pressure tolerance test in a 83-year-old female patient suffering from low tension glaucoma.

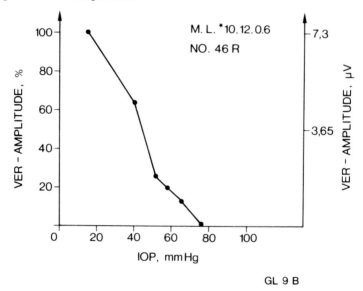

Fig. 3B. Amplitude/pressure curve corresponding to the original registration in Fig. 3A

glaucoma are demonstrated. Under minor artificial intraocular pressure increase the VER-amplitude dropped down to the noise level which was already reached at an IOP of 45 mmHg.

Neuroretinal rim area and pressure tolerance test in ocular hypertension

In 16 consecutive patients suffering from ocular hypertension (no visual field loss in repeated computer perimetry, c/d-ratio < 0.3; normal outflow facility and IOP exceeding 21 mmHg without therapy) the pressure compliance test was performed using steady state evoked potentials (15 Hz). The signals were analyzed by a vector-voltmeter (see refs.[33,23]). Additionally, stereophotographs of the optic disc were taken and these pictures were analyzed by computer assisted planimetry. This study was carried out as a double-center, single masked procedure. The pressure tolerance test was performed at the Department of Ophthalmology of the Ulm University and the stereophotographs – also taken in Ulm –

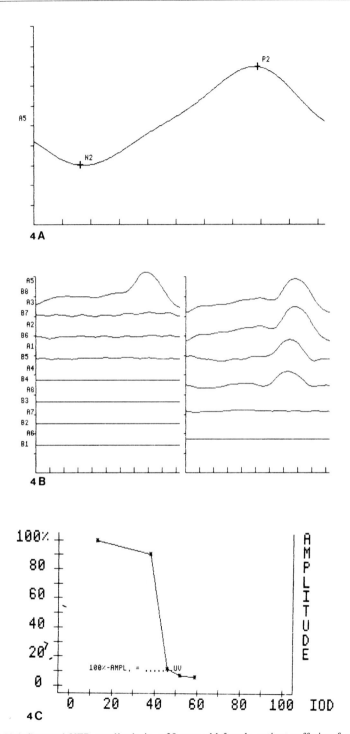

Fig. 4. A: Uninfluenced VER-amplitude in a 29-year-old female patient suffering from low tension glaucoma. The VER-amplitudes were recorded by a stimulation rate of 1.9 Hz and by means of the averaging method. B: Original VER–recordings of the pressure tolerance test corresponding to Fig. 4A. 4A shows the uninfluenced signal and the recordings B8, B7, B6, B5 show the VER-amplitudes under pressure load. C: Amplitude/pressure curve corresponding to the original registrations in 4A and 4B.

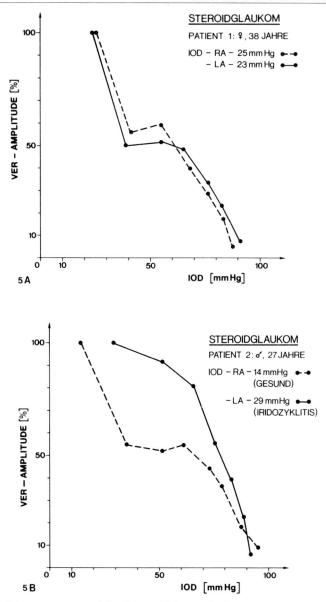

Fig. 5. A: Amplitude/pressure curves of the right and left eye of a 38-year-old male patient suffering from steroid glaucoma in both eyes. The VER recordings were done by a vectorvoltmeter. B: Amplitude/pressure curves of the right and left eye of a 27-year-old patient suffering from a steroid glaucoma in his left eye.

were analyzed at the Glaucoma Center of the University of British Columbia in Vancouver/Canada[21].

In 24 eyes a weakly monotonous or not monotonous behavior of the a/p–curves was found and in seven eyes no intermittent plateau could be observed. Because of a low visual acuity no visual evoked potentials were recordable in one eye. Analysis of the optic disc data showed a pathologically reduced neuroretinal rim in seven eyes and a healthy, normal rim area in 24 eyes.

Because one part of the data has to be characterized as continuous data (neuroretinal rim area) and the other part as bipolar data (slope of the a/p–curves) the biserial–correlation coefficient according to Meyer–Bahlburg[19] was used for statistical analysis. The correlation coefficient was $r = 0.58$ and proved to be statistically significant on the $p = 0.05$ level.

Secondary glaucoma

To investigate different stages of secondary glaucoma only the inclusion criterion : intraocular pressure higher than 21 mm Hg due to variable diseases except POAG or ocular hypertension, was applied. Four patients suffering from pseudoexfoliation syndrome, three patients with steroid glaucoma and three patients with neovascularization glaucoma were examined.

The slope of the a/p–curves was found to be heterogeneous in these ten patients suffering from different kinds and stages of secondary glaucoma. In four eyes the curve characteristic has to be judged as monotonous and in six eyes as healthy, i.e., an intermittent increase or plateau in the a/p-curve was detectable. In spite of the heterogeneous slope of the a/p-curves in this group of patients a correlation between a monotonous a/p-curve and optic nerve damage can be demonstrated. Two patients suffered (see Fig. 5 A,B) from steroid glaucoma and therefore the IOP increase was due to medical therapy. In patient 1 the intraocular pressure ranged from 22–26 mmHg. No visual field loss and no morphological optic nerve damage were detectable. Due to a frequently relapsing iridocyclitis in both eyes this patient had to apply dexamethasone eye drops for about three months. Patient 2 suffered also from a frequently relapsing iridocyclitis but only in his left eye. For five years he has had to apply dexamethasone eyedrops nearly every day. He showed severe cupping of the disc and an advanced visual field loss in his left eye.

As demonstrated in Fig. 5 A, both eyes of patient 1 showed a weakly monotonous a/p-curve, i.e., with regard to the defined evaluation criteria a physiological behavior. However, the a/p-curve of the left eye in patient 2 showed a monotonous slope, while its healthy companion showed a weakly monotonous behavior[27,24].

Discussion

The results presented here show that eyes affected with open angle glaucoma behave in a manifestly different manner than eyes of healthy controls under the conditions of the test procedure described. In the case of glaucomatous eyes the intermittently occurring plateau in the a/p-curve, i.e., a weakly monotonous behavior, is missing. This curve characteristic could be found in 37 consecutively examined glaucoma patients. Therefore, the sensitivity of the method has to be regarded as 81%. For clinical purposes and for routine examinations the specificity, i.e., to identify a healthy eye as being healthy and also the sensitivity, i.e., to identify a glaucomatous eye as being glaucomatous, ranges in an acceptable order of magnitude. Furthermore, the reproducibility of the results was good.

Increases of IOP influence the circulatory perfusion of neural elements within the eye: as a result, the function of these elements is modified and may lead to complete functional disruption (as a result of sufficient increases in IOP). From studies conducted by Bartl[4,5] we know that the electroretinogram, as a measure of retinal function (rods and cones, receptor cells, bipolar cells, and amacrine cells), detects artificial IOP increases far less sensitively than visually evoked cortical potentials. An explanation for these findings may be derived from the considerations put forward by Gafner and Goldmann[12], who believed that an increase in IOP has an unfavorable effect principally on the blood supply in the area of the lamina cribrosa. On the basis of further results described in the literature[35], it may be assumed that in case of IOP increase, the blood supply is first of all influenced in the laminar and prelaminar part of the optic nerve head. This applies to a long, continuous increase as well as to an artificially induced, acute increase in pressure like that induced in the present studies. The principle of a loading test was used here in the same way as the exercise ECG is generally applied in cardiology. With regard to the literature available and to the results of Bartl we consider the prelaminar section of the optic nerve head to be the area where damage occurs. Vascular autoregulation was found in monkey studies conducted by Geijer and Bill[13]. In photopapillometry, under artificially induced IOP increase, Robert and Maurer[28] were also able to find indications for a vascular autoregulation in the optic nerve head. As already demonstrated in earlier studies[23–25] a/p curves of healthy eyes were not subject to a continuous (monotonous) decrease, but rather, after an initial dip, remained flat (weakly monotonous) or even increased in VER-amplitude (not monotonous). These curves did not progress to continuous decline to the noise level until higher IOP values were obtained. A counter or autoregulatory mechanism of the blood vessels in the optic nerve head offers an explanation for this response. Such an autoregulatory mechanism, which maintains a reserve perfusion of the optic nerve head and thus its functional capacity despite increased intraocular pressure is, according to our results, absent in patients with confirmed open angle glaucoma or low tension glaucoma.

A complete interruption of conductivity in the optic nerve head, that is, the decline in VER-amplitudes to the noise level, takes place in healthy subjects and in patients with open angle glaucoma with approximately the same intraocular pressure (critical pressure approx. 80 mmHg). Patients with low tension glaucoma manifest this interruption earlier during IOP loading, like for example 60 mmHg. Anderson[3] posits that in addition to an increase in intraocular pressure, other pathogenetic factors play a part in the origin of glaucomatous damage. Since the type of damage involved is comparable in low tension glaucoma and in open angle glaucoma[17,18] although the damaging force of increased IOP is absent, much points to a vascular origin of LTG[7,8]. Our results show that as a response to pressure loading, mutual factors exist between open angle glaucoma and low tension glaucoma; namely the sign of autoregulation in both forms of glaucoma. The difference in pressure sensitivity – that is, adjustment of functional capacity at IOPs of 60 mmHg (critical pressure) – provides an initial basis for explaining both the pathologic affinity of the two symptoms as well as the increased sensitivity of the optic nerve in low tension glaucoma. This means that intraocular pressures that may be considered normal in other eyes are already capable of disturbing perfusion and of effecting a decline of optic nerve fibers in low tension glaucoma.

When one compares the results presented herein with the ocular hypertensives, a nonhomogeneous distribution emerges. Certain patients of a homogeneous group show an intermittent plateau (weakly monotonous a/p-curve) as a sign of vascular autoregulation; others react in the same manner as those with open angle glaucoma. No indication can be found with regard to patient variation in this group of ocular hypertensives, with exception of the different a/p-curves. If in some ocular hypertensives, the kink in the a/p-curves as a sign of autoregulation is missing, this indicates that one deals with eyes with a characteristic glaucoma. As shown in earlier studies, an eye of this type might be classified as having suspected glaucoma. If, instead, autoregulation is present, we assume that no disease process is at work. This conclusion is supported by the fairly good correlation of the autoregulation–behavior compared to results in optic nerve head analysis.

All patients except one, who were rated as showing a pathologically reduced neuroretinal rim area, react in the pressure tolerance test with a monotonous a/p-curve. In six patients a healthy neuroretinal rim area was found and no sign of autoregulation could be observed in the a/p-curves. This result led to the conclusion that a deficient autoregulation may be a prerequisite for glaucomatous optic nerve damage and may be detected earlier than morphological changes like a reduced neuroretinal rim area. Observations in patients suffering from secondary glaucoma indicate that such a lack of autoregulation may develop with time. The absence of autoregulation in one part of the ocular hypertensives examined may signify a premature transition from simple ocular hypertension to primary open angle glaucoma. Observations during an extended period must show whether patients in whom the sign of autoregulation is absent, actually develop a glaucoma with corresponding optic nerve damage and whether patients with a still intact autoregulatory reserve progress to loss of autoregulation or not.

References

1. Alm A, Bill A: Ocular and optic nerve blood flow at normal and increased intraocular pressure in monkeys: a study with radioactively labeled microspheres including flow determinations in the brain and other tissues. Exp Eye Res 15:15–29, 1973
2. Anderson DR: Ultrastructure of the optic nerve head. Arch Ophthalmol 83:63–73, 1970
3. Anderson DR: The posterior segment in glaucomatous eyes. In: Luetjen–Drecoll E (ed): Basic Aspects of Glaucoma Research, pp 167–190. Stuttgart/New York: Schattauer 1982
4. Bartl G: Das Elektroretinogramm und das evozierte Sehrindenpotential bei normalen und an glaukom erkrankten Augen. Graefes Arch Clin Exp Ophthalmol 207:243–269, 1978
5. Bartl G, Benedikt O, Hiti H: Das elektrophysiologische Verhalten gesunder und glaukomkranker menschlicher augen bei kurzzeitiger intraokularer Druckbelastung. Graefes Arch Clin Exp Ophthalmol 195:201–206, 1975
6. Batschelet E: Introduction to Mathematics for Life Scientists. Berlin: Springer 1971
7. Drance SM: Some factors in the production of low tension glaucoma. Br J Ophthalmol 56:229–242, 1972
8. Drance SN, Sweenly VP, Morgan RW, Feldman F: Studies of factors involved in the production of low tension glaucoma. Arch Ophthalmol 89:457–465, 1973
9. Ernest TJ: Autoregulation of optic– disc oxygen tension. Invest Ophthal Vis Sci 13:101–108, 1974
10. Ernest TJ: Pathogenesis of glaucomatous optic nerve disease. Trans Am Ophthalmol Soc 73:366–372, 1975
11. Ernest TJ: Optic disc blood flow. Trans Ophthalmol Soc UK 96:348–359, 1976
12. Gafner F, Goldmann H: Experimentelle Untersuchungen über den Zusammenhang von Augendrucksteigerung und Gesichtsfeldschädigung. Ophthalmologica 130:357–377, 1955
13. Geijer C, Bill A: Effects of raised intraocular pressure on retinal, prelaminar and retrolaminar optic nerve blood flow in monkeys. Invest Ophthal Vis Sci 18:1030–1042, 1979
14. Hayreh SS: Anatomy and physiology of the optic nerve head. Trans Am Acad Ophthalmol Otol 78:240–254, 1974
15. Hayreh SS: Pathogenesis of optic nerve damage and visual field defects. In: Heilmann K, Richardson KT (eds): Glaucoma – Conceptions of a Disease, pp 104–137. Stuttgart: Thieme 1978
16. Hayreh SS: Structure and blood supply of the optic disc. In: Heilamnn K, Richardson KY (eds): Glaucoma – Conceptions of a Disease, pp 78–103. Stuttgart: Thieme 1978
17. King D, Douglas G, Drance S, Schulzer M, Wijsman K: Comparison of visual field defects in normal tension glaucoma and high tension glaucoma. Am J Ophthalmol 101:204–207, 1986
18. King D, Douglas G, Drance S, Wijsman K: Optic nerve analysis in low tension glaucoma versus high pressure glaucoma. Invest Ophthalmol Vis Sci Suppl 27:41, 1986
19. Lienert GA: Verteilungsfreie Methoden in der Biostatistik. Meisenheim/Glahn: Anton Hain 1973
20. Phelps CD: The pathogenesis of optic nerve damage in glaucoma: a review of the vascular hypothesis. In: Blodi FC (ed): Current Concepts in Ophthalmology, pp 142–161. St. Louis: C V Mosby 1972
21. Pillunat LE, Douglas GR, Stodtmeister R, Drance SM: Pressure compliance of the optic nerve head an neuroretinal rim in ocular hypertension. Invest Ophthalmol Vis Sci 1989, Submitted
22. Pillunat LE, Stodtmeister R: Inzidenz des Niederdruckglaukoms bei haemodynamisch relevanter Carotisstenose. Spektrum Augenheilk 2:28–32, 1988
23. Pillunat LE, Stodtmeister R, Wilmanns I: Autoregulation of ocular blood flow during changes of intraocular pressure. Graefes Arch Clin Exp Ophthalmol 223:219–223, 1985
24. Pillunat LE, Stodtmeister R, Wilmanns I: Early diagnosis of glaucoma by pressure compliance testing of the optic nerve head. Invest Ophthalmol Vis Sci 27:40, 1986
25. Pillunat LE, Stodtmeister R, Wilmanns I: Pressure compliance of the optic nerve head in low tension glaucoma. Br J Ophthalmol 71:181–187, 1987
26. Pillunat LE, Stodtmeister R, Wilmanns I, Christ T: Drucktoleranztest des Sehnerven bei okulärer Hypertension. Klin Mbl Augenheilk 188:39–44, 1986
27. Pillunat LE, Stodtmeister R, Wilmanns I, christ T: Ein neues Verfahren zur Beurteilung des Sehnervenschadens bei okulärer Hypertension. Sitzungsber Rhein Westf Augenärzte 148:93–96, 1987
28. Robert Y, Maurer W: Pallor of the optic disc in glaucoma patients with artificial hypertension. Docum Ophthalmol 57:203–214, 1984
29. Sossi N, Anderson DR: Effect of elevated intraocular pressure on blood flow. Arch Ophthalmol 101:176–182, 1982
30. Stodtmeister R, Pillunat LE: Pressure tolerance test – Clinical technique and specificity. This volume, pp
31. Stodtmeister R, Pillunat LE, Wilmanns I: Der Drucktoleranztest – Eine neuere Technik bei der Differentialdiagnose des Glaukoms, Fortschr Ophthalmol 1989, in press.
32. Stodtmeister R, Pillunat LE, Wilmanns I: Drucktoleranztestung des Sehnervs mit Hilfe gemittelter, visuell ovozierter kortikaler Potentiale. Spektrum Augenhilk 1:311–314, 1987
33. Stodtmeister R, Pillunat LE, Wilmanns I: Der Drucktoleranztest – Eine neuere Technik in der Differentialdiagnose des Glaukoms. Fortschr Ophthalmol 1989, in press
34. Stodtmeister R, Wilmanns I, Pillunat LE: Methodik okulärer Kreislaufdiagnostik. In: Stodtmeister R et al (eds): Okuläre Durchblutungsstörungen, pp 95–101. Stuttgart: Enke 1987
35. Ulrich WD, Ulrich C: Die Saugnapfverfahren in der okulären Kreislaufdiagnostik. In: Stodtmeister R et al (eds): Okuläre Durchblutungsstörungen, pp 80–88. Stuttgart: Enke 1987

DISCUSSION

Juan E. Grunwald : Dr Pillunat, in your double-center study with Vancouver, how did you decide on which eyes did and wich eyes didn't show signs of autoregulation? And in what way was the study single-masked ?

Lutz E. Pillunat : We made the investigation in Ulm and sent the photographs to Vancouver for optic nerve head analysis, while we were assessing the pressure-compliance test. The criterion for the latter was the presence or not of a non-monotonous or weakly monotonous behavior of the curve.

Juan E. Grunwald : Did you know the Vancouver results when you assessed your curves ?

Lutz E. Pillunat : No, and they didn't know our results when they assessed the stereophotographs.

Bernard Schwartz : With regard to the neuroretinal rim measurements, I would like to point out that they represent a mixture of phenomena, and that they do not necessarily reflect well the amount of cupping; they might reflect the amount of pallor, rather. If you have a cup with a gently sloping temporal edge, you are more likely to judge the limits on pallor rather than on the actual geometry of the cup.

Lutz E. Pillunat : We are absolutely aware of this problem. Nevertheless, we decided to use the technique, because it is important to have some hints about the validity of our results before proceeding any further. It wouldn't be conceivable, at this stage, to turn to follow-up studies which would give much more reliable results but only after 10 years or so.

Harry A. Quigley : Is there any correlation between the baseline IOP and the degree of autoregulation as estimated by the test?

Lutz E. Pillunat : No, baseline IOP isn't correlated to the degree of autoregulation and neither to neuroretinal rim defects.

Harry A. Quigley : I wouldn't expect a single IOP measurement to be correlated to neuroretinal rim defects. But, surely, between two subjects beginning your stress test at respectively 15 and 29 mmHg intraocular pressure, you would expect a difference in the response ?

Lutz E. Pillunat : We didn't observe any such correlation. The general shape of the curves would be the same in your example, only one of them would be shifted to the right.

Charles E. Riva : Would it not be better to refrain from calling a certain type of curve an "autoregulation behavior" and to just describe it as a "plateau" ? After all, there is no known relation between blood flow and the amplitude of the visually evoked cortical potentials.

Lutz E. Pillunat : It is true that we do not know exactly what we are measuring. It may be blood flow, or axoplasmic flow or some metabolic disturbance. But we think that it is a sign of autoregulation.

Harry A. Quigley : You wouldn't expect something that occurs within two minutes to be due to changes in axoplasmic flow!

Lutz E. Pillunat : No, we tend to relate it to the blood flow, rather. After all, the behavior is rather similar to Dr Grunwald's results: If you increase the IOP in a single step and leave it there, the amplitude decreases first, and then comes up again within one minute or so.

Harry A. Quigley : And for how long does each step last in your normal, multiple step test ?

Lutz E. Pillunat : Around 15 to 20 seconds.

Harry A. Quigley : Is this long enough to get a stable value, in the light of what you have just said about the amplitude decreasing and then rising again ?

Lutz E. Pillunat : I do not think that it is a stable situation, in the physiologic sense at least, but this is the method that gives the best results. It would be possible, of course, to make each step last much longer but this would make the test extremely long, long enough for a tonographic effect, at least.

PATTERN REVERSAL ELECTRO-ENCEPHALO-DYNAMOGRAPHY AND PATTERN REVERSAL ELECTRO-RETINO-DYNAMOGRAPHY IN THE ASSESSMENT OF OPTIC NERVE HEAD AND RETINAL AUTOREGULATION

Wulff-D. Ulrich, Christa Ulrich, Bernd Gerewitz and Helmut Teubel

Department of Experimental Ophthalmology, Eye Clinic of the Karl-Marx-University, Leipzig, GDR

Abstract

The principle of pattern reversal Electro-Encephalo-Dynamography (pr EEDG) is described as a noninvasive method to examine ocular autoregulation. EEDG examinations of healthy subjects show preservation of normal ocular function at reduced ciliary perfusion pressure suggesting the existence of effective autoregulation in the eye including the optic nerve head. The characteristic EEDG curve of autoregulation in normal eyes is composed of a steady part representing an autoregulative capacity covering 15 to 20 mm Hg and a declining (amplitude) or rising (latency) part starting from the critical point. Pattern reversal Electro-Retino-Dynamogram (pr ERDG) has the same characteristic as the pr EEDG in respect of ciliary perfusion pressure.

The results from 124 patients show that in primary open angle glaucoma with visual field defects and cupping of the disc, ocular autoregulation and pressure tolerance are strongly diminished or even abolished, while in glaucoma patients without detectable visual field defects and with normal papillae one can find any stage between normal and significantly disturbed autoregulation. The results from 32 patients suffering from low tension glaucoma damage: (1) impaired autoregulation, (2) decreased ciliary perfusion pressure, (3) impaired autoregulation combined with decreased ciliary perfusion pressure, and (4) primary loss of glial tissue of the papilla.

1. Introduction

Blood flow in a tissue or an organ depends both on perfusion pressure and on vascular resistance.

The peripheral resistance is determined by the given vascular pattern, its specific properties in the organ concerned, and by the fluid properties of the blood. Peripheral resistance, as has been shown for various tissues and organs, can be varied under certain conditions to keep the blood flow constant. The mechanism providing constant blood flow to a tissue or an organ despite varying perfusion pressure over a certain range is referred to as autoregulation.

It was desirable to find a method by which alterations of circulation in the eye and optic nerve head could be detected in humans. Since the determination of blood flow in the eye or even in separate regions of the eye will pose considerable problems, we chose other ways of obtaining an insight into the autoregulative behavior of the human eye.

2. Principle of the EEDG method

What we needed was
– a method to determine ocular perfusion pressures,
– a method to change ocular perfusion pressure in a definite and reproducible and simple manner, and
– a parameter which could be used to assess quantitatively any changes in the blood supply of the eye and the optic nerve head.

2.1. Determining perfusion pressures

The newly developed oculo–oscillo–dynamographic (OODG) method was used to determine ocular perfusion pressures[1-3]. Here we concentrated on ciliary perfusion pressure as the ciliary arterial system appears to respond more sensitively to IOP changes, especially in glaucoma patients, than the retinal system.

2.2. Suction cup oculopression

A suction oculopressor (SOP) according to Ulrich and Ulrich[4,5] was used to produce defined changes in IOP and hence in perfusion pressure. Our very light suction cups will adhere to the bulb even at very low negative pressures, provided, of course, that the connecting hoses are supported in a suitable manner. A negative pressure of approximately 10–20 mm Hg is sufficient, which corresponds to an IOP rise of 2.5 to 5.0 mm Hg.

The method of artificial IOP elevation is important for obtaining reproducible results (Table 1). Impression dynamometry[30] is unpleasant for both patient and doctor, and is often difficult to perform. It causes considerable displacement of the bulb, affects orbital circulation, and makes it difficult to obtain uninfluenced and undisturbed visual evoked cortical potentials (VECP).

Table 1. History of VECP pressure tolerance tests

Authors	VECP stimulation technique	Methods of elevating IOP and determining pp$_{cil}$
Fox, Blake and Bourn 1973[6]	flash	finger pressure
Benedikt, Bartl et al. 1974[7]	flash	impression dynamometer acc. to H. K. Müller
Bartl, Benedikt et al. 1975[8] Bartl 1978[9]		
Ulrich 1976[10] Ulrich et al. 1980[11]	flash	suction cup acc. to Ulrich, Ulrich (VECP-Dynamography)
Ulrich et al 1982 a,b,c, 1984[12-15]	pattern reversal	suction cup and OODG acc. to Ulrich, Ulrich (ElectroEncephalo-Dynamography, EEDG)
Pillunat, Stodtmeister et al. 1985,	pattern reversal	suction cup and OODG acc. to Ulrich, Ulrich 1986 [16,17]
Ulrich, Ulrich et al 1986 a,b[18,19]	pattern reversal	EEDG

2.3. Pattern reversal VECP

As a criterion for assessing changes of blood supply to the eye and the optic nerve head we chose the VECP (Table 1) proceeding in a similar way as Fox et al.[6] and the working group Benedikt, Bartl et al.[7-9]. While luminance (flash) stimulation was used in earlier studies, we later employed (since 1982, Table 1) pattern reversal stimulation since the VECPs obtained in this way are of substantially lower variability.

2.4. The EEDG method

This VECP dynamographic method we termed electro-encephalo-dynamography (EEDG), analogous to electro-retino-dynamography (ERDG, Wulfing[20]). EEDG is a

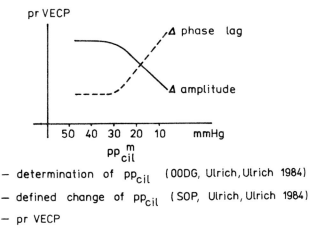

Fig. 1. Principle of electro–encephalo–dynamography (EEDG) to examine ocular autoregulation and to determine pressure tolerance (pp_{cil} ciliary perfusion pressure).

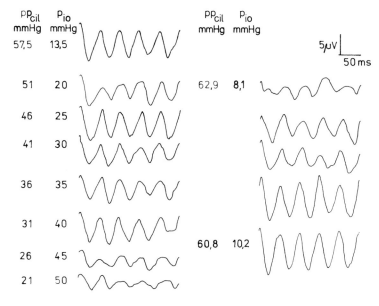

Fig. 2. EEDG of a 32-year-old male healthy subject. Left: pr VECP during stepwise decrease of ciliary perfusion pressure (increase of IOP). Right: Recovery after the period of increased IOP (pp_{cil} mean ciliary perfusion pressure, p_{io} IOP).

combination (Fig. 1) of OODG, SOP and pr VECP. It permits determining VECP amplitude and latency changes with a stepwise decrease of ciliary perfusion pressure. It is an objective noninvasive diagnostic procedure which can be repeated at any time.

3. Ocular autoregulation

In earlier papers[18,19] we have proved that an effective autoregulation of the blood supply, also to the optic nerve head, exists in human eyes. Autoregulation in the anterior part of the optic nerve had been postulated to exist in primates by Geijer and Bill[21] after originally contradictory results[22] obtained by the particle distribution method. In further studies[19,23,24]

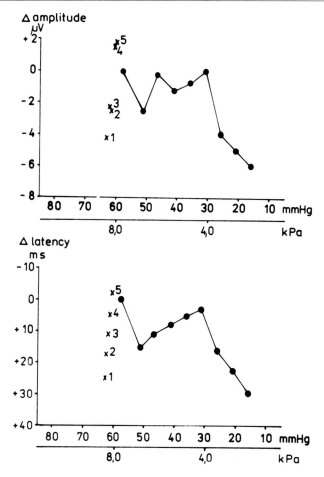

Fig. 3. Evaluated VECP amplitudes and latencies versus ciliary perfusion pressure of the 32-year-old male healthy subject of Fig. 2. The numbered crosses represent amplitude and latency during recovery.

we found that in patients with primary open angle glaucoma as well as in patients with low tension glaucoma, autoregulation is disturbed and ciliary perfusion pressure altered, resulting in a decrease of ocular pressure tolerance.

3.1. Ocular autoregulation in healthy subjects

To test whether there is a general pattern of ocular autoregulative behavior, a group of 26 healthy subjects was examined[18]. Additional pr ERG studies were made at various artificially elevated IOPs (pr ERDG) in combination with pr EEDG to extend the analysis of ocular autoregulation.

3.1.1. EEDG in healthy subjects: Fig. 2 shows an EEDG of a healthy person and Fig. 3 the evaluated VECP amplitude (above) and latency (below) plotted against ciliary perfusion pressure, *i.e.*, with increasing IOP, the steady-state VECP's remain relatively uninfluenced over a wide range. After the first ciliary perfusion pressure decrease of 6.5 mm Hg you see a little alteration of the VECPs that recover quickly and remain unchanged over a range of about 20 mm Hg. Then the amplitude of the VECP diminishes and a phase lag of the VECPs appears.

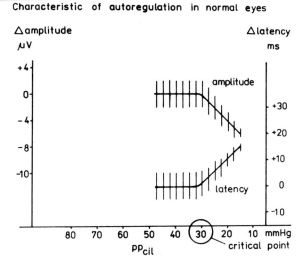

Fig. 4. Schematic diagram of characteristic ocular autoregulative behavior of healthy subjects.

EEDG examinations of healthy subjects resulted in the general pattern of autoregulative behavior shown in Fig. 4. When the ciliary perfusion pressure decreases, the pr VECP amplitude and latency are preserved until the ciliary perfusion pressure reaches about 30–35 mm Hg. Below 30 mm Hg the amplitude decreases and the latency increases rapidly.

The preservation of normal organic function at reduced ciliary perfusion pressure above a critical point at approximately 30 mm Hg mean ciliary perfusion pressure suggests the existence of autoregulation of the blood flow. The normal mean ciliary perfusion pressure in humans is about 45 to 50 mm Hg. (In most of our studies the VECP results are related to the mean effective ciliary perfusion pressure (pp_{mcil}) calculated by the Wetzler-Boeger equation (see[4]).

Since a reduction of ciliary perfusion pressure to approximately 30 mm Hg does not result in any pr VECP changes, one can draw the conclusion that a range of about 15 to 20 mm Hg is covered by autoregulation (autoregulative capacity).

3.1.2. pr ERDG and pr EEDG in healthy subjects: It has been pointed out in several publications[25–29] that the pr ERG shows amplitude and latency disturbances in glaucoma patients at an early stage. Here the question arises whether early glaucoma damage may be primarily due to disturbance in retinal circulation and not in the anterior part of the optic nerve. If the pr ERG turned out to be more resistant to circulatory disturbance than the pr VECP, then this would be in conformity with the widely accepted hypothesis that it is the ciliary arterial supply to the anterior part of the optic nerve which is the first and the main part where ischemia appears in glaucoma.

However, as we can see from Fig. 5, where the latencies obtained by simultaneous recording of pr ERDG and pr EEDG are shown for comparison, the ERDG and the EEDG characteristics in respect of ciliary perfusion pressure are much the same. But how can that be explained?

The pr ERG shows alterations at the same ciliary perfusion pressure as the pr VECP. If it were true that the pr ERG originated in the ganglion cells of the retina, then the pr ERG would have to depend on the retinal circulation exclusively. But as a dependence on the ciliary circulation can be observed it could just as well be assumed that such retinal layers as are supplied by the ciliary system, and thus subjected to ciliary circulatory disturbances during IOP rises, must also be involved in the generation of the pr ERG.

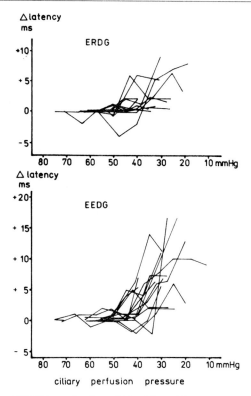

Fig. 5. Pr ERDG and pr EEDG latencies from 14 healthy subjects, shown related to systolic ciliary perfusion pressure instead of calculated mean ciliary perfusion pressure for convenience. Therefore the critical point is shifted to higher values.

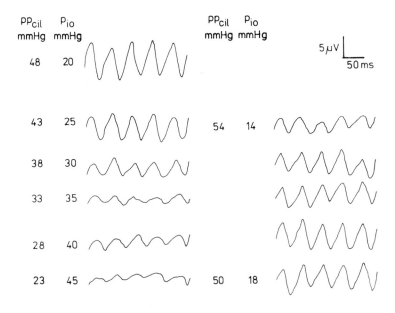

Fig. 6. EEDG of a 57-year-old female patient with primary open angle glaucoma with visual field defects and cupping of the disc (pp_{cil} ciliary perfusion pressure, p_{io} IOP), Abbreviations as in Fig. 2.

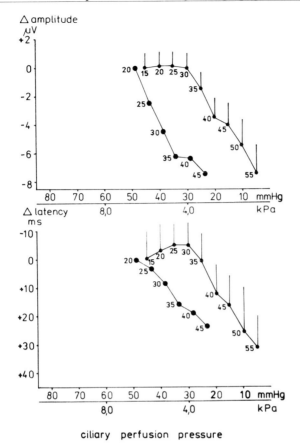

Fig. 7. Evaluated VECP amplitudes (above) and latencies (below) versus ciliary perfusion pressure of the 57-year-old female patient of Fig. 6, compared with the data from 26 healthy subjects.

Irrespective of this open question the amplitude and latency changes of the VECP in the EEDG yield information on the whole circulatory system of the eye, *i.e.*, of all circulatory regions involved, including the optic nerve head. The characteristic behavior of the VECP found at diminished ciliary perfusion pressure depends on retinal and choroidal circulation as well as on the circulation in the region of the optic nerve head. It represents the autoregulative capacity of the system in general, and if there is a weakest point in the blood supply, then it will reflect primarily the autoregulation at that point. And if that weakest point is the optic nerve head, then our results reflect autoregulation of the blood circulation in this region.

3.2. Ocular autoregulation in primary open–angle glaucoma

Fig. 6 shows an EEDG taken from a 57-year-old female patient with progressive primary open-angle glaucoma with visual field defects and cupping of the disc, and Fig. 7 the corresponding evaluation of amplitude and latency versus ciliary perfusion pressure. Decreasing ciliary perfusion pressure by only 5 mm Hg reduces the VECP markedly and continuously without any sign of recovery, which means there is no autoregulative reaction.

Figs. 8 to 10 show the EEDGs of a 48-year-old female patient with primary open-angle glaucoma with a cup/disc ratio of 0.3 in the right eye and 0.6 in the left. While the potentials elicited in the right eye (Fig. 8a) remain relatively unchanged during IOP rise,

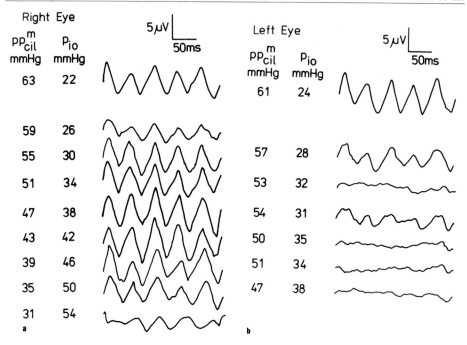

Fig. 8a, b.. EEDGs of a 48-year-old female patient with primary open angle glaucoma with a cup/disc ratio of 0.3 in the right eye (Fig. 8a) and 0.6 in the left eye (Fig. 8b) (pp_{mcil} mean ciliary perfusion pressure p_{io} IOP).

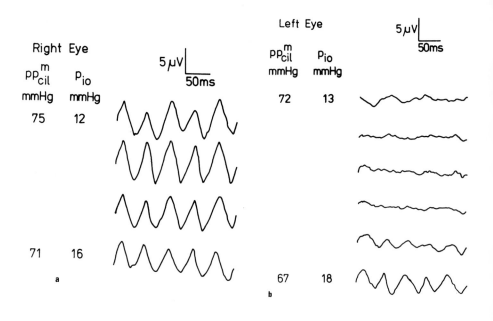

Fig. 9a, b.. EEDG recovery in the 48-year-old female patient of Fig. 8. Abbreviations as in Fig. 8.

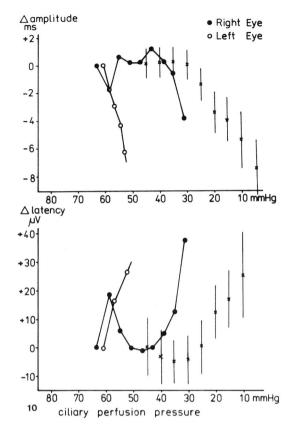

Fig. 10. Evaluated VECP amplitudes and latencies of the patient of Fig. 8. Abbreviations as in Fig. 8.

those elicited in the left eye (Fig. 8b) are distinctly reduced at an IOP rise by no more than 4 mm Hg and are almost extinguished after a rise of 8 mm Hg.

The recovery of the potentials is also quite different. While on the right (Fig. 9a) they recover immediately, on the left (Fig. 9b) they recover only after several minutes.

Fig. 10 shows amplitudes and latencies of the patient plotted against ciliary perfusion pressure, compared with the data from 26 healthy subjects. There is no autoregulation in the left eye, and the ciliary perfusion pressure is shifted to higher values (shifted to the left). In the right eye the ciliary perfusion pressure is also increased. There is autoregulation. The curve, however, is shifted to the left, *i.e.*, it deviates from the normal characteristic. The same applies to the latencies. In both eyes the outflow resistance is raised, on the left side distinctly more than on the right.

As this case demonstrates, the impairment of autoregulation may be very different in the eyes of one patient.

The results from 124 patients (Tables 2 and 3) show that in primary open-angle glaucoma with visual field defects and cupping of the disc, ocular autoregulation and pressure tolerance are strongly diminished or even abolished, while in glaucoma patients without detectable visual field defects and with normal papillae one can find any stage between normal and significantly disturbed autoregulation.

3.3. Ocular autoregulation in low tension glaucoma

The EEDG of a 39-year-old female patient suffering from low tension glaucoma (Fig.

Table 2. Primary open angle glaucoma with visual field defects and cupping of the disc

n	Autoregulatory capacity	Ciliary perfusion pressure (pp$_{cil}$)	Pressure tolerance	Outflow resistance
23	strongly reduced	increased	reduced	increased
5	strongly reduced	normal	reduced or absent	increased
26	absent	increased	absent	increased
2	absent	normal	absent	increased

Table 3. Primary open angle glaucoma without visual field defects and without cupping of the disc

n	Autoregulatory capacity	Ciliary perfusion pressure (pp$_{cil}$)	Pressure tolerance	Outflow resistance
22	normal	normal	normal	increased
18	normal	increased	normal	increased
16	reduced	increased	normal	increased
7	reduced	normal	reduced	increased
4	strongly reduced	increased	reduced	increased
1	strongly reduced	normal	strongly reduced	increased

11) with a cup/disc ratio of 0.8 and visual field defects show a complete lack of autoregulation. At as small an elevation of the IOP as from 14 to 20 mm Hg the VECPs are extinguished. Outflow resistance is normal.

A comparison of the EEDG results with clinical findings (Table 4) indicates four possible causes of the development of low tension glaucoma damage: (1) impaired autoregulation, (2) decreased ciliary perfusion pressure, (3) impaired autoregulation combined with decreased ciliary perfusion pressure, and (4) primary loss of glial tissue of the papilla[24].

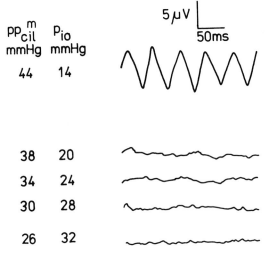

Fig. 11. EEDG of a 39-year-old female patient with low tension glaucoma (pp$_{mcil}$ mean ciliary perfusion pressure, p$_{io}$ IOP).

Table 4. Ocular autoregulation and ciliary perfusion pressure in low tension glaucoma

n	Autoregulation (autoregulatory capacity)	Ciliary perfusion pressure (pp_{cil})	Visual field defects	Cup/disc ratio
3		reduced	+++	1.0/1.0/1.0
10	absent (O)	normal	++++++++++	0.9/1.0/1.0/0.8/ 0.8/0.8/0.9/0.9/0.9
2		increased	++	1.0/0.9
4	reduced or	reduced	++++	0.9/0.9/0.7/0.9
7	strongly reduced	normal	+——+++	0.8/0.7/0.7/0.6/0.9/0.9/0.8
0	(< 9 mmHg)	increased		
4	slightly reduced	reduced	++–+	0.8/0.8/0.7/0.9
2	(10 to 14 mm Hg)	normal	—	0.7/0.8
2		increased	—	0.5/0.6
3	normal	reduced	+++	0.6/0.7/0.6
3	(> 14 mm Hg)	normal	——	0.8/0.8/0.7
0		increased		

+ typical visual field defects observed
– no visual field defects observed

4. Conclusion

4.1 The characteristic curve of autoregulation in normal eyes (Fig. 4) is composed of the following parts:
– a steady part representing the autoregulative capacity covering 15 to 20 mm Hg;
– a declining (amplitude) or rising (latency) part starting from the critical point at approximately 30 to 35 mm Hg mean ciliary perfusion pressure.

4.2. In primary open-angle glaucoma (Fig. 12) the curve may reflect any stage between normal behavior and complete loss of autoregulation. The different stages in the development of impaired autoregulation are marked with numbers:
1. autoregulation is still normal,
2. the steady part is extended to the left while the characteristic of the curve remains normal,
3. the whole curve begins to shift to the left, the critical point moves to higher ciliary perfusion pressure values and the steady part contracts, *i.e.*, the autoregulative capacity drops,
4. and 5. the steady part of the curve has disappeared denoting complete loss of autoregulation. A further shifting of the curve is seen.

4.3. In low tension glaucoma (Fig. 13) the curve has only a short (1) or no (2 and 3) steady part at all which means loss of autoregulation. In most cases the declining part of the curve coincides with that of the normal curve or is somewhat shifted to the right, indicating very low ciliary perfusion pressure.

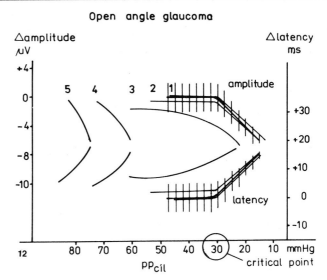

Fig. 12. Schematic diagram of ocular autoregulative behavior in primary open angle glaucoma (pp_{cil} mean ciliary perfusion pressure).

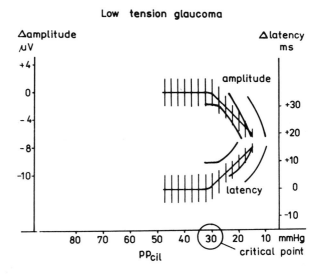

Fig. 13. Schematic diagram of ocular autoregulative behavior in low tension glaucoma (pp_{cil} mean ciliary perfusion pressure).

References

1. Ulrich WD, Ulrich Ch: Einsatz der Okulo–Oszillo–Dynamographie (OODG) für Patientenuntersuchungen. Boucke–Report Tübingen 1984
2. Ulrich WD, Ulrich Ch: Oculo–oscillo–dynamography: A diagnostic procedure for recording ocular pulses and measuring retinal and ciliary arterial blood pressures. Ophthalmic Res 17:308–317, 1985
3. Ulrich WD, Ulrich Ch: Okulo–Oszillo–Dynamographie, ein neues Verfahren zur Bestimmung des Ophthalmikablutdruckes und zur okulären Pulskurvenanalyse. Klin Mbl Augenheilk 186:385–388, 1985
4. Ulrich WD: Grundlagen und Methodik der Ophthalmodynamometrie (ODM), Ophthalmodynamographie (ODG) und Temporalisdynamographie (TDG). Abhandlungen aus dem Gebiete der Augenheilkunde. Sammlung von Monographien Bd 44. Leipzig: VEB Georg Thieme Verlag 1976
5. Ulrich WD, Ulrich Ch: Ein neuer Okulopressor. Fortschr Ophthalmol 82:490–492, 1985

6. Fox R, Blake R, Bourn JR: Visual evoked cortical potential during pressure-blinding. Vision Res 13:501–503, 1973
7. Benedikt O, Bartl G, Hiti H, Mandl H: Die Änderung der elektrophysiologischen Antwort am menschlichen Auge bei kurzzeitiger Erhöhung des intraokularen Druckes. Albrecht v Graefes Arch Ophthalmol 192:57–64, 1974
8. Bartl G, Benedikt O, Hiti H, Mandl H: Das elektrophysiologische Verhalten gesunder und glaukomkranker menschlicher Augen bei kurzzeitiger intraocularer Druckbelastung. Albrecht v Graefes Arch Ophthalmol 195:201–206, 1975
9. Bartl G: Das ERG und das evozierte Sehrindenpotential bei normalen und an Glaukom erkrankten Augen. Albrecht v Graefes Arch Ophthalmol 207:243–269, 1978
10. Ulrich WD: VER–Dynamographie. In: Ulrich WD; Grundlagen und Methodik der Ophthalmodynamometrie (ODM), Ophthalmodynamographie (ODG) und der Temporalisdynamographie (TDG). Abhandlungen aus dem Gebiete der Augenheilkunde. Sammlung von Monographien Bd 44, pp 115–117. Leipzig: VEB Georg Thieme Verlag 1976
11. Ulrich WD, Bohne BD, Reimann J, Wernecke KD: VEP and intraocular pressure. In: Barber C: Evoked Potentials, pp 251–255. Nottingham: Potentials 1978
12. Ulrich WD, Bohne BD, Niederländer C, Ulrich Ch: Einfluß des künstlich erhöhten Augeninnendruckes auf das pattern reversal VECP. Ein Beitrag zur individuellen Funktionsprognose des Glaukoms. 4. Glaukomsymp. Görlitz 1982, Kongreßbericht pp 14–20
13. Ulrich Ch, Ulrich WD: Die Bedeutung des okulären Perfusionsdruckes für die Diagnostik, Einstellung und Therapiekontrolle des Glaukoms. 4. Glaukomsymp. Görlitz 1982, Kongreßbericht pp 38–40
14. Ulrich WD, Bohne BD, Wernecke KD, Kästner R, Reinmann J: Electro–encephalo–dynamography (EEDG) – A new diagnostic procedure? Docum Ophthalmol Proc Series 31:104, 1982
15. Ulrich WD, Ulrich Ch: An electrophysiological approach to the diagnosis and treatment of glaucoma. Dev Ophthalmol 9:140–146, 1984
16. Pillunat L, Stodtmeister R, Wilmanns J, Christ Th: Autoregulation of ocular blood flow during changes of intraocular pressure. Albrecht v Graefes Arch Ophthalmol 223:219–223, 1985
17. Pillunat L, Stodtmeister R, Willmanns J, Christ Th: Drucktoleranztest des Sehnervenkopfes bei okulärer Hypertension. Klin Mbl Augenheilk 186:39–44, 1986
18. Ulrich WD, Ulrich Ch, Bohne BD: Relation between ciliary perfusion pressure and pattern reversal visual evoked cortical potentials. An electro–encephalo–dynamographic investigation. Ophthalmic Res 18:260–264, 1986
19. Ulrich WD, Ulrich Ch, Bohne BD: Deficient autoregulation and lengthening of the diffusion distance in the anterior optic nerve circulation in glaucoma: An electro–encephalo–dynamographic investigation. Ophthalmic Res 18:253–259, 1986
20. Wulfing B: Clinical electroretinodynamography. A diagnostic aid in occlusive carotid artery disease. Acta Ophthalmol suppl 73:1–81, 1963
21. Geijer C, Bill A: Effects of raised intraocular pressure on retinal, prelaminar, laminar and retrolaminar optic nerve blood flow in monkeys. Invest Ophthal Vis Sci 18:1030–1042, 1979
22. Alm A, Bill A: Ocular and optic nerve blood flow at normal and increased intraocular pressure in monkeys (Macaca irus). Exp Eye Res 15:15–29, 1973
23. Ulrich WD, Ulrich Ch, Petzschmann Ä. Richter S, Ulrich A: Okuläre Autoregulation beim primären Weitwinkelglaukom. Fortschr Ophthalmol 85:470–473, 1988
24. Ulrich WD, Ulrich A, Petzschmann Ä, Ulrich Ch: Okuläre Autoregulation und ziliarer Perfusionsdruck beim Niedrigdruckglaukom. Folia Ophthalmol 13:333–337, 1988
25. Wanger P, Person H: Pattern–reversal electroretinograms in unilateral glaucoma. Invest Ophthalmol Vis Sci 24:749–753, 1983
26. Papst N, Bopp M, Schnaudigel OE: Pattern electroretinogram and visually evoked potentials in glaucoma. Albrecht v Graefes Arch Clin Exp Ophthalmol 222:29–33, 1984
27. Van Lith G, Ringens P, De Heer LJ: Pattern electroretinogram in glaucoma. Dev Ophthalmol 9:133–139, 1984
28. Trick GL: PRRP abnormalities in glaucoma and ocular hypertension. Invest Ophthalmol Vis Sci 27:1730–1736, 1986
29. Korth M, Storck B, Horn F, Jonas J: Muster–evozierte Elektroretinogramme (M–ERG) normaler und glaukomatös erkrankter Augen Fortschr Ophthalmol 84:385–387, 1987
30. Weigelin E, Lobstein A: Ophthalmodynamometrie. Basel: Karger 1962

DISCUSSION

Tom van den Berg : Dr Ulrich, in some of your curves the amplitude at the first point with elevated pressure was slightly higher than the baseline. Even if autoregulation was active, you might expect the amplitudes to be equal or lower, but not higher!

Wulff D. Ulrich : The variability is important in the first points. Sometimes you see a small increase and sometimes a small decrease in amplitude.

Tom van den Berg : Then this is just variability. You don't interpret these results as signs of autoregulation, do you?

Wulff D. Ulrich : No, it is just variability of the response.

Harry A. Quigley : Could you tell us what was the reversal rate and the sizes of the testing field and of the checks?

Wulff D. Ulrich : Well, here is the complete technical data. Stimulating field: 12; check size: 25 minutes of arc; reversal rate: 10 Hz; average luminance of cathode ray tube: 50 cd/m^2; contrast: 20%; 64 reversals were averaged. This is all the information you need to reproduce the experiment, I think.

Harry A. Quigley : Very well. Now may I ask you a question about your results: did you find any difference in the baseline amplitude, without artificial IOP elevation, I mean, between normals and glaucoma patients with visual field defects ?

Wulff D. Ulrich : There is one known difference, and this is that in glaucoma patients with visual field loss, you find that amplitude tends to decrease faster with decreasing contrast. This is the reason why we use 20% contrast to start with, because differences between glaucoma patients and normals are more clear. Sometimes, though, we had to raise the contrast back to 50%, because the baseline amplitude was very low.

Harry A. Quigley : But then, are the amplitudes in the glaucoma patients lower? If that is indeed the case, their signal-to-noise ratios are poorer and that can make interpretation difficult.

Wulff D. Ulrich : Amplitudes aren't lower in our group. In most cases they are the same, within the limits of variability, which is very high as you know. The only difference is that in glaucoma patients the amplitude has a tendency to drop when the contrast of the screen is lowered. So in some of our glaucoma patients, a contrast of 20% was already affecting the amplitude and we had to raise it to 50% to get a good baseline signal.

Harry A. Quigley : In how many of your patients did you have to raise the contrast?

Wulff D. Ulrich : We had to do that mainly in the glaucoma group with visual field defects and cupping. About 30 to 40% of the patients, I would say.

Harry A. Quigley : But can you, then, compare patients tested at 50% contrast with normals tested at 20%? Wouldn't you have to test some normals also at 50% ?

Wulff D. Ulrich : No, it doesn't change anything. We are not studying contrast. The purpose of the contrast adjustment is to get the lowest contrast with a good, stable baseline.

Richard Stodtmeister : Dr Ulrich, I would like to comment on your choice of parameters: you have plotted the curves of amplitude versus ciliary perfusion pressure. However, ciliary perfusion pressure is only an estimate. Moreover, if we assume the presence of autoregulation, then we do not know exactly how ciliary perfusion pressure behaves. I think that plotting amplitudes versus IOP instead is simpler, easier to understand and requires less assumptions.

Wulff D. Ulrich : I think that plotting the amplitude as a function of ciliary perfusion pressure is a better approach to the actual phenomenon you want to study, which is the blood supply to the optic nerve head. And the blood supply depends directly on perfusion pressure, not on intraocular pressure. The only objection to using perfusion pressures is the possible presence of a tonographic effect, but we have considered that: we measured the IOP before and after the experiment and made the necessary correction.

Charles E. Riva : What is the IOP corresponding, for instance, to a perfusion pressure of 30 mmHg ?

Wulff D. Ulrich : Around 30 to 35 mmHg.

Maurice E. Langham : It seems to me that the interpretation of this test depends very much on knowing what the actual IOP is at every measured point. And there is evidence that the tonographic effect is far from negligible. How exactly did you correct for that ?

Wulff D. Ulrich : We measure the IOP before we install the suction cup and just after taking it off, and assume that the IOP decrease is linear. We know that it isn't exactly linear, but it is a close approximation. At one point or another you have to make some compromise and I do not think that this is a critical one.

Maurice E. Langham : On the contrary, I think that very important errors can be involved.

Wulff D. Ulrich : No, this is very unlikely. You see, these are very small steps of IOP incrementation: 4 or 5 mmHg or so. It isn't as if you had a single step to 50 mmHg.

Erik L. Greve : But it may be that the tonographic effect is different in normals and in glaucoma patients. Have you considered that ?

Wulff D. Ulrich : Yes, we did, because it is an important problem and a difficult one. We have studied that before, in combination with other experiments, and we made our corrections according to our previous experience and results.

Richard Stodtmeister : Dr Ulrich, I would like to ask what were your criteria for glaucoma, because you mentioned "glaucoma patients without visual field defects and with normal optic nerve heads". How do you define, then, glaucoma ?

Wulff D. Ulrich : Our main criterion for open-angle glaucoma was abnormally high outflow resistance. This is not the case for low-tension glaucoma, where the outflow resistance is normal.

George L. Spaeth : Dr Ulrich, I would like to ask you what makes you so convinced that when you increase the IOP, the drop in the visually evoked cortical potentials is due to a drop in perfusion pressure. After all, you would get a similar drop if you put a clamp on the optic nerve head, and this isn't very different from what you are doing when you increase the IOP: you apply some extra pressure to the optic nerve head.

Wulff D. Ulrich : I have no definite answer to your question, Dr Spaeth. When you raise the IOP, you put of course some pressure on the optic nerve head, but you also decrease the perfusion pressure. And the results seem consistent with this hypothesis, so I believe it to be true. But we can't prove it yet and that's what we are concentrating our efforts on.

Richard Stodtmeister : An Italian group has just published* the results of a study involving increase of the IOP while the perfusion pressure remained constant. And they concluded that a decline of function is due to perfusion pressure changes and not to IOP changes.

Harry A. Quigley : It is very likely, George, that this method indeed reflects blood flow in some way or another. If you wait long enough at each pressure step, you find something that Dr Anderson studied in monkeys a few years ago**: when the perfusion pressure drops to around 25 mmHg, the electrophysiological responses both for the outer and inner retina drop off, and so do probably the cortical potentials. This is true not only of the pattern ERG which reflects the activity of the inner retina but also of the flash ERG which is heavily dependent on the choroidal circulation. Now whether we can in fact measure the true perfusion pressure in the eye and not make a rough estimation, that's another story.

Juan E. Grunwald : One more thing concerning George's question: we can't be sure that this technique really reflects blood flow, but the correlation with the results of other techniques is remarkable: the fact that the curve breaks at 30-35 mmHg pressure, the fact that with small pressure increments the amplitudes first drop and then come back after one minute, and so on. You wouldn't have this

Editors' notes:

* Siliprandi R, Bucci MG, Canella R, Carmignoto G: Flash and pattern electoretinograms during and after acute intraocular pressure elevation in cats. Invest Ophthalmol Vis Sci 29: 558-565, 1988

** Gerstle CL, Anderson DR, Hamasaki DI: Pressure effect on ERG and optic nerve conduction of visual impulse. Short-term effects in owl monkeys. Arch Ophthalmol 90 :121-124, 1973

last effect, for instance, if the phenomenon was only pressure-dependent, because the IOP stays constant. But there was one more thing I wanted to ask Dr Ulrich. From the two tests, pattern-ERG and pattern-VECP, which is the most suitable for this purpose? Which is the most sensitive to IOP elevation ?

Wulff D. Ulrich : This isn't an easy question. They both give curves with similar characteristics. Technically speaking, pattern-ERG is more difficult because the signal is weaker and therefore you have to average over more sweeps. But as to which method is more sensitive, I can't say. We were unable to compare them directly, because it is very difficult to record simultaneously VECP and ERG while at the same time you are raising the IOP.

PATTERN VISUAL EVOKED POTENTIALS UNDER ARTIFICIAL INTRAOCULAR PRESSURE INCREASE IN GLAUCOMA: METHODOLOGICAL CONSIDERATIONS

Thomas J. T. P. van den Berg, Frans C. C. Riemslag, George N. Lambrou and Hank Spekreijse

The Netherlands Ophthalmic Research Institute and The Laboratory of Medical Physics and Informatics of the University of Amsterdam, AMC, Meibergdreef 15, 1105 AZ Amsterdam, The Netherlands

Abstract

Stodtmeister and colleagues have reported, among other things, that the amplitude change of the steady state pattern reversal Visual Evoked Potential (VEP) as a function of IntraOcular Pressure (IOP) increase, induced with a section cup, can be used as an early diagnostic tool for glaucoma. We evaluated this so-called pressure tolerance test since there exists a great need for such a relatively quick test. IOP was increased in steps of about 10 mmHg until the VEP was abolished. Since it was found that application of the suction cup could also influence the optics of the eye, this was also tested in the following way: After pressure was released the VEP amplitude had to return to the initial value in about one minute. Seven normals and 18 glaucoma patients were tested. We could not confirm the initial reports. VEP resistance to pressure increase was observed in both groups until about 60 mmHg. Contrary to Stodtmeister's findings, the controls also did not show an initial drop in VEP amplitude at the first increase in IOP. Such a drop was invoked as if application of the suction cup resulted in optical disturbance of the eye.

The aim of the present study was to evaluate pressure induced changes in visual Evoked Potential (VEP) amplitude as a possible diagnostic tool for clinical use in Dr. Greve's glaucoma department. Studies in our laboratory (see Spekreijse et al.[1] for a review) have shown the VEP to be of interest in a number of eye diseases. Moreover, we found the results of previous studies on this subject reported in the literature to be encouraging.

What differentiates a glaucoma patient from a glaucoma suspect is loss of visual function. It is, therefore, natural that many methods aiming at a positive diagnosis of glaucoma involve testing of the visual function. On the other hand, for prognostic reasons we wish to bring forward signs of the disease, so that we may anticipate and prevent the functional damage which occurs. For this reason, a provocation technique may be useful. For reasons of safety provocation should be not too long. Therefore, a visual function assessment faster than quantitative perimetry is desired. Fortunately, we know that the VEP is often distorted rather early in the disease and by using steady state VEP's, fast recordings are possible. So we could try to bring the VEP distortion forward by a challenge to the system. At this conference we assume the blood flow to be important in the pathogenesis of glaucoma. A challenge would be to reduce the perfusion pressure of the eye by application of a suction cup. (The question then remains as to whether an acute reduction of the blood supply provokes the endangering condition as opposed to chronic reduction.)

The perspectives for this technique seemed to be good, especially after considering the positive reports by Bartl et al.[2], Ulrich et al.[3,4] and Pillunat et al.[5-7]. We chose to follow more or less the procedures of Stodtmeister and Pillunat. We recorded VEP's to 8 or 17 Hz checkerboard reversals with check sizes of 20' to 60', depending on the best response from the subject. Signal analysis consisted of selective filtering at the stimulation frequency, synchronous detection of the response and averaging over 1 to 10 sec, depending on the signal to noise ratio.

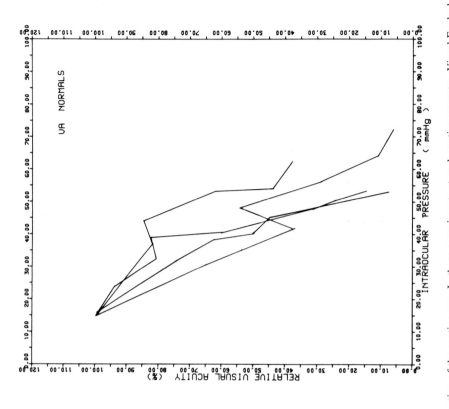
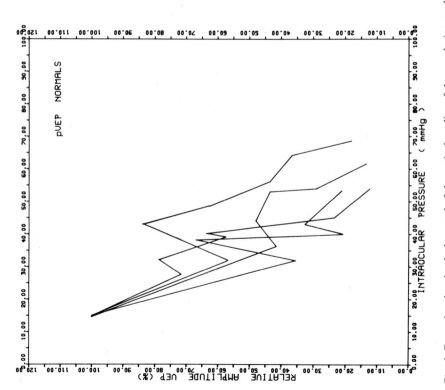

Fig. 1. Examples showing bad control of the optical quality of the eye during application of the suction cup. In these experiments at each suction pressure, Visual Evoked Potential to checkerboard patterns (left: pVEP) as well as Visual Acuity (right: VA), were determined. As suggested by the decline of the VA, optical problems caused the pVEP to drop as soon as the suction cup was applied.

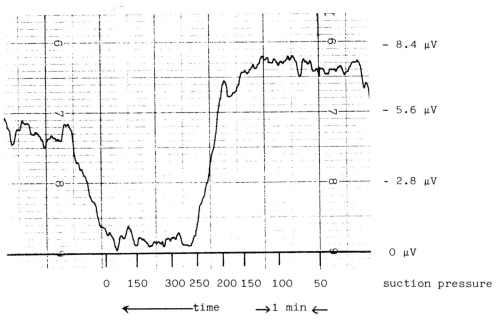

Fig. 2. Example demonstrating resistance of the VEP to increases in suction pressure (and subsequent increases in intraocular pressure), as was found by us in all normal subjects and in 14 out of 18 glaucoma patients.

Our first concern was the early decline of the VEP occurring immediately after the suction cup was placed[5-7]. In the control group, placement of the suction cup immediately caused the VEP to decrease by 50%, although the IntraOcular Pressure (IOP) increased to only about 30 mmHg, a value easily reached during a handstand, a Valsalva maneuver or a prolonged cough. Should we take it that in normals in those conditions the VEP's are indeed halved?

We suspected that there was some other reason than IOP increase for this decline. We wondered whether application of the suction cup to the eye also causes optical disturbance. Since the VEP depends on acute vision, we wondered whether optical disturbance could be of importance. Fig. 1 shows the results from some early experiments in which transient VEP's were used. In these experiments Landolt–C visual acuity (VA) and VEP were alternately measured. Here also we see the VEP decline as soon as the suction cup is placed. However, the VA also declines directly. In fact, the two visual functions seem to decline in parallel. In personal experiments we tried to decide whether optical blurring occurred. Based on our subjective experiences we found indications that optical problems were indeed involved (double vision, blink related blurring, excessive tear production).

These early experiments taught us that it is very important to keep the suction cup completely free from the cornea, something that is not always easy to achieve if the subject looks straight ahead or if the subject has somewhat narrow eyelids. Some subjects do tolerate the suction cup well enough, but others do not, even after proper anesthesia, resulting in extensive tear production and subsequent blurring. Sometimes the suction cup drifts towards the cornea even if it was primarily correctly positioned. To check for optical degradation of the eye we looked for the return of the response after the experiment. The criterion used was that the response should return to normal within one minute after release of the suction cup. This criterion was checked in all subsequent experiments. Experiments were rejected that did not comply with this criterion and in those cases slit-lamp examination often showed abrasion of the cornea.

After exclusion of the experiments that did not comply with this criterion, all normal subjects[8] showed the type of behavior as shown in the example of Fig. 2. When the suction cup is placed with a starting pressure of around 50 mmHg to keep it in place, the CEP remains unchanged. The suction pressure is increased in steps of about 50 mmHg and the response remains more or less stable until 200 mmHg (IOP~60 mmHg). Then the response drops quickly to noise level. When the pressure is released (in this case in two steps) the response quickly returns to normal. This case in fact shows the worst recovery that was accepted. On the other hand, the signal to noise ratio was among the best we obtained.

However, more or less the same behavior was found for most of the glaucoma patients[8]. Eight out of ten Low Tension Glaucoma patients (LTG) and six out of eight POAG or 'Medium Tension glaucoma' patients (MTG) showed also more or less stable VEP's for IOP's to about 60 mmHg. This "plateau" was at the same level as the reference value as for the normals. Then, at some IOP value, the VEP's dropped to noise level. This critical IOP value seemed to be somewhat higher (!) and more variable for the patient group as compared to the control group. In the two patients who showed deviant behavior in both glaucoma sub groups, the VEP amplitude dropped directly after insertion of the suction cup. It should always be remembered, however, that in these cases the response returned within one minute after pressure release.

How can we interpret these findings in terms of vulnerability of the system? Apart from the four deviant patients we see that up to a certain point the VEP is resistant to increased IOP levels. The VEP seems, therefore, to be resistant to a decrease in perfusion pressure. As regards the basis of this resistance, we can only speculate. Maybe the relevant blood supplies have over-capacity, so that a mild decrease in blood flow does not result in deficient metabolic exchange. Maybe blood flow autoregulation causes the observed stability. Grunewald's results suggest, however, that autoregulation copes with only 5–15 mmHg. Reserve metabolites in and around the cells could also be considered, but this seems unlikely since pressure blinding is known to occur within 10 sec or so, whereas the duration of these experiments is in the order of minutes.

With respect to application of this test as an early glaucoma diagnostic tool it is odd to see that glaucoma patients tended to have higher resistance than normals. Taking into consideration that our normal subjects were younger than most patients, this seems to indicate that the test does not expose increased vulnerability of the system. Moreover, Pillunat et al.[5] have found curves of POAG patients to lie above the normal curves. All this seems to indicate that in the case of glaucoma there is no increased susceptibility to acute IOP increase, or that the VEP does not reflect this susceptibility. On the other hand, in four out of 18 cases we did find VEP loss as soon as the IOP was raised. It may be that these patients are different from the others in some way, related to the pathogenesis of their disease but we could find no evidence to that effect. For example, not all were more progressed stages (nor the reverse). The number of patients was too limited to allow definite conclusions.

In conclusion, our experience with this technique left us skeptical as to its applicability in glaucoma. However, the different behavior noted in four patients calls for more study before more definite conclusions can be drawn.

Acknowledgements

Patients were referred for this study by Drs. Greve and Geijssen, who also volunteered to participate as normal subjects. We appreciated particularly the hospitality of Dr. Stodtmeister, who spent two days instructing us on his technique, at his laboratory in Ulm.

References

1. Spekreijse H, Apkarian PA: The use of a system analysis approach to electrodiagnostic (ERG and VEP) assessment. Vision Res 26:195–219, 1986
2. Bartl G, Benedikt O, Hiti H, Mandl H: Das elektrophysiologische Verhalten gesunder und glaukomkranker menschlicher Augen bei kurzzeitiger intraocularer Druckbelastung. Albrecht v. Graefes Arch Klin Exp Ophthalmol 195:201–206, 1976
3. Ulrich W–D, Ulrich C: An electrophysiological approach to the diagnosis and treatment of glaucoma. Dev Ophthalmol 9:140–146, 1984
4. Ulrich W–D, Ulrich C, Bohne B–D: Deficient autoregulation and lengthening of the diffusion distance in the anterior optic nerve circulation in glaucoma: An electro–encephalo–dynamographic investigation. Ophthalm Res 18:253–259, 1986
5. Pillunat LE, Stodtmeister R, Wilmanns I, Christ T: Autoregulation of ocular bloodflow during changes in intraocular pressure. Graefe's Arch Clin Exp Ophthalmol 223:219–223, 1985
6. Pillunat LE, Stodtmeister R, Wilmanns I, Christ T: Drucktoleranztest des Sehnervenkopfes bei okularer Hypertension. Klin Mbl Augenheilk 186:39–44, 1986
7. Pillunat LE, Stodtmeister R, Wilmanns I: Pressure compliance of the optic nerve head in low tension glaucoma. Br J Ophthalmol 71:181–187, 1987
8. Van den Berg TJTP, Spekreijse H, Reimslag FCC, Lambrou GN: An evaluation of the pressure tolerance test. In preparation.

DISCUSSION

Charles E. Riva : What was exactly the time course of your experiment, Dr van den Berg? How long did each pressure step last ?

Tom van den Berg : Initially we used very long steps, of 40 or 50 seconds. But with experience, we were able to lower them to 20 seconds per step.

Harry A. Quigley : Did you check retinoscopically for induced astigmatism ?

Tom van den Berg : Not retinoscopically, but we checked the refraction when we suspected something to be wrong with it, and also examined the eyes at the slit lamp, whenever we had indications that the suction cup had "maltreated" the cornea.

Juan E. Grunwald : I can partly answer your question, Harry. Every time that we use the suction cup, I look at the fundus, ophthalmoscopically. Usually the picture is good and sharp, although occasionally you may get a less good picture, on the same subject sometimes.

Harry A. Quigley : But you don't record cortical potentials, Juan. When you want to record cortical potentials it is absolutely critical that you have a sharp image, especially with small check sizes like here. Is it possible to blink normally with a suction cup on ?

Tom van den Berg : No, although some patients do manage to close their eyes, more or less completely, in a spasm of the eyelids.

Harry A. Quigley : When we want to be sure that the cornea is well-protected and will not dry up, we use a hard contact lens. Don't you think that it might be of some help, in this case ?

Tom van den Berg : Yes, it is an alternative. We didn't try it, though.

Richard Stodtmeister : I think that all these problems are important at the beginning, but that most of them are solved with experience. Our patients do complain, occasionally, of some itching or burning sensation on placing the cup, but they consider it as absolutely tolerable. They even prefer this examination to visual field testing! As for corneal abrasions, they are really exceptional. The most severe side-effect is conjunctival hemorrhage, which occurs in about 1% of the cases. Finally, as far as optical factors are concerned, induced astigmatism is less than one diopter. The blurring that some patients describe is rather linked to posterior pole ischemia since it varies with time: it comes and goes. We think that it is the subjective counterpart of the VECP amplitude reduction.

Erik L. Greve : Tom, would you say that the "plateau" was a constant finding in normal patients?

Tom van den Berg : I really can't say. There is certainly an important drop at the beginning, and then a more-or-less constant response over a more-or-less wide range of intraocular pressures. But whether this is really a drop followed by a plateau or whether it has something to do with the disturbance caused by placing the cup, I can't say. The fact remains, however, that in most cases the curves show an approximately stable situation for patients as well as for normals for small pressure increases, and then a rather abrupt drop. Whether this is autoregulation or not, I do not know, so I would rather call it reserve capacity. The eye has, therefore, a reserve capacity against IOP increase, which doesn't seem to be reduced in glaucoma patients, as a rule. This is the main point I wanted to make. As for the mechanism of this reserve capacity, I think that the question is still open.

Bernard Schwartz : Did you investigate the intraindividual variability of the method ?

Tom van den Berg : Yes, we did, and the results are quite reproducible.

Harry A. Quigley : Can you give us a figure ?

Tom van den Berg : I would say that the intraindividual variability is of the order of 10%; not more than 20% anyway. I am speaking of course about a few young, healthy and well-informed volunteers; ourselves, as a matter of fact.

Harry A. Quigley : Then there was no age-matching between the controls and the patients. Don't you think that the response may be age-related ?

Tom van den Berg : Yes, that might of course be a problem and explain some part of the variability. But there are many other factors intervening at that point, eye volume, scleral rigidity and so on. Not to mention that studying the response against IOP and not against perfusion pressure like Dr Ulrich does, may also be a source of variability.

Richard Stodtmeister : We have our objections to that last point, relating the response to perfusion pressure, that is. To do that, you need to measure the arterial supply pressure, by compressing some of the central ophthalmic artery branches, whether you do it by ophthalmodynamometry or by oculo-oscillo-dynamography. But what you measure, in that way, is the pressure of the ophthalmic artery at the point where it gives off the central retinal artery or the posterior ciliary arteries. And this is very far away from the point where the damage is supposed to occur.

Harry A. Quigley : I would rather think that Dr Ulrich has a point in measuring perfusion pressure, especially in patients with poor carotid inflow. If, by doing ophthalmodynamometry, you discover a glaucoma patient whose central retinal artery collapses at 30 mmHg, then I think everyone will agree that this is a vascular phenomenon having nothing to do with his original glaucoma, although it does make the prognosis much worse. And of course this is reflected in this experiment, which is an electrophysiologic ophthalmodynamometry, in a way.

Tom van den Berg : Yes, sure!

Yves C.A. Robert : May I just ask: isn't it dangerous to raise the intraocular pressure so high in low-tension glaucoma patients ?

Erik L. Greve : This is a very frequent question. Stephen Drance says no, it isn't dangerous, and is very positive about it.

Discussion

Tom van den Berg : Moreover, we always check for the recovery of the cortical response after removal of the suction cup and it has never failed to come up swiftly, unless there was some problem with the cornea.

Harry A. Quigley : I would rather put it this way: the potential risk is less important than the potential information to be gathered, and therefore is acceptable, provided the patient consents with that. But I have another question to ask: what was, in your experiment, the mean IOP where the response dropped to zero, in normals and in low-tension glaucoma patients ?

Tom van den Berg : If I remember well, it was about 60 mmHg for the normals and 65 mmHg for the low-tension glaucomas. So the differences we found were really small. If you combine that with the variability of the curves, I don't very well see how we can use this data for prognosis in individual glaucoma patients.

V. FLUORESCEIN ANGIOGRAPHY

CONTRIBUTIONS AND LIMITATIONS OF FLUORESCEIN ANGIOGRAPHY IN UNDERSTANDING GLAUCOMA; OR, "WHERE DO WE GO NEXT?"

George L. Spaeth

Service and Research Laboratories, Wills Eye Hospital / Thomas Jefferson University, Ninth and Walnut Streets, Philadelphia, PA 19107–7559, USA

In 1977 a monograph was published which detailed the contributions of fluorescein angiography to the understanding of the pathogenesis of optic nerve damage glaucoma[1]. Relatively little has changed in the field since that time. The reason for this is clear. The technological limitations of fluorescein angiography, combined with the extreme variability of patients and the heterogeneity of the condition "of glaucoma" have severely limited the value of fluorescein angiography in the diagnosis and management of individual patients. An understanding of the various mechanisms of glaucoma is interesting, but our ultimate goal is effective treatment. In this regard, fluorescein angiography at present is, in the simplest terms, of no substantial assistance.

This is not to say that fluorescein angiography is not of substantial assistance in understanding glaucoma and that research in the field is inappropriate or should not continue. An analogy can be drawn to the water drinking test. There is no doubt that the intake of fluid and the osmotic make-up of what is ingested affects intraocular pressure[2-4]. However, the water drinking test is, in fact, of no value in helping predict the natural history of individual patient's clinical course, and that is the major diagnostic challenge in glaucoma. Fortunately, for patients there was a sufficiently large number of individuals who did not believe that abnormalities of blood flow played any primary role in the pathogenesis of glaucoma, and the test itself was sufficiently cumbersome that fluorescein angiography never became a common methodology of studying, diagnosing, or treating patients with or considered suspect for glaucoma.

However, it is worthwhile reviewing some of the conclusions of several early studies, and reexamining them in the light of time, to determine whether or not any were valid. Though there have been several leading investigators, I will here consider primarily my own work.

Fluorescein angiography, performed in a highly standardized manner, obtaining photographs around every half second, was performed in 50 normal controls between the ages of 19 and 83, in 87 patients considered to be primary open-angle suspects, in 62 patients with definite primary open-angle glaucoma, in 32 patients with a variety of other types of glaucoma, and in 16 cases having an entity considered a sub-group to the "low-tension glaucoma" (in which intraocular pressure was in the range usually considered normal, but patients had progressive optic nerve and visual field damage were characteristic-localized pseudo-pit, optic disc hemorrhages, and dense paracentral scotomatas). In this study, a wide variety of several parameters were investigated, including systemic blood pressure, ophthalmodynamometric pressures, arm-to-tongue circulation time, the time for fluorescein to fill or to appear in various ocular structures (the choroid, the retinal arteries, the retinal veins, the disc), whether there was staining of the optic disc, whether there was peripapillary hyperfluorescence, etc. The patient groups were comparable with regard to age, sex and race. Regarding the normals and the primary open-angle glaucoma groups, the mean age was 48, the percentage of women slightly exceeding that of men, and white patients comprising 80% of the group. This was also true in all other investigative groups.

In reviewing the data, I could find nothing in the way of a systematic error to explain away the statistically significant differences that were found. It is pertinent to summarize the results:

The higher the intraocular pressure, the longer it took for fluorescein to fill the disc, make an intraretinal transit, or fill the choroid. This applied in patients with primary open–angle glaucoma and in primary open-angle glaucoma suspects, but not in patients with secondary glaucoma or in normals. The differences between the two groups were significant and the relationship between pressure and filling time was direct and highly significant with a p value of less than 0.01.

When considering the relationship between the state of control of disease and the various hemodynamic variables, there is a direct correlation between "retinal vein filling time" and the state of control, retinal vein filling time being 8.9 seconds and the patients are considered to be certainly controlled, 9.4 in those probably controlled, 11.1 in those probably uncontrolled, and 12.2 in those certainly uncontrolled. The differences were highly significant (Table 1).

Table 1. Relationship between state of control of disease and hemodynamic variables

	CC	PC	PUC	CUC*
Intraretinal transit time**	2.1	2.3	2.7	2.8
Disc filling time	1.8	1.4	2.5	1.7
Retinal artery filling time	1.5	1.8	2.2	2.3
Retinal vein filling time	8.9	9.4	11.1	12.2

*CC = Certainly controlled
PC = Probably controlled
PUC = Probably uncontrolled
CUC = Certainly uncontrolled
**Time given in seconds

When correlating diagnosis in the presence or absence of disc staining, it was noted that 3% of the normals showed either a mild or moderate stain, 8% of the glaucoma suspects, 54% of the patients with secondary glaucoma, 34% of those with low–tension glaucoma, and 42% of those with primary open-angle glaucoma. The differences between the groups were highly significant (Table 2).

Table 2. Correlation between disc staining and diagnosis percentage of each group

	NC	GS	OG	LTG	POAG*
No stain	97	92	46	66	58
Mild stain	3	8	36	14	29
Moderate stain	0	0	18	20	13
Total	100	100	100	100	100

On considering the areas in which hypoperfusion was present, this was noted to differ in the various diagnostic groups, there being virtually no selectivity in the patients with secondary glaucomas, moderate limitation to the inferotemporal and superotemporal areas in patients with primary open–angle glaucoma, and extreme selectivity in patients with "low-tension glaucoma" (100% having involvement of the inferotemporal portion and an additional 67% having involvement of the superotemporal portion as well, with no involvement of the nasal areas (which were involved in the other glaucomas (Table 3).

Table 3. Cross–tabulation: region of decreased disc perfusion compared to diagnosis (percentage of decrease)

Disc fluorescence	NC	GS	OG	LTG	POAG
Area 1	0	4	0	0	17
Area 11	10	5	27	30	69
Area 2	0	18	18	67	50
Area 12	0	9	18	35	17
Area 3	0	18	20	100	70
Area 13	4	9	28	100	70
Area 4	0	20	14	0	25
Area 14	0	5	9	0	8
Area 5	0	20	9	0	25
Area 15	0	4	0	0	17

In considering the number of regions of the disc that showed hypoperfusion compared to the diagnosis, there was an average number of nil in those who had no glaucoma, one in the glaucoma suspects, two in those with secondary glaucomas, three in those with low-tension glaucoma, and five in those with primary open-angle glaucoma (Table 4).

Table 4. Number of regions of disc showing hypoperfusion compared to diagnosis (average number of regions of hypoperfusion)

NC	GS	OG	LTG	POAG
0	1	2	3	5

Ophthalmodynamometry was of little apparent benefit in relation to diagnosis, state of disease, intraocular pressure, or controlled disease with one exception. It was noted that in patients with primary open-angle glaucoma, the phenomenon of disc blanch occurred more frequently at a lower pressure than in any of the other types of glaucoma. Disc blanch was defined as the level of pressure at which the optic disc became blanched in comparison to the level of pressure at which the retinal vessels collapsed.

Staining of the optic disc was directly and highly correlated with the state of control of the disease, the stage of disease, and the state of disc perfusion, being more prominent in those with more advanced disease, more uncontrolled disease, and poorer disc perfusion. The correlation was highly significant with a $p < 0.001$.

The presence of visual field loss was highly correlated with all the circulation times, with a $p < 0.001$ for all circulation times with the exception of retinal vein filling time, which was less significant ($p < 0.02$).

There was a high correlation between decreased perfusion of the optic disc and the presence of disc staining, the stage of disease, the control of disease, the presence of visual field loss, and circulation times (with $p < 0.001$).

There was a high correlation between the amount of pallor of the optic disc and decreased circulation time of the disc ($p < 0.001$).

There was a direct and high correlation between the intraocular pressure following fluorescein angiography and various circulation times, most specifically the time to fill the optic disc (Table 5). There are interesting differences and correlations between various circulation times in this regard. The intraretinal transit time had a $p < 0.03$ whereas the disc filling time had $p < 0.001$ (Table 6).

Age	Normal	Chronic OAG	Difference
40–49	1.1 ± 0.4	2.8 ± 2.3	$p=0.001$
50–59	1.3 ± 0.3	1.9 ± 1.5	$p=0.01$
60–69	1.5 ± 0.7	2.3 ± 3.1	$p=0.01$
70–79	1.2 ± 0.5	2.2 ± 1.4	$p=0.001$

* mean± standard deviation

Table 6. Findings in various diagnostic categories

	NC	GS	OG	LTG	POAG*
IOP (mm Hg)	15	23	30	18	24
Arm–tongue circulation time	14	15	17	17	13
Disc filling time	1.2	1.5	1.6	1.5	1.6
Intraretinal transit time	2.0	1.9	2.7	2.1	2.7
CD ratio (horizontal)	0.4	0.6	0.5	0.6	0.8

*NC = Normal controls
GS = Glaucoma suspect
OG = Other glaucomas
LTG = Low tension glaucoma
POAG= Primary open-angle glaucoma

There appeared to be no escaping of the conclusion that increased intraocular pressure was accompanied by prolongation of certain circulation times, most specifically filling the optic disc. Furthermore, it was obvious that there was retardation of passage of dye through the optic disc that was related to diagnosis, stage and control of disease. An interesting finding was the similarity of presence of disc staining in patients with both primary open-angle glaucoma and low-tension glaucoma, suggesting that this finding, so characteristic of patients with advanced glaucoma, was a factor of something similar in the two diseases, rather than a response that was directly correlated to the intraocular pressure level itself.

A distinction was made between "delay of perfusion" and "hypoperfusion". In the former, there was some slowing of the perfusion, but eventually filling, whereas in the latter the area under examination was consistently underperfused with fluorescein. It was interesting that the major changes occurred with regard to disc hypoperfusion and not regarding delay.

This study did not direct itself to whether or not abnormalities in perfusion of the optic nerve were secondary to earlier changes in the optic disc, or were primary, causing other changes in the optic disc. That vitally important question still needs to be answered.

However, fascinating patterns, or subgroups, appeared when the individual angiograms were analyzed. This individual analysis did not permit statistical analysis, but the patterns were so clear-cut that it seems imprudent to ignore them.

It was obvious that there were patients with marked persisting elevation of intraocular pressure, definite glaucoma, but no apparent abnormality of blood flow. This was a quite routine finding in patients with secondary glaucomas. There was also a group of patients in whom lowering intraocular pressure was followed by a dramatic improvement in the blood flow and in the intensity of perfusion as well as in the completion of perfusion of the optic disc. In some patients, this was an incremental phenomenon, in that lowering intraocular pressure partially resulted in some improvement in circulation, whereas lowering it further resulted in a further improvement. This was dramatically seen in one patient in whom the intraocular pressure was lowered approximately 20 mm Hg to around 20 with a marked improvement, but with persisting hypoperfusion, yet when intraocular pressure was lowered to 14 mm Hg, the circulation times became normal, the areas of hypoperfusion decreased, though one area of hypoperfusion persisted.

Perhaps of greatest interest in this regard was one family in which three members of the family were all affected, but to differing degrees (Table 7). One brother had a low-tension glaucoma with advanced nerve and field loss despite intraocular pressures below 21, his sister had ordinary primary open-angle glaucoma with elevated pressure and moderate disc and field damage, and the youngest brother had "ocular hypertension" with pressures in the 30s, a large cup, but no detectable visual field loss. The disc filling times in these patients showed an abnormal time in the patient with the low-tension glaucoma, a borderline time in the patient with the ordinary open-angle glaucoma, and a normal time in the patient with ocular hypertension. Furthermore, lowering the intraocular pressure was associated with a significant improvement in the disc filling time in all patients, but in the low-tension glaucoma patient, even though there was an improvement, the times were still abnormal (Table 7).

The conclusion, as mentioned before, seemed undeniable. There is a relationship between insufficiency of blood flow and glaucoma, and furthermore, this relationship is related to the level of intraocular pressure. However, there are patients in whom this relation is prominent and others in whom it is virtually absent. Additionally, lowering of

Table 7. Circulation times in three members of one family

Pt	IOP(mm Hg)	DX	Choroidal	Disc	Retinal artery
A	12	LTG	3.2	2.8	2.0
	24		5.4	4.7	3.4
B	22	POAG	2.0	2.0	1.6
	12		2.0	1.4	1.2
C	25	GS	1.6	1.6	2.0
	21		0.4	0.8	0.8

intraocular pressure improves blood flow in some patients and in some tissues. The problem, however, is that the noise of the system is so great, the variability between patients is so great, the blending of diagnostic entities so great, and the technology position so poor, that the use of fluorescein angiography in the individual patient is at this time (utilizing present standard techniques) of little or no apparent benefit (Table 8).

There are, however, so many other intimations of abnormality of blood flow in patients with glaucoma that it seems highly appropriate to make a major effort to establish a method sufficiently sensitive and specific to be applicable to individual patients (Tables 1–7). In my opinion, no present method has accomplished this. I doubt that without major modifications any present method can.

In my opinion, the most fruitful area for future research has to do with stereoscopic, high resolution, video angiography. Unfortunately, progress in this area has been disap-

Table 8A. Fluorescein angiography in glaucoma

Of great help in understanding what is happening to glaucoma
Of little or no help in individuals at present

Table 8B. Fluorescein angiography in glaucoma

Specific numbers of little help – too much noise
Rate of flow hard to determine
Not a benign test
Not an easy technique, especially in glaucoma patients

pointingly slow. It seems likely that the techniques are now available. What is needed are funds, commitment, and time and most importantly, correlation of findings with the clinical course of the disease.

References

1. Spaeth GL: The Pathogenesis of Nerve Damage in Glaucoma: Contributions of Fluorescein Angiography. New York: Grune & Stratton 1977
2. Becker B, Christensen RD: Water–drinking and tonography in the diagnosis of glaucoma. Arch Ophthalmol 56:321, 1956
3. Krupin T, Podos SM, Becker B: Effect of optic nerve transection on osmotic alterations of intraocular pressure. Am J Ophthalmol 70:214, 1970
4. Spaeth GL: The water drinking test. Arch Ophthalmol 77:50, 1967

This paper is disacussed together with the other papers on fluorescein angiography on page 261 ff.

FLUORESCEIN ANGIOGRAPHY:
Its contribution to evaluation of the optic disc and the retinal circulation in glaucoma

Bernard Schwartz

Department of Ophthalmology, Tufts University School of Medicine and New England Medical Center Hospitals, 750 Washington Street, Box 450, Boston, MA 02111, USA

Abstract

Various studies using fluorescein angiography for evaluation of the optic disc and the retinal circulation in glaucoma have been reviewed. Techniques have been developed not only to qualitatively evaluate the fluorescein angiogram, but also its measurement using either microdensitometry or image analysis of the optic disc and the retinal circulation. Absolute fluorescein filling defects, *i.e.* those which persist throughout the entire angiogram cycle, have been noted to be larger in number and in area in ocular hypertensives and open-angle glaucoma eyes compared to normals and primarily occur in the wall of the optic disc cup. These defects correlate with the degree and site of visual field loss, and also are associated with age and increased blood pressure.

Filling defects appear to be specific for glaucomatous eyes and eyes with ischemic optic neuropathy, and are not apparent in eyes which have glaucoma-like discs, such as high myopic eyes and eyes with increased optic disc cupping and pallor due to neurological disease. Follow-up studies indicate that with the appearance of visual field loss or a glaucomatous change in the disc, new or larger fluorescein filling defects are observed. Once present, they appear to be relatively stable. Measurements of fluorescein defects by 2-point photofluorometry suggest that the defects represent areas of a smaller vascular bed together with narrower vessels and increased permeability of the vessels. Fluorescein angiography used to evaluate the retinal circulation indicates a decrease in rate of filling of the arteries and veins in ocular hypertensives and open-angle glaucomas compared to normals. In particular with the progression of visual field loss and optic disc changes in ocular hypertensive eyes, a decrease in retinal venous circulation has been noted.

Introduction

Fluorescein angiography provides a clinical method to evaluate the circulation of the optic disc. The appropriate technique for performing fluorescein angiography involves the use of filters that block the pseudofluorescence of the optic disc.[36] Since the early studies (Hayreh and Walker in 1967[17] and Oosterhuis and Gortzak-Hoorstein in 1970[28]) demonstrated circulation abnormalities in the optic disc in glaucoma, a number of observers have used this technique to study the circulation of the optic disc in both ocular hypertension and glaucoma[3,4,6,8,9,12,14,19,22,29,39,42]. We have developed qualitative techniques to adequately evaluate fluorescein angiograms of the optic disc[36] as well as quantitative techniques to measure the fluorescein filling defect with two point photofluorometry[37] and to measure the defect and the circulation parameters of the retina using computerized image analysis[25]. The purpose of this presentation is primarily to review our studies of these techniques for studying both the optic disc and the retinal circulation in glaucoma.

This study was supported in part by a grant from Research to Prevent Blindness, Inc., New York, NY, USA

Fluorescein angiography of the optic disc in ocular hypertension and glaucoma

1. Definition of fluorescein angiographic defects

Our initial studies showed filling defects of the optic disc, both in ocular hypertension and glaucoma, as discrete areas.[36]

The term "defect" essentially refers to a filling defect that is observed in the arterial or early arterio-venous phase (Fig. 1). Two types of defects were defined. The absolute defect, *i.e.* an area of the disc that demonstrates total hypofluorescence and non-filling throughout all phases of the fluorescein angiogram, and the relative filling defect which refers to an area of the disc that either fills more slowly (time delay) than other areas of the disc or never achieves total fluorescence (intensity) compared to other areas of the disc. Since the relative filling defect may be a physiological phenomenon, we primarily confined the remainder of our studies to a description and measurement of absolute defects.

2. Characteristics of absolute defects in normal, ocular hypertensive and open angle glaucomatous eyes

The absolute defects tend to increase in number per optic disc from normal (0.62) to ocular hypertensive (0.80) to glaucomatous eyes (1.59)[36]. Thus usually in open angle glaucomatous eyes, more than one area of the disc is involved as an absolute defect, compared to normal or ocular hypertensive eyes. The absolute defects in normal eyes tended to be small and central, and located where the vessels originate centrally in the disc. The absolute defects in glaucomatous eyes and ocular hypertensive eyes were located

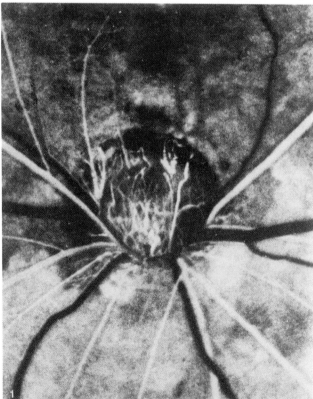

Fig. 1. Absolute fluorescein filling defects at 12 and 6 o'clock in glaucomatous eye in early arterio-venous phase. [Reprinted by permission,[36] © 1977 American Medical Association]

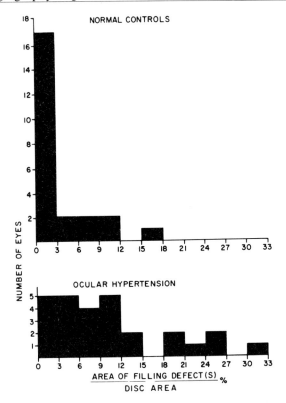

Fig. 2 Histograms of frequency distribution of percent area of fluorescein filling defects in normal (top) and ocular hypertensive eyes (bottom). [Reprinted by permission[23], © 1977 American Medical Association]

more superiorly and inferiorly in the optic disc especially closer to the disc margin than to the center[10,34] (Fig. 1). The absolute defects in glaucomatous eyes are on the average larger than ocular hypertensive or normal eyes[23,27]. The frequency distribution of areas of fluorescein defects in ocular hypertensive eyes is significantly different than in normal eyes, with larger areas of filling defects in ocular hypertensive eyes compared to normal eyes[23] (Fig. 2).

The 50th percentile for normal eyes was 1.1 for area of fluorescein filling defect as percentage area of the disc, while in ocular hypertensive eyes, it was 7.3.

In ocular hypertensive eyes, significant positive correlations were observed for the areas of filling defect with age and systolic blood pressure, with the area of defect increasing with age, and increasing with systolic blood pressures[23]. No such significant correlations were observed in normal eyes.

The above studies primarily evaluated the fluorescein angiographic defects on 2-dimensional photographs of the optic disc. By comparing stereo photographs of the optic disc with the fluorescein angiogram, the location of the absolute fluorescein filling defect could be assigned to the rim, wall or floor of the cup. The wall of the cup had a significantly greater percentage of filling defects in glaucomatous eyes than in ocular hypertensive or normal eyes. The floor of the cup had more filling defects in normal eyes than in glaucomatous eyes. Also, the involvement of the wall of the cup with fluorescein filling defects increased with the degree of visual field loss in glaucomatous eyes. These observations suggest that the wall of the cup is more often the site of vascular damage, especially in relation to field loss in glaucoma, and not the floor of the cup.

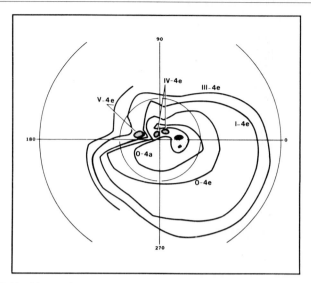

Fig. 3. Visual field with superior arcuate scotoma, paracentral scotomas and nasal step. Filling defect (dark area) in superior part of disc corresponds with site of field loss. However, there is an additional defect near the inferior pole of disc, shown in blind spot, which does not correspond to any field loss. [Reprinted by permission[10], © American Medical Association]

3. Correlation of absolute filling defects with visual field loss

In glaucomatous eyes, with increasing visual field loss, there was a greater number of optic discs seen with absolute defects[10,36]. Furthermore, the location of the field loss corresponded to the location on the disc of the absolute defect[10] (Fig. 3). Also, a significant negative correlation between the area of fluorescein angiographic defect and the amount of visual field loss has been shown, that is, the larger the area of defect, the greater the visual field loss[27] (Fig. 4). This relationship has been confirmed by others[2,6,30,39,44].

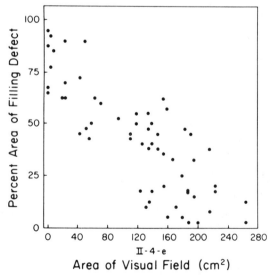

Fig. 4. The relationship between percent area of filling defect and area of intact visual field for the II-4-e- isopter for glaucomatous eyes. [Reprinted by permission[26]]

4. Correlation of absolute fluorescein filling defects with nerve fiber layer loss

Photographs of the retinal nerve fiber layer and of fluorescein angiograms of the optic disc of 31 open angle glaucoma eyes and 43 ocular hypertensive eyes were evaluated for nerve fiber layer defects and absolute fluorescein filling defects.[27] All of the glaucomatous eyes showed both defects. Of the 43 ocular hypertensive eyes, 9% had only nerve fiber layer defects, 19% had only fluorescein defects, 14% had both defects and 58% had neither defect. The percent area of fluorescein filling defect of the optic disc increased with severity of the nerve fiber layer defect in glaucoma and ocular hypertension. Thus this study confirms the relationship of fluorescein angiographic defect with visual field loss and also with nerve fiber layer loss. The association of fluorescein angiographic defects with nerve fiber layer loss is less certain in ocular hypertensive eyes than in glaucomatous eyes.

5. Specificity of absolute fluorescein filling defects

The specificity of these fluorescein filling defects was studied in patients who had optic discs resembling glaucoma, such as high myopic eyes[46], patients with optic nerve atrophy due to chiasmal or pituitary tumors, and patients with sectorial or ischemic optic neuropathy due to vascular hypotension.[40] Absolute fluorescein filling defects were found to occur only in patients with open-angle glaucoma and in those patients with sectorial or ischemic optic neuropathy. Thus absolute filling defects appear to be specific for these entities and fluorescein angiography of the optic disc may be useful to differentiate open angle glaucoma from other entities that have similar optic discs.

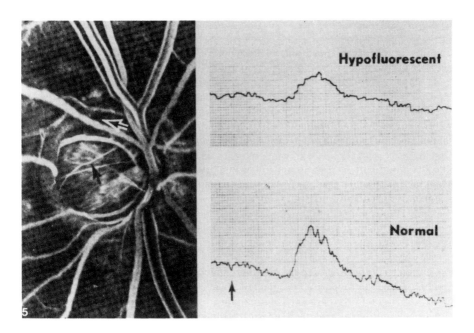

Fig. 5. Left: Fluorescein angiogram of right optic disc showing absolute filling defect superiorly above (white outlined arrow). Normal fluorescent area (black arrow) is shown in central part of disc. *Right*: Two-point fluorophotometer recording showing superior fluorescein curve for filling defect and inferior curve for normal fluorescent area. Vertical arrow at bottom of normal curve indicates time of injection of fluorescein. [Reprinted by permission[37], © 1980 American Medical Association]

6. Quantitative characteristics of absolute fluorescein filling defects

The 2-point fluorophotometry technique was used to analyze quantitatively absolute fluorescein defects in glaucomatous optic discs[37]. With this technique, one fiber optic probe is aligned in the image of the disc obtained with a Zeiss fundus camera onto the fluorescein filling defect area. The other fiber optic probe is placed adjacent to the fluorescein filling defect area in an area that appears to have a normal fluorescein pattern. After the intravenous injection of fluorescein, the fluorescein dye curves of the two areas are compared.

Significant differences were found between the hypofluorescent, or the fluorescein filling defect area and the normal fluorescent areas (Fig. 5). Specifically, the mean transit times, the ascending slopes, the descending slopes, the amplitudes of the fluorescein curves, as well as the areas of fluorescein filling under the curve, were significantly different, and were of lesser magnitude in the fluorescein filling defect areas. Also, the fluorescein defects had a slower and lesser filling of fluorescein and a slower disappearance of fluorescein compared with the normal fluorescent areas.

Age, blood pressure, ocular pressure and percent area of optic disc pallor were significantly correlated with changes in the circulation of the areas of normal fluorescence and hypofluorescence. Specifically, there were significant negative correlations between systolic and diastolic blood pressures and the times required to reach the peak of the fluorescein curve, suggesting the greater the blood pressure, the less time required for the fluorescein to reach its peak. Also, the greater the intraocular pressure, the greater the time required for the fluorescein to reach its peak, and the greater the time for the fluorescein to drain or disappear from the peak of the fluorescein curve to its baseline. These findings suggested a decreased blood flow and a smaller vascular bed, together with narrower vessels in the area of the fluorescein defect.

7. Increased permeability of the optic disc and filling defects in glaucoma

A number of observers have shown that optic discs in glaucoma show increased permeability to fluorescein[30,38,43]. These observations have been primarily made by obtaining "late" photographs following several minutes after the injection of fluorescein, and thus after several transit times of fluorescein through the optic disc vessels (Fig. 6). Increased permeability to fluorescein or leakage shows as an increased accumulation of fluorescein, usually in the bottom of the cup. In addition to these qualitative observations, several attempts have been made to measure the increased permeability. Using 2-point fluorophotometry with fluorescein, we demonstrated in 13 glaucomatous eyes increased permeability directly in the fluorescein defect area[37]. When a combination of indocyanine-green and fluorescein was used, the differential increase in fluorescein is a measure of the permeability of the vessels of the disc[5]. Increased permeability or diffusion of fluorescein into the optic disc was noted in three open-angle glaucomatous eyes, one chronic angle-closure glaucomatous eye and two low tension glaucomatous eyes, but not in seven ocular hypertensive eyes.

8. Follow-up studies of glaucomatous and ocular hypertensive eyes with fluorescein filling defects

Follow-up studies were done on 60 eyes of normals, ocular hypertensives and primary open-angle glaucomas as well as low tension glaucomas[41]. Clinically stable patients did not show any change in their optic disc angiographic filling patterns. However, eyes that developed new visual field defects with increased cupping and pallor correspondingly showed new absolute filling defects. In those eyes with established visual field defects, any further changes in the visual field occurred without obvious changes in the disc fluorescein defect. Surgical lowering of intraocular pressure, with or without a decrease in

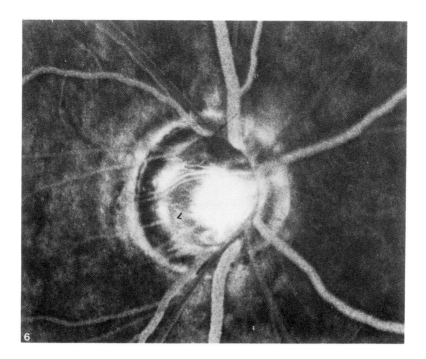

Fig. 6. Glaucomatous eye as in Fig. 1 in late venous phase. Leakage is seen in central and inferior portion of disc as well as boundaries of disc. [Reprinted by permission[36], © 1977 American Medical Association]

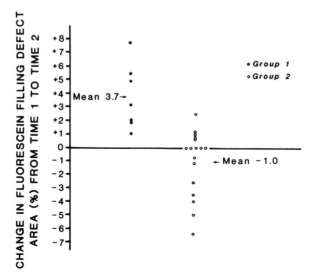

Fig. 7. Changes in fluorescein filling defect area (Time 2 minus Time 1) in group 1 (developed field and/or disc change by Time 2) and in group 2 (no field or disc changes). [Reprinted by permission[45], courtesy of Ophthalmology]

disc cupping and pallor, did not result in any visible improvement of the fluorescein angiographic pattern[22,41]. Furthermore, both we and Spaeth[38] have observed that ocular hypertensive patients who had absolute fluorescein filling defects present before the development of visual field defects, subsequently developed visual field loss that corresponded to the site of the fluorescein defect.

Another follow-up study of 24 ocular hypertensive eyes that had at least two optic disc fluorescein angiograms with a mean of 3.9 years apart, showed that seven eyes which went on to visual field loss or increased optic disc cupping and pallor, showed a significant increase in fluorescein filling defect areas as measured by computerized image analysis[45]. The other 17 eyes which did not develop visual field loss or glaucomatous disc changes showed no significant change in the area of the fluorescein defect (Fig. 7).

It would appear that eyes that develop new visual field defects accompanied by changes in the optic disc show new or larger absolute filling defects, but once absolute fluorescein filling defects are established, optic discs appear to be stable.

Fluorescein angiography in evaluation of the retinal circulation in ocular hypertension and glaucoma

Several techniques have been applied to measure the retinal circulation in ocular hypertension and glaucoma, particularly microdensitometric measurements[35] and image analysis [7,11,13,16,20,31,32,33]. The latter has also been applied to the study of fluorescein angiographic defects in the optic disc[25]. Using these techniques a number of parameters of the retinal circulation can be evaluated, such as the time of first appearance of fluorescein in the retinal veins minus the time of first appearance in the retinal arteries, *i.e.* the transit time through the circulatory bed of the retina; the time at which fluorescein density reaches its peak in the retinal veins minus the time of its peak in the retinal arteries, *i.e.* an estimation of the circulation through the retina; fluorescein filling times, *i.e.* times at which the density of fluorescein peaks in the optic disc minus its first appearance in the optic disc; the time at which the fluorescein reaches its peak in the retinal arteries minus its first appearance in the retinal arteries; the time at which fluorescein reaches its peak in the retinal veins minus its first appearance in the veins; and the time at which the fluorescein reaches its peak in the peripapillary choroid minus its first appearance in the choroid. Similarly, from the plots of the fluorescein curves, the ascending slopes of filling of the retinal arteries, veins, disc and choroid can be determined.

Typical densitometric curves of the filling of the veins, arteries, disc and choroid have been produced both by microdensitometric determination as well as by computerized image analysis (Fig. 8). The arteries fill first, followed by the disc and choroid and subsequently by the veins, which corresponds to the qualitative observations seen in fluorescein angiography. Of particular interest in these studies were the significant differences between normal eyes and ocular hypertensive eyes for the rate of filling of the retinal arteries (Fig. 9) and the retinal veins (Fig. 10), with the vessels filling slower in patients with ocular hypertension. When normal eyes were compared with eyes with primary open-angle glaucoma, a significant difference was observed for the ascending slopes of the retinal veins, with the veins filling slower in glaucomatous eyes. A significant difference between normal and glaucomatous eyes was also observed for the time for the retinal arteries to fill, the value being greater in glaucomatous eyes[15,35] (Fig. 11). With age there was a slower filling of the retinal arteries of the optic disc and the peripapillary choroid. With increased diastolic blood pressure, there was a longer time required to fill the peripapillary choroid. With increased ocular pressure, there was a significantly decreased rate of filling of the retinal veins. Similarly, with increased visual field loss there was a longer time needed for the disc to fill, confirming the findings observed with 2-point photofluorometry of fluorescein filling defects.

All of the above parameters were measured as relative parameters and therefore were

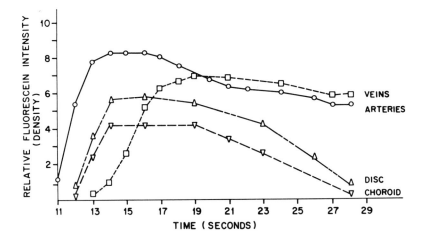

Fig. 8. Densitometric curves of retinal, peripapillary choroid and disc circulations measured throughout the fluorescein cycle. [Reprinted by permission,[35] © 1980 American Medical Association]

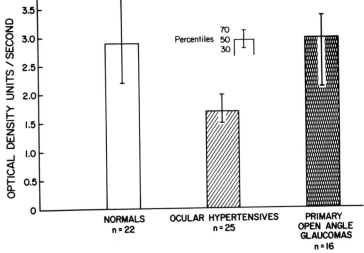

Fig. 9. Ascending slopes of retinal arteries for normals, ocular hypertensives and open-angle glaucomas. [Reprinted by permission,[35] © 1980 American Medical Association]

independent of the time of injection of fluorescein, the rate of circulation from the antecubital vein to the eye, and artifacts in terms of lighting or exposure of the fluorescein angiographic photographs. However, Spaeth[38] and other observers[12] have noted significant delays in the appearance of fluorescein in retinal vessels, disc and choroid in glaucomatous patients in relation to increased intraocular pressure, optic disc abnormalities and visual field loss, by measuring the time from the injection of fluorescein into the antecubital vein to its appearance in the optic disc.

Follow-up observations of ocular hypertensives who went on to glaucomatous optic disc changes or visual field loss confirmed a decreased filling rate of the retinal veins associated with glaucomatous progression[45].

These observations suggest that the retinal venous system is particularly sensitive to increased ocular pressure in relation to filling with fluorescein and presumably blood flow. The decreased rate of venous filling in ocular hypertensive and glaucomatous eyes may be of particular interest since there is an increased prevalence of vein occlusions in ocular hypertensives and open-angle glaucomas[18,24].

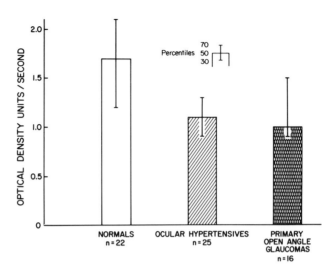

Fig. 10. Ascending slopes of retinal veins for normals, ocular hypertensives and open-angle glaucomas. [Reprinted by permission,[35] © 1980 American Medical Association]

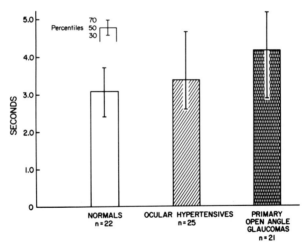

Fig. 11. Peak time minus first appearance time in retinal arteries in normals, ocular hypertensives and open-angle glaucomas. [Reprinted by permission[35], © 1980 American Medical Association]

References

1. Adam G, Schwartz B: Increased fluorescein filling defects in the wall of the optic disc cup in glaucoma. Arch Ophthalmol 98:1590-1592, 1980
2. Azzolini C, Brusini P: Fluorescein angiography of the optic disc and visual field defects in open-angle glaucoma at the initial stage. In: Heijl A, Greve EL (eds): Proceedings of the 6th Int. Visual Field Symposium, Dordrecht: Dr. W. Junk Docum Ophthalmol Proc Series 42:415-419,1985
3. Batrachenko JP: Fluorescein angioretinography in primary glaucoma. Vestn Oftalmol 83(3) 22-26, 1970
4. Begg IS, Drance SM, Goldman H: Fluorescein angiography in the evaluation of focal circulatory ischaemia of the optic nervehead in relation to the arcuate scotoma in glaucoma. Canad J Ophthalmol 7:68-74, 1972
5. Ben-Sira I, Loebl M, Schwartz B, Riva CE: In vivo measurements of diffusion of fluorescein into the human optic nerve tissue. International Symposium on Fluorescein Angiography. Docum Ophthalmol Proc Series 9:311-314, 1976

6. Bonnet M, Baserer T, Grange JD: Angiographie fluorescéinique de la papille dans l'hypertension oculaire et le glaucome (Etude de 62 globes). J Fr Ophtalmol 2:239-246, 1979
7. Brancato R, Del Caro L, Ravalico G, Sicuranza G: The computerized elaboration of fluoroangiographic data on retinal vascularization. Docum Ophthalmol Proc Series 9:117-123,1976
8. De Laey JJ: Fluorescein angiography of the optic disc and the peripapillary choroid in intraocular hypertension. Fluoro Angiographic Study of the Choroid in Man. Bull Soc' Belge Ophtalmol 174:55-77, 1977
9. De Laey JJ: Semiologie fluorescéinique de la papille. J Fr Ophtalmol 5:639-648, 1982
10. Fishbein S, Schwartz B: Optic disc in glaucoma: topography and extent of fluorescein filling defects. Arch Ophthalmol 95:1975-1979, 1977
11. Fonda S, Melli M, Neroni M, Sargentini A, Torlai F, Peduzzi M: Recent developments in eye fundus imaging for clinical application: television fluoroangiography and new technologies. Graefe's Arch Clin Exp Ophthalmol 220:66-70, 1983
12. Forofonova TI, Suprun AV: Fluorescence angiography in the evaluation of blood circulation in the posterior segment of the eye in symptomatic hypertension and incipient glaucoma. Vestn Oftalmol (pt 3):31-34, 1975
13. Friberg TR, Rehkopf 0G, Warnicki JW, Eller AW: Use of directly acquired digital fundus and fluorescein angiographic images in the diagnosis of retinal disease. Retina 7(4):246-251, 1987
14. Geijssen HC, Hayreh SS, Greve EL, Phelps CD: Fluorescein angiography in varicus types of open-angle glaucoma. Invest Ophthalmol Vis Sci (Suppl) 26:42, 1985
15. Goldmann H, Cabernard E: Fluorescein in the human optic disc. II. The fluorescein appearance rate. Albrecht v. Graefes Arch Klin Exp Ophthal 200:123-131, 1976
16. Greene M, Thomas AL: Quantitative television fluoroangiography – optical measurement of dye concentrations and estimation of retinal blood flow. IEEE Trans on Biomed Engin BME-32:402-406, 1985
17. Hayreh SS, Walker WM: Fluorescent fundus photography in glaucoma. Am J Ophthalmol 63:982-989, 1967
18. Hitchings RA, Spaeth GL: Chronic retinal vein occlusion in glaucoma. Br J Ophthalmol 60:694-699, 1976
19. Hitchings RA, Spaeth GL: Fluorescein angiography in chronic simple and low-tension glaucoma. Br J Ophthalmol 61:126- 132, 1977
20. Jung F, Kiesewetter H, Korber N, Wolf S, Reim M, Muller G: Quantification of characteristic blood-flow parameters in the vessels of the retina with a picture analysis system for video-fluorescence angiograms: initial findings. Graefe's Arch Clin Exp Ophthalmol 221:133-136, 1983
21. Laatikainen, L: Fluorescein angiographic studies of the peripapillary and perilimbal regions in simple, capsular and low-tension glaucoma. Acta Ophthalmol (Kbl) Suppl. 111, 1971.
22. Laatikainen L, Mäntylä P: Effects of a fall in the intraocular pressure level on the peripapillary fluorescein angiogram in chronic open-angle glaucoma. Acta Ophthalmol 52:625-633, 1974
23. Loebl M, Schwartz B: Fluorescein angiographic defects of the optic disc in ocular hypertension. Arch Ophthalmol 95:1980-1984, 1977
24. Luntz MN, Shenker HI: Retinal vascular accidents in glaucoma and ocular hypertension. Surv Ophthalmol 25:163-167, 1980
25. Nagin P, Schwartz B, Reynolds G: Measurement of fluorescein angiograms of the optic disc and retina using computerized image analysis. Ophthalmology 92:547-552, 1985
26. Nanba K, Schwartz B: Fluorescein angiographic defects of the optic disc in glaucomatous visual field loss. Proc Fifth International Visual Field Symposium, San Francisco. Docum Ophthalmol Proc Series 35:67-73, 1983
27. Nanba K, Schwartz B: Nerve fiber layer and optic disc fluorescein defects in glaucoma and ocular hypertension. Ophthalmology (in press), 1988
28. Oosterhuis JA, Gortzak-Hoorstein M: Fluorescein angiography of the optic disc in glaucoma. Ophthalmologica 160:331-353, 1970
29. Piccolino FC, Capris P, Selis G: Fluorangiografia della papilla nell'ipertensione oculare e nel glaucoma. Boll Ocul 60:761-771, 1981.
30. Piccolino FC, Selis C, Peirè D, Parodi CC, Ravera G: Fluorescein filling defects of the optic disc and functional evolution in glaucoma. In: Heijl A, Greve EL (eds): Proc 6th Int Visual Field Symposium, Dordrecht: Dr W. Junk Publishers. Docum Ophthal Proc Series 42:421-428, 1985.
31. Piccolino FC, Zingirian M, Parodi CC: Electronic image analysis in retinal fluoroangiography. Ophthalmologica (Basel) 179:142-147, 1979
32. Prünte C, Niesel P: Quantification of choroidal blood-flow parameters using indocyanine green videofluorescence angiography and statistical picture analysis. Graefe's Arch Clin Exp Ophthalmol 226:55-58, 1988
33. Prünte Ch, Niesel P: Indocyaningrün-Videofluoreszenzangio- graphie und statistische Bildanalyse als Methode zur Quantif izierung der Chorioidaldurchblutung. Klin Mbl Augenheilk 192:414-416, 1988
34. Schwartz B: L'emploi de l'angiographie fluoresceinique de la papille dans l'evaluation des patients atteints de glaucome chronique et d'hypertension oculaire. Bull Mém Soc Fr Ophtalmol 93:378-382, 1981

35. Schwartz B, Kern J: Age, increased ocular and blood pressure, and the retinal and disc fluorescein angiogram. Arch Ophthalmol 98:1980-1986, 1980
36. Schwartz B, Rieser JC, Fishbein SL: Fluorescein angiographic defects of the optic disc in glaucoma. Arch Ophthalmol 95:1961-1974, 1977
37. Sonty S, Schwartz B: Two-point fluorophotometry in the evaluation of the glaucomatous optic disc. Arch Ophthalmol 98:1422-1426, 1980
38. Spaeth C: The Pathogenesis of Nerve Damage in Glaucoma: Contributions of Fluorescein Angiography. New York: Grune & Stratton 1977
39. Szecsi K, Safran AB: Correlation entre l'aspect de la papille, l'angiographie fluoresceinique, l'examen en lumière anerythre et le champ visuel dans les cas de glaucome et d'hypertension intra-oculaire. Bull Mém Soc Fr Ophthalmol 92:229-238, 1980
40. Talusan E, Schwartz B: Specificity of fluorescein angiographic defects of the optic disc in glaucoma. Arch Ophthalmol 95:2166-2175, 1977
41. Talusan ED, Schwartz B, Wilcox LM: Fluorescein angiography of the optic disc: a longitudinal follow-up study. Arch Ophthalmol 98:1579-1587, 1980
42. Tenner A: Fluoreszenzangiographie der Papillenregion beim Glaukom. Adv Ophthalmol 32:35-51, 1976
43. Tsukahara S: Hyperpermeable disc capillaries in glaucoma. Adv Ophthalmol 35:65-72, 1978
44. Tsukahara S, Nagataki S, Sugaya M, Yoshida S, Komuro Y: Visual field defects, cup-disc ratio and fluorescein angiography in glaucomatous optic atrophy. Adv Ophthalmol 35:73-93, 1978
45. Tuulonen A, Nagin P, Schwartz B, Wu D–C: Increase of pallor and fluorescein filling defects of the optic disc in the follow-up of ocular hypertensives measured by computerized image analysis. Ophthalmology 94:558-563, 1987
46. Yoshihara M, Yamaji S, Yamasowa K: Fluorographic findings on high myopia. Report 3. On optic disc vascularity. Folia Ophthalmologica Jpn 27:361-365, 1976

This paper is discussed together with the other papers on fluorescein angiography on page 261 ff.

LOW TENSION GLAUCOMA
Correlation between fluorescein angiographic findings and progression

H. Caroline Geijssen and Erik L. Greve

Academic Medical Center, University of Amsterdam, The Netherlands

Abstract

This study compares the fluorescein angiograms of patients with progressive (*n*=25) and non–progressive (*n*=34) low tension glaucoma (LTG). The LTG's were subdivided into four groups: myopic (MLTG: seven progressive and four stable), focal ischemic (FILTG: seven progressive and four stable), senile sclerotic (SSLTG: four progressive and six stable) and finally a group of miscellaneous (miscLTG: seven progressive and 17 stable). The follow–up period was at least three years (mean 114.8 months, *i.e.*, 9.5 years, for progressive LTG and 89.5 months, *i.e.*, 7.5 years, for non–progressive LTG).

The mean intraocular pressure (IOP) for the progressive LTG was 19.3 ± 2.4 mmHg. For the non–progressive LTG the IOP was 18.5 ± 2.8 mmHg.

The arterial filling times were not different. The venous filling times were longer for the progressive MLTG and FILTG. These differences were found between the subgroups and between progressive and non–progressive LTG within one subgroup. The results were not statistically different.

The choroidal filling time was significantly longer for the progressive MLTG and FILTG together as compared to their non–progressive group members. The progressive SSLTG had a longer choroidal defect filling time than the non–progressive SSLTG.

This study suggests that vascular risk factors may be related to progression of at least some types of LTG.

Introduction

Most patients do not develop glaucomatous damage at statistically normal intraocular pressure levels. Some patients however have glaucomatous damage of the optic nerve head and typical nerve fiber bundle defects while their intraocular pressures are statistically normal. This disease we call Low Tension Glaucoma (LTG) or Normal Tension Glaucoma.

The pathogenesis of low tension glaucoma remains controversial. Although the intraocular pressure may be raised within the normal statistical range of intraocular pressures, this provides an insufficient explanation for all LTG. There are indications that vascular factors play a role in the pathogenesis of at least some types of low tension glaucoma[1,2]. Vascular insufficiency related signs of the optic nerve head, such as splinter–hemorrhages and peripapillary atrophy are frequently seen in glaucoma[3-5]. Splinter–hemorrhages were observed with a greater frequency in LTG than in POAG[6,7]. They may precede visual field deterioration. Tuulonen *et al.*[8] on the other hand, did not find a difference in visual field progression in patients with or without a splinter–hemorrhage. Peripapillary atrophy was more frequently observed in LTG than in patients with ocular hypertension[4].

Several papers have been devoted to the results of fluorescein angiography in patients with glaucoma. Most of these studies deal with primary open angle glaucoma (POAG) and ocular hypertension (OH); a few papers are concerned with the fluorescein angiographic findings in LTG. Spaeth[9] described longer filling times in LTG as compared to POAG. This author stressed the differences in the filling defects of the optic nerve head in POAG and LTG. On the bases of these findings, he described what he called a hyperbaric type of glaucoma and ischemic type of glaucoma. We have demonstrated a slow filling of the choroid, delayed filling of the watershed zone and a long arterial phase in LTG[10].

Laatikainen found narrower retinal arteries and veins in LTG than in POAG and normal controls[11]. In her study 75% of LTG cases had a sectorial or peripapillary choroidal filling defect. The high tension glaucomas had only sectorial choroidal filling defects.

To our knowledge, no studies have appeared in the literature on the relation between progression and fluorescein angiographic findings in LTG, with the exception of one preliminary paper from our own group. In this preliminary study on the use of fluorescein angiography in LTG, we have presented evidence that there may be some relation between fluorescein angiographic findings and progression[12]. Talusan et al.[13] reported on the prognostic value of fluorescein angiography in patients with ocular hypertension. Recently Tuulonen et al. described a long venous filling time in patients with progressive ocular hypertension[14].

Not all LTG are progressive. Progression was noted in 40% of cases of LTG by Anderton et al.[15] and by Levene[1]. The progression may occur in sudden episodes in 60% of the cases. The average period of non-progression is in the order of four years.

Until now it has been impossible to predict which LTG patients will show a progressive course and which ones will not.

There is no uniform opinion on the effect of treatment of progression in LTG. Most authors agree that medical treatment does not have much effect in LTG[1]. We have suggested that a stable and low intraocular pressure as obtained by filtering surgery may be beneficial to LTG[16].

It seems probable that there are several pathogenetic mechanisms operating in LTG. It would therefore be interesting if one could distinguish different types of LTG. We, amongst others, have suggested that there are such subgroups in LTG. A subdivision of LTG may be particularly helpful if these different subgroups have a different prognosis. A study of prognostic factors in the large, heterogeneous group of LTG may mask certain factors that can be brought out by separation of the subgroups.

We have shown that the tendency to progress is greater in at least one subgroup of LTG: myopic LTG[17]. Progression was more frequently found in this subgroup than in a group of miscellaneous LTG.

If vascular factors play a role in LTG it may be worthwhile to study whether these factors have any prognostic value in LTG. In this study we have again asked the question whether progression can be predicted on the basis of a vascular deficiency as demonstrated by the fluorescein angiogram. We therefore examined the fluorescein angiograms and the visual fields of 59 patients with LTG, in order to find out whether there were differences in fluorescein angiographic behavior in progressive and non-progressive LTG.

All patients were followed for at least three years.

Definition of the glaucoma patients

We have defined LTG as a disease which is characterized by the co-existence of glaucomatous visual field defects and a typically glaucomatous excavation in a patient whose intraocular pressures are on average below 22 mmHg. An isolated pressure of 26 mmHg in a diurnal tonometry curve was accepted. The anterior chamber angle should be open on gonioscopy.

We have defined the following subgroups:
Focal Ischemic Low Tension glaucoma (FILTG)
Myopic Low Tension Glaucoma (MLTG) and
Senile Sclerotic Low Tension Glaucoma (SSLTG).

The group of FILTG patients can be distinguished from the large group by a typical appearance of the optic nerve head: in this type of disc there is a focal defect of the nerve fiber rim of the disc while most of the remainder of the rim is intact[18]. This so called "focal notch" is most frequently seen at the lower part of the disc.

A patient with MLTG is characterized by the presence of a typical, obliquely implanted myopic disc and myopic peripapillary change[19]. These patients may also have myopic choroidal changes but no signs of degenerative myopia. Patients with a myopia more than S–8.0 were not included in the study. High myopic glaucomas with degenerative changes in the fundus are a special group.

The patients with SSLTG have been described by us as a separate group within the large group of LTG patients. They are characterized by a typical pale, sloping excavation with a sort of "moth-eaten" appearance of the disc tissue. Furthermore, there is extensive peripapillary atrophy and choroidal sclerosis[2].

All patients who did not show the characteristic signs of the three above-mentioned groups were entered in a group called miscellaneous LTG (miscLTG).

Material and methods

All patients had an extensive ophthalmological examination including gonioscopy, diurnal pressure curve without treatment, visual field examination, fluorescein angiography and stereo-disc-photography. Intraocular pressures were measured in the diurnal curve at 9.00, 12.00, 15.00 and 17.00 hrs. Visual field examination was performed with the aid of the Rodenstock Peritest, the Tubinger Perimeter, Scopimeter, the Friedman Visual Field Analyzer or the Humphrey Field Analyzer. Automated perimetry has been used in our department since the late seventies. During the transitional period the visual fields of each patient have been monitored with both manual and automatic perimetry. Judgement of progression is based on several visual fields with the same perimeter. The visual fields were analyzed by an external observer. From all patients, consecutive series of visual fields were available, which made a trend analysis possible. Details of the method have been described by de Jong *et al.*[16]

The method of fluorescein angiography that we have used, has been described in a previous paper[12]. In the same paper the criteria for the different phases of the angiogram were explained. Neither our method nor the criteria are different from those used in general by other investigators[9,21,22].

The moment at which the choriocapillaris was filled entirely, including choroidal filling defects, was used as the end point of the choroidal defect filling time. In contrast, the end point of the choroidal filling time was taken as the moment of the maximum level of filling of the choriocapillaris. All patients had at least one readable fluorescein angiogram. In total 59 patients with LTG met these criteria: 24 patients with miscLTG, 14 patients with FILTG, 11 patients with MLTG and ten patients with SSLTG. The mean follow-up period for the total group was 8.35 years (100.2 months). The range was between four and 23.75 years (48 and 285 months).

Results

Of the 59 patients, 25 showed progression of the visual field during the follow-up period of at least three years. Of these 25 progressive patients, seven were in the group with miscLTG, seven in the group with FILTG, seven in the group with MLTG and four in the group of SSLTG; see Table 1. The mean follow–up period was 114.8 months (standard deviation: 51.7 months). The range for the progressive group was between 51 and 266 months and the range for the non-progressive group was between 48 and 285 months. These differences were not statistically significantly different.

The mean intraocular pressure in the group of patients with visual field progression (19.3 ± 2.4 mmHg) was not significantly different from the mean intraocular pressure in the non-progressive group (18.5 ± 2.8 mmHg).

Table 1. Number of patients with FFA. Follow–up ≥3 yrs

	With visual field progress	Without visual field progress
miscLTG	7	17
FILTG	7	7
MLTG	7	4
SSLTG	4	6
Total	25	34

miscLTG = miscellaneous low tension glaucoma; FILTG = focal ischemic low tension glaucoma; MLTG = myopic low tension glaucoma; SSLTG = senile low tension glaucoma

Table 2. Arterial filling time (seconds). Follow-up ≥3 yrs

Subgroup	No.	With visual field progress	STD	No.	Without visual field progress	STD
miscLTG	7	2.06	0.98	17	2.44	0.98
FILTG	7	2.47	0.53	7	2.13	0.37
MLTG	7	3.01	1.31	4	2.18	0.38
SSLTG	4	1.95	0.32	6	2.88	1.28
Total	25	2.42	1.01	34	2.42	0.89

Table 3. Venous filling time (seconds). Follow-up ≥3 yrs

Subgroup	No.	With visual field progress	STD	No.	Without visual field progress	STD
miscLTG	6	8.88	3.01	17	8.72	2.45
FILTG	7	7.50	1.20	7	8.54	2.76
MLTG	7	12.11	6.11	4	9.58	0.48
SSLTG	4	10.58	2.61	6	8.57	2.03
Total	24	9.70	4.26	34	8.76	2.33

Arterial filling times

There were no differences in the arterial filling time between the progressive and the non–progressive LTG, neither in the total group nor in the subgroups (Table 2).

Venous filling times

In the total group of LTG the mean venous filling time for the progressive group is longer than for the non-progressive group. This difference however is not statistically significant (Table 3). In the subgroups the venous filling times for the progressive MLTG and SSLTG, are not only longer than their non-progressive group members but also longer than the filling times of the progressive LTGmisc and FILTG (Table 3). Again these differences only show a tendency but are not statistically significant.

Choroidal filling times

The choroidal filling time is longer for the progressive patients than for the non-progressive patients in the total group. These differences are not statistically significant. As can be seen from Table 4 the progressive FILTG and MLTG have longer filling times than their non-progressive group members.

Only when the progressive MLTG and progressive FILTG are taken together and compared with their non-progressive group members, the difference reaches statistical significance.

The choroidal defect filling time in progressive SSLTG compared to non-progressive SSLTG is however markedly different. The progressive SSLTG had a mean choroidal filling time of more than 14 s. The end point was usually even later than the last

Table 4. Choroidal filling time (seconds). Follow–up ≥ 3 yrs

Subgroup	No.	With visual field progress	STD	No.	Without visual field progress	STD
miscLTG	7	6.08	2.13	14	6.44	2.12
FILTG	7	8.34*	2.84	7	5.44	3.10
MLTG	6	9.27*	2.19	4	5.38	1.81
SSLTG	4	6.30	2.52	6	7.68	2.01
Total	22	7.71	2.80	31	6.32	2.46

* FILTG + MLTG $p < 0.01$

photograph of the series taken with 1 s intervals. The non-progressive SSLTG had a mean choroidal filling time of 9.1 s.

Discussion

The intraretinal transit time - comparable to our arterial filling time - and venous filling time, as found in a group of miscellaneous glaucoma patients ($n=197$) and normal controls ($n=50$) by Spaeth[9], do not substantially differ from our results. The intraretinal transit time (Spaeth) was 2.0 ± 0.3 s. The mean venous filling time for the whole group (glaucomas and controls) was in the same range as our findings (9.7 ± 1.6 s.). Spaeth however did not compare progressive and non-progressive glaucomas. Slow venous filling times have been associated with progression in ocular hypertension[8].

In SSLTG the venous filling time is longer in the progressive patients than in the non-progressive patients (not statistically significant). In MLTG the venous filling time and the choroidal filling time are both longer in the progressive patients. Although the choroidal filling time in progressive and non-progressive SSLTG is not significantly different, the choroidal defect filling time is clearly longer in the progressive SSLTG group than in the non-progressive SSLTG patients. One is tempted to conclude that there is some similarity in SSLTG and in MLTG, from the point of view of choroidal disease.

It is interesting that the FILTG show only a longer choroidal filling time. In FILTG a slower venous circulation was not observed in the progressive patients.

Although we found differences in the filling times in progressive and non-progressive LTG in some subgroups most of these differences did not reach statistical significance. Only the combination of FILTG and MLTG shows a statistically significant longer choroidal filling time in the progressive group. The difference in the choroidal defect filling time in SSLTG is most marked.

The lack of statistical significance is most probably due to the small numbers in the progressive and non-progressive group and due to the large standard deviation. Also it should be realized that the routine method of fluorescein angiography is a rather crude method[23] where the time between the photographs is usually in the order of one second. A better definition of the beginning and end of the different phases could lead to more significant differences between the subgroups. In an earlier paper we reported on a relation between the arterial filling time and progression[12]. We could not confirm this finding in the present study. This could be due to a different composition of the group.

One of the interesting aspects of this study is that we could show that there may be differences between identifiable subgroups of LTG. We have reported earlier that one should think in terms of a spectrum of glaucoma patients. On the one hand, there are the true pressure glaucomas and on the other hand, there are the glaucomas where the intraocular pressure plays only a minor part in the pathogenesis. As an example we have presented senile sclerotic glaucoma[20]. This study shows that by separating several subgroups it is possible to demonstrate that at least in some patients with LTG, vascular disturbances may be related to progression. Further refinement of the definition of the subgroups and in particular refinement of the methods for examination of blood flow in the optic nerve head may lead to a clinically useful prognostic indicator based on vascular insufficiency. In another study we have shown that progression may be different in different subgroups of LTG[17]. This is a further reason for separating the subgroups.

We conclude from this study that there is at least an indication that vascular factors play a role in the progression of some patients with LTG. Our findings suggest that slow venous filling times, slow choroidal filling times and slow choroidal defect filling times are also associated with progression in established LTG.

Our findings are possibly useful for the individual patient when the filling times are extremely long. The standard deviation of filling times even in the different subgroups is often too large to allow a more subtle differentiation between progressive and non–progressive glaucomas. However, these findings will certainly stimulate us to continue the search for a better definition of vascular risk factors.

References

1. Levene RZ: Low tension glaucoma: Critical review and new material. Surv Ophthalmol 24:621–664, 1980
2. Demailly P, Cambien F, Plouin PF, Baron P, Chevallier B: Do patients with low tension glaucoma have particular cardiovascular characteristics? Ophthalmologica 188:65–75, 1984
3. Anderson DR: Relationship of peripapillary haloes and crescents to glaucomatous cupping. Glaucoma Update III, pp 103–106. Krieglstein GK (ed). Berlin/Heidelberg: Springer–Verlag 1987
4. Buus DR, Anderson DR: Peripapillary crescents and halos in normal–tension glaucoma and ocular hypertension. Ophthalmology 96:16–19, 1989
5. Heyl A, Samander C: Peripapillary atrophy and glaucomatous visual field defects. Docum Ophthalmol Proc Series 42:403–409, 1985
6. Gloster J: Incidence of optic disc hemorrhages in chronic simple glaucoma and ocular hypertension. Br J Ophthalmol 65:452–456, 1981
7. Suzanna R, Drance SM, Douglas GR: Disc hemorrhages in patients with elevated intraocular pressure. Occurrence with and without field changes. Arch Ophthalmol 97:284–285, 1979
8. Tuulonen A, Takamoto T, Wu D, Schwartz B: Optic disc cupping and pallor measurements of patients with a disc hemorrhage. Am J Ophthalmol 103:505–511, 1987
9. Spaeth GL: The Pathogenesis of Nerve Damage in Glaucoma: Contributions of Fluorescein Angiography. New York: Grune and Stratton, 1977
10. Geijssen HC, Hayreh SS et al: Fluorescein angiography in various types of Open Angle Glaucoma. Suppl to Invest Ophthalmol Vis Sci 26:42 (abstract) 1985
11. Laatikainen L: Fluorescein angiographic studies of the peripapillary and perilimbal regions in simple, capsular and low tension glaucoma. Acta Ophthalmol suppl 111:9–83, 1971
12. Geijssen HC, Greve EL: Progressive low tension glaucoma and fluorescein angiography. Glaucoma Update III, pp 77–83. Krieglstein GK (ed). Berlin/Heidelberg: Springer–Verlag 1987
13. Talusan ED, Schwartz B, Wilcox LM Jr: Fluorescein angiography of the optic disc. A longitudinal follow–up study. Arch Ophthalmol 98:1577–1587, 1980
14. Tuulonen A, Nagin P et al: Increase of pallor and fluorescein filling defects of the optic disc in the follow–up of ocular hypertensives measured by computerized image analysis. Ophthalmology 94:558–563, 1987
15. Anderton SA, Coakes RC et al: The nature of visual loss in low tension glaucoma. Docum Ophthalmol Proc Series 42:383–386, 1985
16. De Jong N, Greve EL et al: Results of filtering procedure in Low Tension Glaucoma. Int Ophthalmol 13–1/2:131–139, 1989
17. Geijssen HC, Greve EL: Myopic Low Tension glaucoma and visual field progression. In preparation.
18. Spaeth GL: Low Tension Glaucoma: its diagnosis and management. Docum Ophthalmol Proc Series 22:263–287, 1980
19. Greve EL, Furuno F: Myopia and glaucoma. Albrecht von Graefes Arch Klin Exp Ophthalmol 213:33–41, 1980
20. Geijssen HC, Greve EL: The spectrum of primary open angle glaucoma. I: Senile sclerotic glaucoma versus high tension glaucoma. Ophthalm Surg 18:207–213, 1987
21. Schwartz B, Rieser JC, Fishbein SL: Fluorescein angiographic defects of the optic disc in glaucoma. Arch Ophthalmol 95:1961–1974, 1977
22. Hayreh SS, Walker WM: Fluorescent fundus photography in glaucoma. Am J Ophthalmol 63:982–990, 1967
23. Hayreh SS: Glaucoma. Conceptions of a Disease, Pathogenesis, Diagnosis and Therapy, pp 127–128. Heilman K, Richardson KT (eds). Stuttgart: Georg Thieme Publ 1978

DISCUSSION

Douglas R. Anderson : I would first like to ask a question on something Dr Schwartz said. He spoke about increased permeability and leakage of fluorescein into the disc. Is that real leakage from the disc capillaries or diffusion from the nearby choroid ?

Bernard Schwartz : It is leakage from the disc capillaries.

Harry A. Quigley : How can you be sure about that, Bernie? You only see fluorescein molecules appearing in the disc area. How do you know where they are coming from ?

Bernard Schwartz : We have studied fluorescein leakage with the 2-point fluorophotometry* and the 2-dye technique**. And we were anxious ourselves, of course, to know where the fluorescein was coming from. But Dr Riva can certainly explain that better.

Charles E. Riva : What we did was to inject at the same time indocyanine green and fluorescein. After about 10 seconds both dyes appear in the disc but then, while indocyanine green decreases, fluorescein will slowly increase. This is due to fluorescein diffusing from the choroid. But in some cases you have a faster increase of fluorescein at some points of the disc. This is fluorescein leaking from disc capillaries.

Harry A. Quigley : Does indocyanine green diffuse from the choriocapillaris into the interstitial space under normal circumstances ?

Charles E. Riva : No, it stays inside the vessels. And that was the whole idea about the 2-dye technique: to use simultaneously two dyes, of which one diffuses and one doesn't.

Harry A. Quigley : But you didn't find any leakage of indocyanine green, did you? This is probably because nothing was leaking out of the capillaries, otherwise indocyanine green would have leaked out, too. The staining with fluorescein was probably due to diffusion from the choroid.

Charles E. Riva : No, I think that even with increased permeability of the vessels, indocyanine green would still stay inside them.

Harry A. Quigley : How big is the indocyanine green molecule compared to fluorescein ?

Editors' notes

* Sonty S, Schwartz B: Two-point fluorophotometry in the evaluation of the glaucomatous optic disc. Arch Ophthalmol 98: 1422-1426, 1980.

** Ben-Sira I, Loebl M, Schwartz B, Riva CE: In vivo measurements of diffusion of fluorescein into the human optic nerve tissue. International Symposium on Fluorescein Angiography. Doc Ophthalmol Proc Series 9: 311-314, 1976

Charles E. Riva : It isn't a question of size. It is rather due to the fact that indocyanine green is bound to plasma protein while fluorescein is free.

Harry A. Quigley : Well, I still think that the increase in fluorescence that you saw in your experiments is due to diffusion from the choroid. In a normal disc there is a certain amount of nerve tissue through which any fluorescein molecules coming from the choroid must diffuse before you see them. And you are also looking through a higher thickness of tissue so that there is some staining, though not much. Now in a glaucomatous disc there is a more or less important loss of nerve tissue so that the molecules can diffuse faster and you can also shine your light on them and see them better, too. You said, Bernie, that in your 2-point technique you monitored the rise of fluorescence in two different points of the disc and that one was faster. Did you look if that wasn't always the one nearer the disc rim ?

Bernard Schwartz : The two points were almost adjacent to each other, so that if there was a diffusion from the choroid the dye would appear more or less simultaneously. Their only difference was that one was within a localized defect and the other next to it. Moreover, the 2-point fluorophotometry technique is very short-lasting. It measures fluorescence only within the first transit cycle, and that is rather short for diffusion from the choroid.

Harry A. Quigley : We have all seen fluorescein leaking from retinal vessels and it doesn't look like that at all: what you see is a fluorescent cloud coming out of a capillary bed, sometimes you can even individualize the leaking point.

Juan E. Grunwald : Well, it depends on how much fluorescein is leaking. And if the rise is in the first transit cycle, then there isn't enough time for the dye to diffuse from the choroid.

Charles E. Riva : In some glaucoma eyes the fluorescence rose very fast to very high levels and stayed there. All this in the first passage.

Harry A. Quigley : But weren't those the eyes with almost no rim left? In which case you would have no diffusional distance whatsoever: you would see the dye coming straight in from the choroid.

Bernard Schwartz : No, some of the eyes with the behavior that Dr Riva just described had good rims.

George L. Spaeth : I do not think that we can solve these problems now. What this discussion points out, is that the differences demonstrated by Dr Schwartz are rather difficult to quantitate and to interpret. Maybe this is a shortcoming of the technique or maybe we need to study it better. But I think that at this point we should just move on.

Gisbert Richard : I would like to emphasize the fact that in fluorescein angiography it is the first few seconds that are the most important. Sometimes, of course, you can pick up signs of circulatory disturbances a little bit later but, as a rule, you have to follow very carefully the filling process during the first few seconds. And to do that you need a much higher rate of photography than one picture per second. A second important point is, I think, that it is very difficult to determine the maximal filling by eye: if you repeat the assessment a number of times you realize that you have an important variability, and therefore you need image processing if you want to get reproducible readings. It is much better, I think, to study the time of fluorescein appearance in a sector or at a given point, if you have to do it by eye.

Erik L. Greve : We have reached the same conclusion and are going to come with exactly the same proposal, in our presentation in the last session.

Sohan S. Hayreh : I think that fluorescein angiography has given us very useful information on a substantial number of issues. But, like any technique, it has its pitfalls and limitations, of which one must be well aware. First of all, the interpretation of an angiogram is primarily a matter of expertise and that's where flaws come in, in quite a number of studies. Second, the way you do the angiogram will determine what sort of data you can expect to extract out of it. If you take your pictures every two or three seconds, much of the information will remain hidden, which would be there to see if you took them every quarter of a second. Last, but by far not least, is the question of what does disc fluorescence represent. People's ideas aren't very clear about that, and it is thought to somehow reflect the vascularity of the disc. But its significance varies with time: as long as the surface capillaries aren't filled, it reflects the deep ciliary circulation; but once the surface layer has filled, then it reflects the retinal circulation. I have confirmed that in experimental studies by cutting selectively the posterior ciliary arteries or the central retinal artery. However, when I did cut both systems, there still was fluorescence to be seen in some discs, coming from the retrolaminar part of the optic nerve head. So one should be very cautious and not jump to conclusions judging from the overall fluorescence of the disc, at least in standard angiograms. It may be that new techniques, such as video-angiography will come up with better performances in that respect.

Bernard Schwartz : How exactly was visual field progression defined in the low-tension glaucoma study ?

Erik L. Greve : Knowing all the problems due to long-term fluctuation we have been very careful with that point. Diagnosis of progression was based either on the trend over a series of visual fields, or on the presence of so dramatic deterioration between two examinations that it was clearly far beyond long-term fluctuation.

Harry A. Quigley : Was the assessment qualitative or quantitative? I mean if I wanted to reproduce your study using your own criteria, would I be certain that I would judge progression as you did? Or is it like we have all done in most of our studies, looking at the visual field and saying: "Clinically I would say this person has progressed"?

Erik L. Greve : I guess you would describe it as a very careful clinical judgement. What do you say, Carol ?

Caroline H. Geijssen : Yes, although I would stress the fact that it is very well standardized in our clinic and therefore quite reproducible, in spite of the variations in the visual field due either to long-term fluctuation or, sometimes to an operation.

Harry A. Quigley : You are both aware, of course, of the United States low-tension glaucoma study, which tries to wrestle with this problem so that all clinics participating will have the same standards for progression. It is bothersome of course to do three visual fields in the beginning to have a reliable baseline but, as we found out in our nerve fiber layer study, it is absolutely vital. And if we didn't do a second field for confirmation when we suspected progression, we would have misinterpreted a substantial amount of cases.

Erik L. Greve : This is precisely the reason why we based our judgement on a series of fields. And I do not think that we introduced any uncontrollable parameters there because, to stay on the safe side, we were really very strict and excluded all patients where the diagnosis of progression wasn't clear-cut and unquestionable.

Bernard Schwartz : I would like to moderate the pessimistic view that George Spaeth has given us of the clinical usefulness of fluorescein angiography, by adding a few words on its indications in glaucoma today. Primarily we use it in patients with glaucoma-like discs where we can't confirm the diagnosis because their IOP is borderline and, for some reason – high myopia for example – we can't obtain a reliable visual field. Secondarily, we use it to evaluate ocular hypertensives, in conjunction with nerve fiber layer photography. If in either of the two investigations we detect an abnormality, then we are more inclined to treat.

Erik L. Greve : I agree with you, Bernie. I think, moreover, that anyone who can demonstrate correlation between fluorescein angiography and progression, has a very firm point to make. Your work with Anja Tuulonen is a hint in that direction. We had hoped to come with better results than we did, but the statistics did not rise to the expectations. Still, I believe that the information is in the angiograms and that we should analyze them with less crude tools.

VI. VIDEO – ANGIOGRAPHY

VIDEOANGIOGRAPHY: A NEW TECHNIQUE FOR THE QUANTIFICATION OF THE RETINAL CIRCULATION

Gisbert Richard

University Eye Hospital, Mainz, FRG

Key words: Videoangiography; retinal circulation time; image analysis; retinal blood flow; choroidal circulation; fluorescein

Abstract

Using the new method of videoangiography it is possible to quantify retinal and choroidal circulation in the one area of the body where vessels are constantly observable under physiological conditions. The enabling factor is a study of fluorescein-filling in the blood vessels during slow-motion playback of the angiogram. The progress of choroidal filling can be exactly followed, so that different, precisely defined sectors and retinal and choroidal circulation times are determinable. This means the arterial, capillary and venous circulatory phases of the retina can be isolated at will for study. The way for this method is opened by a division of the overall circulation interval of a bolus through the retinal vessel into arterial, early venous and late venous circulation times. A method is presented that allows the quantitative determination of the blood flow in retinal arteries in human beings. Television fluorescein angiograms are used as input. This method does not need any gauge procedures since all the necessary information is taken from the image itself. Also, the patients' eye movements do not introduce errors because their influence is removed by the computer program.

Introduction

The study of physiological and pathological hemodynamics in the retinal and choroidal blood vessels requires that the intervals between photography be shorter than in conventional serial fluorescein angiography. Videoangiography offers this possibility, and our goal in the last years has been to improve the image quality of this method to the point where high-quality pictures are possible with slight brightness stress for the patient.

Although this method was first developed for routine use in the clinic, it soon became evident that it opens up completely new possibilities for scientific research.

Videoangiographical technique

Computer-assisted videoangiography is an improved method of fluorescein–angiography developed and introduced into clinical practice by us[1]. The fluorescein angiogram is recorded continuously, the patient suffers little discomfort and the picture quality is good.

Soon to be added to the system is a continuous digital display with increased precision in measuring the flow of fluorescein. The result is an even wider application for videoangiography in research and clinical practice.

In videoangiography a specially-developed adapter makes it possible to use a highly sensitive residual light amplification (low-light) camera, so that much less light is required for videoangiography than for conventional sequential angiography.

The examination unit consists of the following parts: A video camera is coupled to a diagnostic camera with the special adapter. A brightness control allows light intensity to be adjusted continuously during the videoangiography. The video camera signal is fed

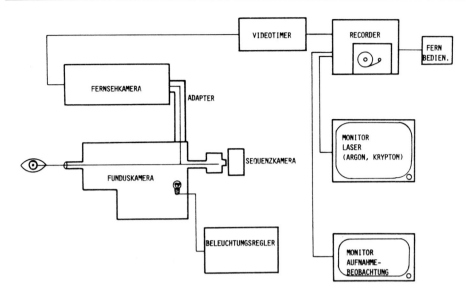

Fig. 1. Videoangiographical system.

through a video timer and a computer to a monitor, where the picture appears with a patient code and a time signal. A video recorder simultaneously stores the picture on tape for a later frame-by-frame or slow-motion evaluation. The angiography can be observed both in the central monitor and in a control monitor, where an instant camera stands ready to photograph individual frames. A simple switchover allows a miniature camera to make sequential pictures of the angiography simultaneously with the video recording.

Advantages of videoangiography over sequential angiography

The angiographic pictures are stored on videotape and are immediately available for playback whenever desired. Since film development is not required, both patient and physician are spared waiting till a later date to discuss the pictures. Each phase of the angiogram can be studied at actual speed, in slow-motion, or frame-by-frame and can be recorded on polaroid film. The ease of recording opens new opportunities for medical training. A further monitor can be placed directly beside the laser, allowing the therapist to refer instantly to the actual intraocular situation while lasering. The quality of the picture can be adjusted at will at any time during the angiography.

The unpleasant flashes – characteristic of sequential angiography – are eliminated. Particularly at the beginning of a conventional angiogram these flashes often cause rapid blinking by the patient, so that the all-important first few seconds of the angiogram are photographed either poorly or not at all. With videoangiography this problem is solved.

Retinal circulation times

Slow-motion analysis of videoangiography introduces a new degree of precision into assessment of the retinal circulation times: it permits an accurate determination of the flow-rate of fluorescein through the retinal vessels.

The use of this method has led us to divide the overall retinal circulation time into three subcategories: (1) arterial circulation time; (2) early venous circulation time, and (3) late venous circulation time.

Arterial circulation time

The arterial circulation time is defined as the interval between the arrival of fluorescein at a point in the temporal vessels four disc diameters away from the disc and its arrival at the disc itself. This means the velocity of arterial flow can be determined in millimeters per second: this in turn serves as a criterion for the condition of the arterial circulation. We took the disc as a standard because its diameter (1.5 mm) is independent of refraction and other factors. It therefore serves as an objective unit measurement. The arterial circulation time for the arteria temporalis superior in our healthy controls averaged 0.62 s, for the arteria temporalis inferior 0.65 s. The arteria temporalis superior filled generally a little earlier than the arteria temporalis inferior.

Early venous circulation time

The early venous circulation time is defined as the interval between the arrival of fluorescein at the disc and the onset of the laminary venous border flow at the disc. The average early venous circulation time for both vena temporalis superior and inferior was 3.44 s in our healthy controls.

Late venous circulation time

The late venous circulation time is defined as the interval between the arrival of fluorescein at the disc and the complete filling of the vena temporalis superior and inferior at the disc. The average late venous circulation time for the healthy controls ($n=100$) was 7.87 s.

Choroidal circulation times

Because of its ability to capture images rapidly, videoangiography permits an analysis of circulation times with a precision of 1/50 second[1,2]. This opens the way to an analysis of choroidal circulation. The goal of this paper is to draw a demarcation line between physiological and pathological filling of the choroid. This is a presupposition to define the syndrome of primary choroidal occlusion and to describe its clinical findings[8].
These techniques have been used to analyze the hemodynamics of the eye in open angle glaucoma and low tension glaucoma[6,7].

Quantitative measurement of retinal blood flow, by application of digital image–processing methods to videoangiograms

In the following sections we will briefly describe the individual steps of data processing needed to produce the desired result.

Data preparation. Firstly, the data has to be processed by the digital image method. Each individual image is divided into 512 - 512 picture elements (pixels) with a depth of eight bits. This means that an intensity value between 0 and 255 is given to each pixel. There is no information loss in the process of analogue to digital conversion because the dynamic range of the recording camera is only about seven bits. Within the frame of the TV norm used the camera takes 25 of these full images per second. The computer program can carry out the complete process of eye-movement corrections automatically.

Flow in an arterial vessel. The flow through a branchless artery can be simply calculated by the formula

$$F = (D/2)^2 \cdot \pi \cdot L/T$$

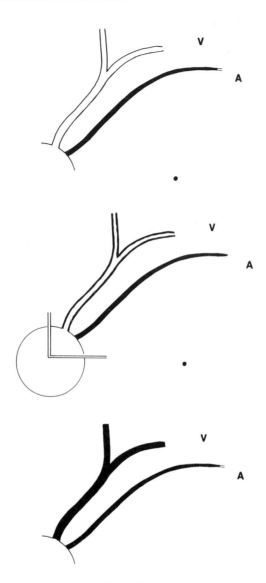

Fig. 2. Top: Arterial circulation time. Middle: Early venous circulation time. Bottom: Late venous circulation time.

where D = diameter of the vessel, L = length of the part concerned, T = flow-time over the length L. It is assumed that the diameter of the vessel is almost constant over the length L. An example is shown in Fig. 3. The flow is studied between the regions A and B. L can be simply read from the image. The determination of the diameter D, and especially of the flow-time F, needs more effort and will be shown in the following. The flow-time T can be calculated from the time-dependent intensity curves of the regions A and B. Fig. 2 shows these time curves normalized to one pixel area. These curves depend on many parameters (injection velocity, resampling of the injection bolus in the lung, amount of fluorescein, blood pressure amplitude, camera sensitivity, other nonlinear interferences of the data recording process, etc.). However, their shape has to be nearly identical for all parts of one artery except for the time shift between different parts. To calculate this time shift T properly, the curves have to be corrected for the local background defined by the

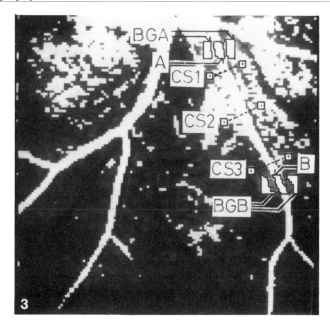

Fig. 3. Retinal arteries: the proximal (A) and distal (B) region and corresponding background (BGA, BGB) are marked. Three cross-sections (CS1, CS2, CS3) are defined.

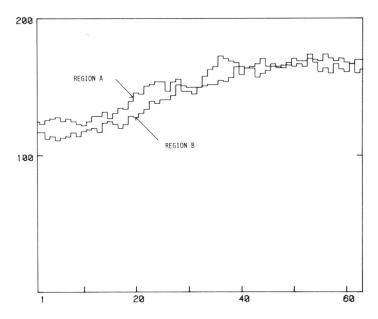

Fig. 4. Intensities (arbitrary units) as functions of time (frames, 1 frame = 0.04 s) for regions A and B in Fig. 1.

regions BGA and BGB in Fig. 1 and normalized in such a way that both curves fill the same dynamic range. The latter can be simply achieved by subtracting the minimum of each individual curve and then dividing by the maximum. Now the two curves are iteratively shifted against each other in time direction. For each individual shift the sum of the absolute differences between the intensities, normalized to the overlapping range, is calculated. This sum has a minimum for the time shift.

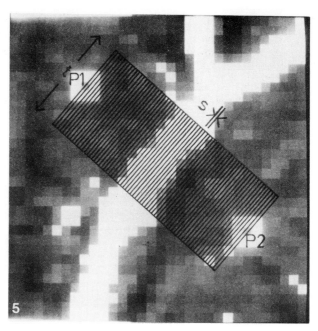

Fig. 5. Extraction process to calculate a cross–section of a vessel.

From Fig. 5 it can be seen how the vessel diameter D is calculated. The two points P1 and P2 are interactively set using the cursor. Also, the thickness T and the slit widths have to be defined interactively. Typical values are t = 10 and s = 0.1 pixel units. The program now calculates for each individual slit the pixel fractions falling into that slit. These fractions are multiplied by the corresponding intensity values and summarized over the slit. From the resulting vessel profile the vessel width can be easily determined. Normally, this cross-section is taken at different locations of the vessel (see Fig. 3) and the mean over the results is taken. The whole procedure requires some numerical effort. However, it allows a calculation of D with an accuracy of about 0.2 pixel units.

In the example shown, the flow-time from A to B is four frames, *i.e.*, 0.16 s, the vessel diameter is D = 0.13 mm within a mean error of only 5% for the different locations. The velocity is 13.5 mm/s and the total flow comes out to be 0.18 µl/s.

With the method presented here the retinal blood flow in human beings can be well determined. Up to now, however, there has been an uncertainty in the results, typically 25%. This error is due to the time resolution of the TV camera being 0.04 s, corresponding to the TV norm. To reach a higher resolution, the recording velocity has to be increased by using other hardware equipment, which will be built up in the near future. However, the method itself, especially the logical structure of the computer programs, is not affected by these hardware changes.

References

1. Richard G: Die klinische Anwendung der Viodeoangiographie der Retina. Klin Mbl Augenheilk 185:119, 1984
2. Richard G: Differentiation of retinal circulation times by videoangiography. Ophthalmologica (Basel) 191:161, 1985
3. Richard G, Darrelmann O, Kreissig I, Schubring G, Weber J: Videoangiographische Unterteilung der Netzhaut–Kreislaufzeit. Ihre Bedeutung für die Diagnostik von Durchblutungsstörungen der Netzhaut. Fortschr Ophthalmol 81:592, 1984

4. Richard G, Kreissig I: Der Einfluβ der Lasertherapie bei Retinopathia diabetica auf die Hämodynamik der Netzhautgefäβe. Klin Mbl Augenheilk 186:107, 1985
5. Preuβner PR, Richard G, Darrelmann O, Weber J, Kreissig I: Quantitative measurement of retinal blood flow in human beings by application of digital image-processing methods to television fluorescein angiograms
6. Richard G: Videoangiographie. Ecomed: Landsberg 1988
7. Richard G, Hackelbusch R, Schmidt KH, Schäfer M: Untersuchung zur Haemodynamik des Auges bei Glaucoma chronicum simplex und low tension Glaucom– eine videoangioglraphische Studie. Fortschr Ophthalmol 85:367, 1988
8. Richard G, Jean B: Primary choroidal occlusion. Acta XXV Concilium Ophthalmologicum, 1726 – 1730. Kugler & Ghedini Publications, Amsterdam/Berkeley/Milano, 1987

DISCUSSION

Bernard Schwartz : I was very impressed by Dr Richard's presentation of a technique which is – all of us will agree, I guess – very promising for the future. We had attempted a similar conceptual approach a few years ago, with a much cruder technique of course, plotting the "dye-curves" of the retinal vessels and calculating their slopes, the first-appearance times and other parameters*. Some of the parameters are pressure-dependent while some others are not and, anyway, I think that there is a lot of information to be gathered through this approach. That's why the contribution of video-angiography is likely to be very important.

Erik L. Greve : Gisbert, how exactly did you define your choroidal circulation time ?

Gisbert Richard : The starting point is when fluorescein first appears in a sector. The ending point is when all the sector has filled, *i.e.* when there aren't any unstained spots any more. This is the only way you can judge choroidal filling by eye; trying to pick the maximum fluorescence is extremely difficult.

Charles E. Riva : I think that the first-appearance time is a very tricky parameter to measure, especially in the large retinal vessels. One should keep in mind that between a main arterial and a main venous branch there are a number of possible ways for the blood and the dye to flow. First appearance times reflect only the shortest of these paths and therefore, the circulation of a small area around the optic nerve head. If you want to get some information about the whole retina, you have to measure the whole curve of vessel fluorescence. We studied that, a few years ago, and we found that with increasing IOP this curve gets flatter and flatter. But this is pure hydrodynamics and not of very much value for studying the physiology of the circulation.

Christian Prünte : Moreover, to get any information from those dye curves, there are quite a number of parameters that you must control by standardizing your method. Variations in the speed of injection, for instance, will cause variations of the bolus form and, therefore, of your dye-curves.

Gisbert Richard : I absolutely agree with you. However, the technique allows a very good insight into the retinal and choroidal filling process, at a fraction of the cost of more sophisticated devices. And by adding image processing on top of video-angiography, I think that we can greatly improve our results.

Sohan S. Hayreh : This is absolutely true. However, I don't think that first-appearance times can be of very much help. There are very many parameters influencing it, and the intra-individual variability is enormous. You can inject a given patient in exactly the same way ten times: you may well get ten different values.

Charles E. Riva : Allow me to disagree with that. If you pushed a catheter into the vena cava, you would get perfectly reproducible results. And even without such an extreme measure, you can increase reproducibility by having a strict

---

* *Editors' note*: Schwartz B, Kern J: Age, increased ocular and blood pressure and the retinal and disc fluorescein angiogram. Arc Ophthalmol 98: 1980-1986, 1980

protocol for injection. But you know how these things are usually done: if you don't find a good vein in the elbow, you inject in the wrist; or maybe in the back of the hand... you can't expect reproducibility in that way !

Sohan S. Hayreh : This isn't entirely true. When fluorescein angiography was still a novelty, I used to put a catheter up to the vena cava, like you said. And my results weren't that reproducible. I think that it is much safer to forget about arm-retina times and to concentrate on the very first few seconds of fluorescein filling. There can be short filling delays in some parts of the choroid, but you have to be very fast to pick them up. And, with routine angiography at least, you can't be sure to pick them up at every examination. It is the same as with the watershed zones: their presence is evidence, their absence is not.

Gisbert Richard : That's right, and this is precisely where video-angiography can be of help, in analyzing the filling of the retinal vessels or of the choroid. I am not talking about the optic nerve head, with which things are entirely different: it is so hard to analyze that one should rather study the filling of the peripapillary choroid.

CHOROIDAL ANGIOGRAPHY

Christian Prünte

University Eye–Clinic, Munich, FRG

Introduction

In the last years it has been suggested that disorders in ocular blood circulation may play a role in the origin of glaucoma damage. In 1985 Phelps and Corbett[1] found that 47% of their patients with low-tension glaucoma suffered from migraine. This suggested for the first time that vasospastic events might play a role in the pathogenesis of low-tension glaucoma. In 1986 Gasser et al.,[2] and in 1988 Drance et al.[3] found a correlation between low-tension glaucoma and disturbances of blood-flow in the finger. In 1987 Flammer et al.[4] suggested that choroidal vasospasms can cause glaucoma-like visual field defects.

Choroidal perfusion is of great importance in various diseases of the eye. The avascular outer retinal layers, including the photoreceptors, are entirely supported by the choroidal circulation. Moreover, the optic nerve head, which is of great importance in the origin of glaucoma damage, is supported by vessels stemming from the choroidal circulation.

Fluorescein fundus angiography does not give sufficient information about choroidal circulation because fluorescein dye leaks readily from the highly fenestrated choriocapillaris and the emission wave length of fluorescein with its peak at 545 µm is relatively short, so that nearly complete absorption occurs in the pigment epithelium and macular xanthophyll. The introduction of indocyanine green (ICG) fluorescence angiography[5,6] has made it possible to examine choroidal circulation in human patients. This method provides only a poor resolution of morphological details because a lot of vascular layers are projected into one picture. Since examining pictures of the angiograms alone is not sufficient, it was necessary to find a method for quantification of choroidal blood flow by picture analysis of ICG video–fluorescence angiograms[7].

Method

A normal unmodified 30° Zeiss fundus camera with an external light supply (projector lamp and fiber optics) is used. The exciter and barrier filters are specially made by Zeiss.

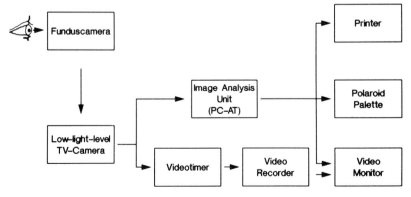

Fig. 1. Block diagram of the complete instrumental set-up.

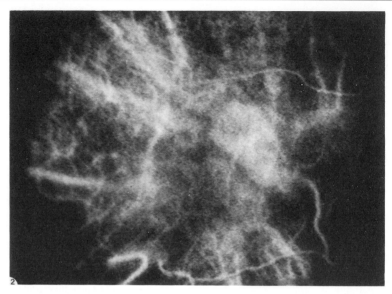

Fig. 2. Arterial filling phase of a normal subject. Sections of choroidal arteries are visible.

Using this method, retinal light exposition is below 3 mW/cm^2. The fundus camera is directly linked to a low-light-level TV camera. From the TV camera the images are directly stored in a PC-AT with a temporal resolution up to eight pictures/s. Parallel to this the film is stored on 3/4 inch videotape. The picture analysis is made automatically by the PC–AT after determining special parameters such as size and position of the measuring field in the angiogram. The complete instrumental set-up is presented in the block diagram of Fig. 1.

The angiograms are obtained by injecting a solution prepared by dissolving 6 mg ICG in 0.5 ml distilled water, immediately followed by injection of 5 ml 0.9% NaCl solution in the cubital vein.

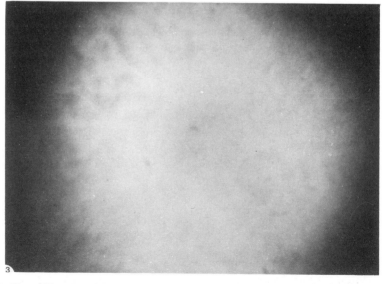

Fig. 3. Capillary filling phase of a normal subject. Uniformly white image of the dye-filled choriocapillaris.

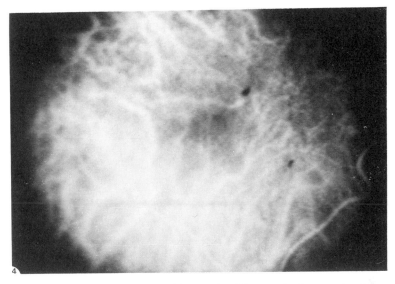

Fig. 4. Capillary filling phase of a patient with age-related dry macular degeneration. Large choroidal vessels are visible through the dye–filled capillary layer.

When performing an ICG angiography in a normal subject in the arterial filling phase, short sections of arterial choroidal vessels are visible (Fig. 2). With the beginning of capillary dye-filling, the picture becomes increasingly blurred. At the peak of capillary filling there is a uniformly white picture (Fig. 3). Because fluorescence of ICG dye is a surface activity[8], it is not possible to look through the capillary layer and regard dye-filled larger vessels. If there is a rarefaction of the choriocapillaris, the capillary network is less dense and it is possible to look through this layer and recognize larger choroidal vessels at the peak of capillary filling as shown in Fig. 4 in a patient with dry age–related macular degeneration. The contrast of the larger vessels against the background at the peak of capillary filling correlates with the extent of rarefaction of the choriocapillaris. In the venous filling phase short sections of choroidal veins can be recognized, as demonstrated in Fig. 5.

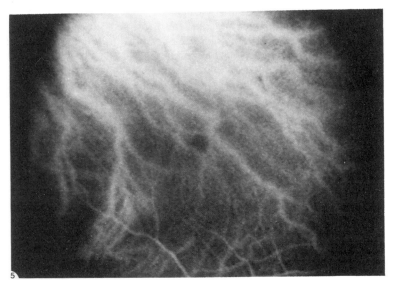

Fig. 5. Venous filling phase of a normal subject. Sections of choroidal veins are visible.

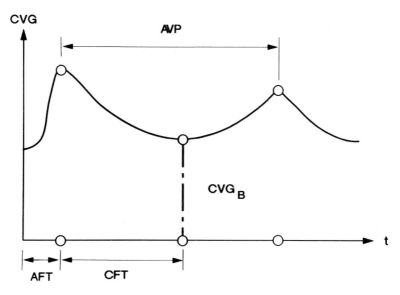

Fig. 6. Typical graph of the coefficient of variance of grey values (CVG) and determination of parameters of choroidal blood flow from this graph.

For the picture analysis, the grey values of all video points in a measuring field of any desirable size and position in the angiogram are determined. The resolution is 256 grey levels. For these video points the mean grey value (MV), the standard deviation of grey values (SD) and the coefficient of variance of grey values

$$CVG = \frac{SD \times 100}{MV}$$

are calculated. The CVG quantifies the contrast of large vessels against their background and is independent of the brightness of the picture. This means that parameters like changes in illumination, pupil diameter, the concentration of the dye in the bolus and the bolus form do not influence the CVG value. The graph of the CVG (Fig. 6) for the time of dye passage assumes a typical form with two maximum values at the peak of arterial filling (arteries are visible with best contrast) and the peak of venous filling (veins are visible with best contrast) and a minimum value at the peak of capillary filling (nearly no contrast of big choroidal vessels against their background). From this graph we can determine the following parameters (Fig. 6) of the choroidal perfusion in the measuring field: The mean arterial filling time (AFT) from the first appearance of the dye to the peak of arterial filling, the mean capillary filling time (CFT) from the peak of arterial to capillary dye filling, the mean arterio-venous passage time (AVP) from the peak of arterial to venous dye-filling and the coefficient of variance of grey values at the peak of capillary filling (CVG_B) which corresponds with the amount of perfused capillaries in the choroid.

Results

Fig. 7 demonstrates the results for a normal subject when the intraocular pressure is increased artificially by a spring dynamometer. With increasing intraocular pressure the AFT increases linearly. This corresponds with the opinion that there is no autoregulation in the choroid to adjust blood flow if the perfusion pressure decreases. Very interesting is the fact that the amount of perfused capillaries (CVG_B) increases with rising IOP. This occurs mainly in the range between 15 and 25 mm Hg. A feasible explanation is the

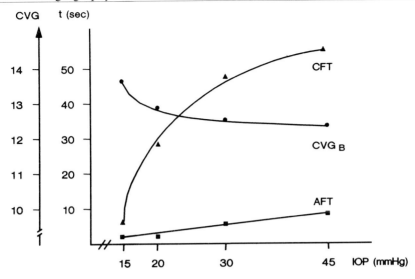

Fig. 7. Values for parameters of choroidal blood flow in a normal subject at increasing intraocular pressure.

possibility that there are more capillaries perfused at the same moment when blood velocity decreases. This fact should cause a linearly increasing CFT. The form of the CFT graph in combination with the CVG_B graph supports the possibility of regulation in the capillary network without any hint whether this is active or passive. There seems to be a more homogeneous blood flow in the capillary network when the total blood supply to the choroid decreases.

Another interesting fact is that choroidal vasospasms can cause glaucoma–like visual field defects, as the following case demonstrates. The patient was a 17- year-old female who experienced an increasing loss of visual acuity from 10/10 to 3/10 and increasing visual field damage of the right eye for six months, verified by several visual field examinations using the Octopus perimeter program G1. The optic disc appeared normal and the highest intraocular pressure ever measured in the right eye was 17 mm Hg. The left eye had a similar visual loss. She had a history of frequent cold hands and feet and migraine headaches. Capillaroscopy of the nailfold of the finger showed a tendency to vasospasms. The ICG angiogram showed a marked reduction of perfused choroidal capillaries with a CVG_B of 28.2 (normal values between 7 and 15) and with shortened CFT (1.0 sec) and AVP (1.5 sec) compared with normal subjects. The visual field examination performed on the same day showed an MD of 10.0 and a CLV of 29.7[9].

Forty–five minutes after a single administration of 20 mg Nifedipine there was an evident improvement of the CVG_B (17.7), corresponding to an increased amount of perfused capillaries and the improvement of visual field indices (MD = 1.8; CLV = 3.8). We also found increased filling and passage times (CFT = 1.5 sec; AVP = 2.0 sec) which remained slightly pathologic. After one week treatment with 20 mg Nifedipine, twice daily, the visual acuity improved from 3/10 to 6/10. These results, confirmed by examinations in other patients, demonstrate that choroidal vasospasms can cause visual field defects. The fact of reduced filling and passage times under vasospastic conditions may be caused by an increased blood flow through arterio-venous shunts in the choroid if the overall capillary diameter is reduced. Fryczkowski demonstrated dilated arterio-venous shunts in vascular casts of the human choroid in diabetes at the 1988 ARVO meeting[10].

These results show mechanisms for regulation in the choroid which may play a role in the pathogenesis of glaucoma. But we need more results using this and other methods for quantification of ocular blood flow to find indications for a participation of ocular perfusion disorders in the development of glaucoma damage.

References

1. Phelps CK, Corbett JJ: Migraine and low–tension glaucoma. A case–control study. Invest Ophthalmol Vis Sci 26:1105, 1985
2. Gasser P, Flammer J, Guthauser U, Niesel P, Mahler F, Linder HR: Bedeutung des vasospastischen Syndroms in der Augenheilkunde. Klin Monatsbl Augenheilk 188:398–399, 1986
3. Drance SM, Douglas GR, Wijsman K, Schulzer M, Britton RJ: Response of blood flow to warm and cold in normal and low–tension glaucoma patients. Am J Ophthalmol 105:35–39, 1988
4. Flammer J, Guthauser U: Behandlung chorioidaler Vasospasmen mit Kalziumantagonisten. Klin Monatsbl Augenheilk 190:299–300, 1987
5. Kogure K, David NJ, Yamanouchi U et al: Infrared absorption angiography of the fundus circulation. Arch Ophthalmol 83:209–214, 1970
6. Flower RW, Hochheimer BF: A clinical technique and apparatus for simultaneous angiography of the separate retinal and choroidal circulations. Invest Ophthalmol 12:248–261, 1973
7. Prünte C, Niesel P: Quantification of choroidal blood–flow parameters using indocyanine green videofluorescence angiography and statistical picture analysis. Graefe's Arch Clin Exp Ophthalmol 226:55–58, 1988
8. Flower RW: Injection technique for indocyanine green and sodium fluorescein dye angiography of the eye. Invest Ophthalmol 12:881–895, 1973
9. Flammer J, Jenni F, Bebie H, Keller B: The octopus glaucoma G1 program. Glaucoma 9:67–72, 1987
10. Fryczkowski AW, Walker J, Chambers B, Davidorf F: The human choroid. ARVO Meeting, Sarasota, May 1st – 6th, 1988

DISCUSSION

Sohan S. Hayreh : Dr Prünte, there is one thing I do not understand in your technique. You speak about the "peak of capillary filling". How can you define that, since with indocyanine green you only get a uniform haze while the dye flows through the capillaries ?

Christian Prünte : That is right, we don't have enough spatial resolution to see the individual capillaries. But when they are maximally filled, the haze has maximum uniformity. This is what our parameter, CVG, quantifies.

Erik L. Greve : Then the curve you have drawn corresponds to one area only ?

Christian Prünte : Yes, it is for one measuring field.

Erik L. Greve : Which is how large ?

Christian Prünte : It depends on what you want to measure. In this case it was about four degrees across.

Göran O. Sperber : How many pixels would that be ?

Christian Prünte : Around 150 pixels across.

Juan E. Grunwald : Does the intensity of fluorescence depend on the amount of dye present? Or on blood volume ?

Christian Prünte : No, it is only surface activity that you pick up. So CVG is only dependent on the distribution of the dye and not on its amount.

François Delori : Then if you had a lot of capillaries, CVG would drop to zero ?

Christian Prünte : In theory, yes. But in practice there are a number of methodological problems – namely a background noise coming from the video camera – that will keep it above a certain level.

Juan E. Grunwald : What does this level depend upon? Is it related to the IOP ?

Christian Prünte : No, it only depends on the equipment.

Richard Stodtmeister : As I understand it, you assumed that brightness of the fundus is linearly related to dye concentration. Is this a known fact or just an assumption ?

Charles E. Riva : I can answer that, Dr Stodtmeister: unless you start with a very thick layer of blood, it is linear.

Christian Prünte : Moreover, the dye concentration is not important for the calculation of CVG. That's what is nice about this technique.

Sohan S. Hayreh : I am trying to understand the increase of your choroidal filling times when IOP is raised. It could well be that IOP increase causes venous congestion and a slowing down of the circulation through the capillaries, which then appear to fill better because they can't empty fast enough.

Christian Prünte : Exactly, but this may be only one of the intervening factors. There may be other factors, such as capillary width, but I can't say anything about that because we don't have enough resolution.

Erik L. Greve : Well, the only thing you can say is that the filling is more uniform in the area you are measuring.

Christian Prünte : That's right, and this could mean that in normal conditions there are small non perfused areas, while under increased IOP these areas open to the circulation as a result of autoregulation. Of course this is only a preliminary study and it isn't possible to draw any definite conclusions.

Douglas R. Anderson : I think I would rather interpret it as Dr Hayreh does: at normal IOP, some capillaries fill before others and they are already emptying when the late ones just start filling. But if you have venous congestion, the emptying process is slowed down so that more capillaries have the time to fill before the earliest ones are empty.

Christian Prünte : Yes, that's possible.

Charles E. Riva : It makes more sense to me, too.

Erik L. Greve : How do you interpret those changes in arterial and capillary times, in your 17-year old "vasospastic" patient ?

Christian Prünte : Without any treatment, the arterial filling time increases during the vasospastic attck – as it could be expected – while the capillary filling time and the arteriovenous passage time decrease. This last phenomenon is much harder to explain. It might be due to arteriovenous shunts, as I said, but we can't be sure of that. Incidentally, we found similar results in patients with senile macular degeneration, who have a rarefaction of the choroidal capillaries.

Erik L. Greve : Is this lengthening and shortening of your various times, before and after treatment, of any significance ?

Christian Prünte : No, I was just presenting a single case, as an example! We have measured some more patients with similar behavior, up to now, but their number is still too small to get any significant results.

Erik L. Greve : Do you think that there is any chance of improving the indocyanine green pictures ?

Christian Prünte : Probably yes, but not drastically: the anatomy of the vascular bed we are looking at, is a very serious obstacle for obtaining of high-quality pictures.

Gisbert Richard : Did the administration of nifedipine change the IOP ?

Christian Prünte : No, not at all.

Discussion

Gisbert Richard: So you think that the drug can really improve the circulation?

Christian Prünte: Yes, I think so, at least in cases of vasospasm. We have some more results to corroborate this, but they are based on visual field indices only, not on angiographic evidence.

Peter J. Roylance: Was there any other therapy, when you administered the nifedipine ?

Christian Prünte: Only local therapy, a beta-blocker, in the controlateral eye, which had open-angle glaucoma.

Peter J. Roylance: And what were the patient's complaints ?

Christian Prünte: None other than a tendency for vasospasms.

George L. Spaeth: The beta-blocker might be an explanation for the vasospasms.

Christian Prünte: Not necessarily: there are a lot of people, without any therapy, who have cold hands and a tendency for vasospasms in nailfold capillaroscopy.

Douglas R. Anderson: I am a bit puzzled by the magnitude of his visual field change. Do you think that the visual fields were reliable ?

Christian Prünte: Absolutely! He had six visual field examinations before treatment, and another six after.

Erik L. Greve: You know, Doug, Joseph Flammer has shown more examples of vasospastic visual fields with tremendous improvement under treatment.

Douglas R. Anderson: But this is a 10 dB improvement. It is really enormous.

Erik L. Greve: Well, you do have this magnitude of changes in migraine, don't you? Anyway, we need more data before can we make any judgement. So I propose to stop the discussion at this point and to move to the last speaker.

VASCULAR PLEROMETRY OF THE CHOROID.
An Approach to the Quantification of Choroidal Blood Flow Using Computer-Assisted Processing of Fluorescein Angiograms.

George N. Lambrou, Thomas J.T.P. van den Berg and Erik L. Greve

Glaucoma Department, Eye Clinic of the University of Amsterdam, Meibergdreef 9, 1105 AZ Amsterdam, The Netherlands

Introduction

It is generally believed that the blood supply to the optic disc has some role to play in the pathogenesis of primary open–angle glaucoma: for certain authors it is a factor of paramount importance, while for others it is a mere risk factor[1]. Unfortunately, the architecture of the papillary area makes blood flow measurements very difficult: barely 1.5 mm in diameter, the optic nerve head is supplied by vessels stemming from three physiologically dissimilar sources. It is felt, however, that the site of damage is the prelaminar region, supplied by vascular branches originating from the peripapillary choroid. This general belief, as well as data from a previous investigation[2] indicating that the choroidal blood flow is reduced in low-tension glaucoma, encouraged us to undertake a study of the perfusion of the peripapillary choriocapillaris, on the grounds that it shares a common arteriolar supply with the prelaminar region of the optic nerve head.

Choosing an adequate method for the investigation was not an easy task. A technique was required that could safely be used on healthy subjects and glaucoma patients, and that would provide an estimate of blood flow in a very small and specific area of the choriocapillaris. In other words we needed an innocuous, quantitative technique with a high spatial and temporal resolution. From all available methods, choroidal angiography – either with fluorescein or with indocyanine green – comes closest to meeting these requirements. We finally decided to use fluorescein angiography since, to quote Hayreh[3], " [it] can truthfully be said to have made the major contribution so far in the study of the choroidal circulation in health and disease".

A last question remained: how to derive quantitative data from a technique which is essentially qualitative, at least if performed in the traditional way. To deal with this problem, we developed a method for deriving the required information from "high-speed" fluorescein angiograms, based on a modelization of the filling process of the choroidal capillary bed. We termed the method "vascular plerometry", a word coined from the greek root "plero-" meaning "to fill".

Modelization of the angiographic appearance of choriocapillaris perfusion

A. Principle

The basic idea underlying our model is best illustrated by a "mind experiment" depicted in Fig. 1. A glass jar of volume **V** is connected to a tank of much larger volume, by means of an input and an output tube. The system is initially filled with a clear liquid, flowing under the action of pump **P** at a flow rate **F**. Thus, the contents of the jar are constantly refreshed. At a given moment a certain amount of dye is added and immediately brought to a concentration **C** inside the tank, with the help of a stirring device. The result is a sharp

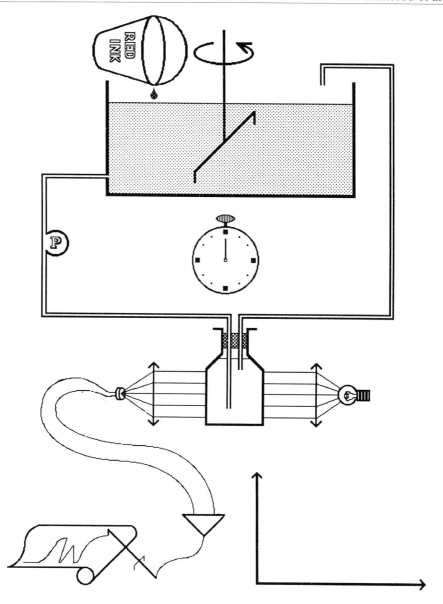

Fig. 1: Set-up for the "mind experiment" described in the text, at time t = 0.

dye front that will travel through the tubes and jar, until eventually the whole system is filled with a solution of dye approximately equal to **C**. The mean dye concentration **c** inside the jar is monitored throughout the process with the help of a light source and of an adequate opto-electronic device.

What will the curve of **c** versus time (**t**) look like? Initially **c** will remain equal to 0 during the time lapse t_0, necessary for the dye front to travel through the input tube. Then, as dye-stained liquid will start flowing in the still dye-free jar, c will start rising steeply. In the meantime, part of the jar contents will be flowing through the output tube back to the tank. As long as **c** is zero (or very close to zero), the outflow of dye will be negligible but, as **c** rises, more and more dye will be carried out of the jar, *slowing down the rate of*

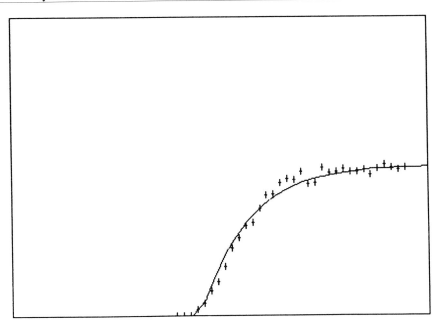

Fig. 2 : Experimental data ("plus"-signs) and theoretical curve according to the jar model (continuous line). Note the irregularities due to the bolus form (local maximum, around t = 44). The time runs from 0 to 60 seconds.

increase of c, which will asymptotically tend to $c_{max} = C$. The resulting curve, depicted in the bottom-right part of Fig. 1, illustrates the behavior of a "leaky integrator" and is entirely described by three parameters: t_0 (the initial latency time, depending only on the characteristics of the inflow system), c_{max} (the final concentration of dye in the whole system), and a "slope" parameter τ which expresses *the ratio of inflow rate to jar volume, i.e. the "perfusion rate" of the jar* (see addendum).

B. Application to fluorescein angiography

The same approach can be used to estimate the perfusion rate of the choriocapillaris, provided that some method is available allowing accurate monitoring of the concentration c of dye in a given elementary area of the fundus. This is possible with fluorescein angiography if certain assumptions are made (see below). Indeed, the amount L of fluorescent light emitted from such an area is directly proportional to:
- the amount E of incident (exciter) light,
- a transmittance coefficient p_1 of the retinal pigment epithelium and media, at the excitation wavelength,
- the "quantum yield" y of fluorescein in blood (*i.e.* the ratio between absorbed (exciter) light and emitted (fluorescent) light,
- the concentration **c** of fluorescein at the site of measurement
- and, finally, to a transmittance coefficient p_2 of the retinal pigment epithelium and media, at the fluorescence wavelength.

From the above parameters, p_1 and p_2 are constant for any given location of the fundus in a given eye, while E can be considered as constant over the duration of the examination. The quantum yield of fluorescein depends on the dye concentration, but its range of variation is small and we can consider it constant, at least at first approximation. Thus we can write:

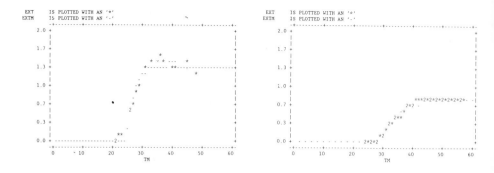

Fig. 3 : Influence of the IOP on the plerometric curve. The same eye was measured first at spontaneous IOP (16 mmHg, left diagram), and, one week later, a second time under artificial IOP increase (40 mmHg, right digram). The decrease in the final level of fluorescence *does not* reflect a slowed-down circulation but, rather, a smaller amount of fluorescein-containing blood in the area of the measurement. Single values are plotted as "*", while figures indicate that "n" symbols are superimposed. Minus-signs form the theoretical, fitted curve. The values of the parameters are: Left diagram : t_o = 24.7, τ = 3.7, D_{max} = 1.37 Right diagram: t_o = 29.0, τ = 6.7, D_{max} = 0.8. The time–scale runs from 0 to 60 seconds.

$$L \sim E \cdot p_1 \cdot y \cdot p_2 \cdot c = k_1 \cdot c \qquad \text{where:} \quad k_1 \sim E \cdot p_1 \cdot y \cdot p_2$$

If an image of the fundus is recorded with an appropriate device (film or video–camera) under appropriate conditions (linear part of the response curve), the film density **D**, or the gray–level **G** recorded at every point will be proportional to the light coming from the fundus, according to the formula:

$$G \text{ (or } D) = k_2 \cdot L$$

Combining the above formulas we can write:

$$G \text{ (or } D) = k_1 \cdot k_2 \cdot c = K \cdot c$$

As **G** and **D** are parameters that can be accurately measured, we can indeed monitor the concentration **c** of dye in a given elementary area of the choriocapillaris. It is therefore possible to apply the model described above to fluorescein angiography.

C. *Approximations and assumptions*

There are, of course, some differences between the ideal situation described above and the actual phenomena taking place in the fundus:
1. The actual dye front is far from being a sharp, single–step increase from zero to maximum dye concentration. Moreover, its form is heavily dependent on the patient's cardiovascular condition at the time of the examination and on the injection itself. This problem can be partially solved by a fast, standardized injection technique and by correcting the measured values with the help of the dye front form, which can be derived from the fluorescence curve of the central retinal artery.
2. In the model, the dye concentration at the site of measurement tends asymptotically to a maximum which is the final concentration within the whole system.

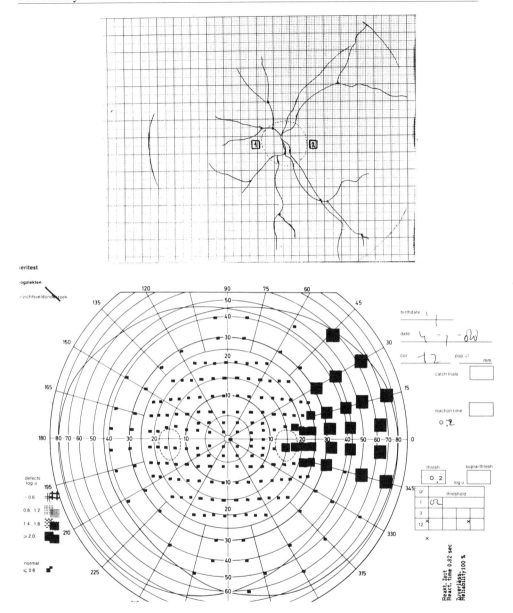

Fig. 4: Visual field of a glaucoma patient and diagrammatic representation of the fundus, showing the location of the measurements. The visual field has been inverted for comfort of orientation. (See the "Examples" section for details).

The actual situation, however, is different: fluorescein concentration in the blood is not constant, but diminishes slowly with time, as the dye leaks out of the vascular system to fill the extracellular space, and as it is cleared by the kidneys. We measured this phenomenon and found it to be between 50 and 100 times slower than the filling process and, therefore, we can safely consider it as insignificant.

3. The "mind experiment" described above is based on Beer's law, which states that the optical density of a dye solution is proportional to the dye concentration. Beer's law, however, doesn't apply to fluorescent dyes because of the so-called

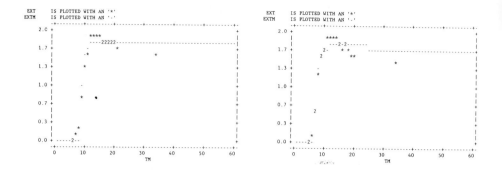

Fig. 5 :Plerometric curves from the two measurement sites of Fig. 4. The values of the parameters are: Temporal site: $t_0 = 13.3$, $\tau = 4.14$, $D_{max} = 1.66$ Nasal site : $t_0 = 12.8$, $\tau = 4.78$, $D_{max} = 1.18$. The time-scale runs from 0 to 60 seconds.

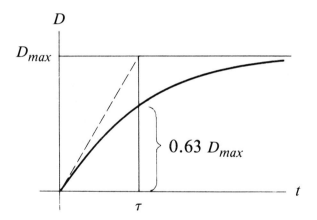

Fig. 6 :Graphic representation of the "leaky integrator" characteristic curve. The tangent at the origin corresponds to the input flow F. The time–constant τ corresponds to the time it would take the dye concentration inside the jar to reach the original dye concentration of the tank, if the dye was stopped from leaving the jar by a selective filter. As it is, it corresponds to the time it takes the dye concentration to reach $1/e = 0.63$ of its final value. The graph actually illustrates film density D over time, on the assumption that $D = K \cdot c$ (see text).

"screening effect": due to the absorption of incident (exciter) light by the fluorescein molecules, the deeper layers of the solution are reached by less light than the surface layers and therefore fluoresce less, even though the dye concentration is the same everywhere. A similar effect is due to the absorption of the blue exciter light by the red blood cells. These facts have led to the fallacious aphorism stating that "the fluorescence of fluorescein in blood is a surface phenomenon". The fallacy lies in the fact that the screening effect is heavily dependent on dye (and red blood cell) concentration and, most important, on the thickness of the screening layers. When only the choriocapillaris and the extracellular space below the retinal pigment epithelium are taken into consideration (*i.e.* a total thickness of 30 to 50 μm, of which only the bottom 20 contain red blood cells), then fluorescence can be considered as roughly proportional to fluorescein concentration.

4. Finally, one might wonder which is the precise choroidal structure approximated by the jar model. As a matter of fact, this question is not really relevant; the relevant issue about choroidal circulation is how fast blood is being refreshed in the choriocapillaris. It is precisely this "refreshment rate" that τ reflects and allows us to assess. Therefore the validity of the reasoning exposed in this paper is independent of the actual anatomical segmentation of the choroid and of the presence or absence of anastomoses.

Examples

Figure 2 shows the "plerometric" curve obtained from the fluorescein angiogram of a 29-year old healthy male volunteer. Fundus pictures were taken at the maximum pace allowed by the fundus camera (one frame per second), starting seconds after a fast antecubital injection of 3 ml of 20% sodium fluorescein. From every frame of the negative, we measured with the help of a magnifyer and of a photocell the mean density D within a 1°-sided square situated 0.5° temporally to the temporal disc edge, free from visible retinal vessels. The values of D versus t are plotted as "+" (plus-signs). By means of a least-squares algorithm, a theoretical curve following our model was fitted to these values. As can be seen from the figure, the experimental data fit the theoretical curve closely, although it is evident that a correction is necessary for the bolus form (small local maximum at approximately 45 seconds).

Figure 3 shows the results of a similar experiment performed on another volunteer, who was examined twice, at a one-week interval. Densitometric measurements were performed on the same site. The conditions of the second examination were identical to the first, except for IOP which was artificially raised from 16 to around 40 mmHg, by means of a scleral suction cup. As a result of reduced perfusion pressure, the choroidal circulation was slowed down during the second examination, which led to an increase in t_o and τ and to a decrease in the final level of fluorescence, reflected by D_{max}.

Figures 4 and 5 show the results of a glaucoma patient. He was chosen because of the strict sectorial distribution of visual field loss (fig. 4a, inverted) and, presumably, of optic nerve fibre damage. The purpose of the experiment was explained to him and he agreed to be submitted to fluorescein angiography, performed in the same way as for the volunteer of Figure 2. Densitometric measurements were obtained from two areas per frame, one near to the site of damage and the other diametrally opposed (Fig. 4b). The plerometric curves are shown in Figure 5. There is a slight deterioration of the flow parameters, although we are unable at the present stage to draw any conclusions from that fact.

Future developments

It is too early to predict what the future developments and the clinical applications of the technique will be. We are actually active with the development of computer-assisted image-processing tools for a less cumbersome and more reliable analysis of the angiographic frames. Our next proposed step is to analyze more "fast angiograms" from volunteers and glaucoma patients, so as to get more insight into the observed phenomena and to refine our approach. At the same time, we will try to adapt the technique for the analysis of video-fluorescein angiograms, which have a much higher temporal resolution and are more comfortable for the patient. We hope, eventually, to develop a semi-automated system allowing fast processing of still-frame and video-angiograms, compatible with clinical research.

ADDENDUM : Derivation of the time–constant τ.

Let us consider the jar model again: The contents of the jar, of volume **V**, are constantly refreshed as fresh liquid flows in and out of the jar, through the corresponding tubes, at a constant flow rate **F**. Over a small time increment **dt**, there will be equal input and output volumes,

$$dV = F \cdot dt$$

The input flow has a constant dye concentration c_{max}. Hence, the amount of dye that will enter the jar over dt will be equal to

$$dq_{in} = c_{max} \cdot dV$$

Similarly, the amount of dye that will leave the jar, carried by the outflow, will be equal to

$$dq_{out} = c \cdot dV$$

In this case, however, the dye concentration **c** isn't constant, but varies with time.

From the above equations we can calculate the net change **dq**, over **dt**, of the amount of dye **q** present within the jar:

$$\begin{aligned}dq &= dq_{in} - dq_{out} \\ &= c_{max} \cdot dV - c \cdot dV \\ &= dV \cdot (c_{max} - c) \quad = \quad F \cdot dt \cdot (c_{max} - c)\end{aligned}$$

Due to the net change **dq**, the concentration of dye in the jar will change as well over time **dt**:

$$dc = dq / V \quad \Rightarrow \quad dq = V \cdot dc$$

Crossing out dq we obtain:

$$V \cdot dc = F \cdot dt \cdot (c_{max} - c)$$

The solution of the above differential equation is the exponential:

$$c = c_{max} \cdot [1 - e^{-\frac{F}{V} \cdot t}] = c_{max} \cdot [1 - e^{-\frac{t}{\tau}}]$$

We see, therefore, that the process behaves as an exponential function with a time constant τ equal to **V/F**, to the reverse, that is, of the "perfusion rate" (Figure 6).

References

1. Minckler DS, Spaeth GL: Optic nerve damage in glaucoma. Surv Ophthalmol 26: 128-148, 1981.
2. Lambrou GN, Sindhunata P, van den Berg TJTP, Geijssen HC, Vyborny P, Greve EL: Ocular pulse measurements in low-tension glaucoma. This volume, pp 115-120
3. Hayreh SS.: The role of fluorescein fundus angiography in the study of the choroidal circulation. Proc First Int Symp on the Choroid. Ittingen, Switzerland, May 11-14, 1986. (Unpublished document)

DISCUSSION

Christian Prünte : Dr Lambrou, I have some problems with your methodology, concerning the bolus form. You said that you intended to derive it from the central retinal artery dye-curve. But this would only be possible if you had the same blood velocity in the two systems, since bolus form depends on blood velocity. Second, the lobule isn't a closed system, while your model is.

George N. Lambrou : No, the lobule isn't a closed system but the model is based only on the input to the lobule, and remains valid as long as this input is unique. I think that we can safely make that assumption for the choriocapillaris.

Erik L. Greve : Moreover the experimental results fit rather well with your model, don't they ?

George N. Lambrou : Yes, they do, but we have to be very cautious about such an argument, since we only have data from a very small number of angiograms.

Charles E. Riva : Have you investigated the effect of pigmentation on your curves?

George N. Lambrou : No, but I do not think that the effect will be of critical importance. There is a pigmentation or rather a transmission parameter in the formula, but it is crossed out during the derivation, if you always do your measurements on the same patient. The method is only designed for intra-individual comparison, anyway.

Charles E. Riva : Yes, but you will see that depending on the pigmentation you will get different curves. We realized this when we were doing our two-dye experiments*. So you will have to correct for that in some way, though I can't see how. Well, there isn't much that can be said at this point; we will have to wait until you have collected more data.

---

* *Editors' note*: Ben-Sira I, Loebl M, Schwartz B, Riva CE: In vivo measurements of diffusion of fluorescein into the human optic nerve tissue. International Symposium on Fluorescein Angiography. Doc Ophthalmol Proc Series 9: 311-314, 1976

Index of Authors

Alm, A.,	65
Anderson, D.R.,	55
Barnes, G.B.,	129
Berg, T.J.T.P. van den,	115, 225, 287
Bill, A.,	73
Delori, F.C.,	155
Dufaux, J.,	137
Farrell, R.A.,	93
Geijssen, H.C.,	115, 255
Gerewitz, B.,	207
Greve, E.L.,	115, 255, 287
Grunwald, J.E.,	147
Hamard, H.,	137
Hamard, P.,	137
Hayreh, S.S.	3
Hendrickson, P.H.,	167
Lambrou, G.N.,	115, 225, 287
Langham, M.E.,	93
O'Brien, V.,	93
Parent de Curzon, A.,	137
Petrig, B.L.,	129
Pillunat, L.E.,	175, 195
Pournaras, C.J.,	129
Prünte, C.,	277
Quigley, H.A.,	83
Richard, G.,	267
Riemslag, F. C. C.,	225
Riva, C.E.,	129
Robert, Y.C.A.,	167
Schilder, P.,	93
Schwartz, B.,	243
Shonat, R.D.,	129
Silver, D.M.,	93
Sindhunata, P.,	115
Spaeth, G.L.,	237
Spekreijse, H.,	225
Sperber, G.O.,	73
Stodtmeister, R.,	175, 195
Teubel, H.,	207
Ulrich, C.,	101, 207
Ulrich, W.D.,	101, 207
Vyborny, P.,	115
Walther, G.,	101